Recent
Advances in
Urologic Cancer

THIS VOLUME
IS ONE OF A SERIES

International Perspectives In Urology

EDITED BY
John A. Libertino, M.D.

NEW AND FORTHCOMING TITLES

McDougal and Persky
TRAUMATIC INJURIES TO THE GENITOURINARY SYSTEM

Javadpour
RECENT ADVANCES IN UROLOGIC CANCER

Jacobi and Hohenfellner
PROSTATE CANCER

DeVere White
ASPECTS OF MALE INFERTILITY

Bennett
MANAGEMENT OF MALE IMPOTENCE

Roth and Finlayson
STONES—CLINICAL MANAGEMENT OF UROLITHIASIS

International Perspectives In Urology

Volume 2

John A. Libertino, M.D.
series editor

Recent
Advances in
Urologic Cancer

Edited by

Nasser Javadpour, M.D.

Urologist in Charge and Senior Investigator
National Cancer Institute
National Institutes of Health
Bethesda, Maryland

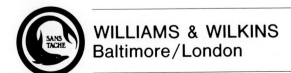

WILLIAMS & WILKINS
Baltimore/London

Copyright ©, 1982
Williams & Wilkins
428 East Preston Street
Baltimore, MD 21202, U.S.A.

Made in the United States of America

Library of Congress Cataloging in Publication Data

Main entry under title:

Recent advances in urologic cancer.

   (International perspectives in urology; v. 2)
   Includes index.
   1. Genito-urinary organs--Cancer. 2. Urology. I. Javadpour, N. II. Series [DNLM:
1. Urologic neoplasms--Diagnosis. 2. Urologic neoplasms--Therapy. W1 IN827K
v. 2 / WJ 160 J41r]
RC280.G4R4   616.99′46   81-10420
ISBN 0-683-04357-9   AACR2

Composed and printed at the
Waverly Press, Inc.
Mt. Royal and Guilford Aves.
Baltimore, MD 21202, U.S.A.

Series Editor's Foreword

Management of tumors of the genitourinary system have become an important aspect of contemporary urologic practice. This is largely a contribution of the 20th century. In light of the importance that uro-oncology has achieved in our time, it seems almost difficult to believe that at the turn of the century urologists were concerned mainly with the management of venereal disease, urinary retention, stones, and the endoscopic control of bladder diseases. In this past decade, major advances have been made in the management of genitourinary malignancies as exemplified by the great strides made in the management of testis tumors.

We, as clinicians, are all too often presented with clinically relevant data in our literature. The basic foundations of uro-oncology are often glossed over. Doctor Nasser Javadpour, the Director of Urology at the National Cancer Institute, and his distinguished colleagues have provided us with a source book of uro-oncology. It provides the practicing urologist an in-depth exposure to protocol design, statistical analysis, advances in tumor markers, the use of electron microscopy and steroid receptors in clinical urology, and the role of immunology and immunotherapy. Doctor Javadpour's discussion of the most recent advances in basic uro-oncology is the foundation on which subsequent textbooks in this series will build. The subsequent uro-oncology textbooks will deal with renal tumors, urothelial tumors, adenocarcinoma of the prostate, and testis tumors.

Doctor Javadpour's book, in addition to providing us with important basic concepts in uro-oncology, also will allow us to more scientifically analyze the current urologic literature. It may also stimulate some of us to think critically about basic uro-oncologic problems and hopefully lead to major contributions in the clinical management of genitourinary malignancies.

JOHN A. LIBERTINO, M.D.

Preface

Over the past decade, advances in urologic oncology have been un-precedented. These advances mostly have been in areas of molecular biology and clinical management of cancer. The importance of basic laboratory research and controlled clinical trials are elucidated by progress in several urologic cancers, including testicular cancer, embryonal rhab-domyosarcoma and Wilms' tumor. The recognition of biases in retrospective studies and realization for the need for randomized clinical trials in comparing the efficacy of various treatments has been the hallmark of these advances. The primary objectives of this book are to summarize the state of the art in urologic cancer by recognized authorities in the field. The articles have been arranged into two parts, the diagnostic advances and therapeutic advances. The diagnostic section includes statistical basis, chromosomal analysis, oncofetoproteins as tumor markers, immunobiology, and diagnostic and interventive radiology as it applies to the urologic cancer. The therapeutic section includes the principle therapeutic modalities including advances in surgery, chemotherapy, and radiotherapy. Two chapters also have been allocated to immunotherapy and utilization of parenteral nutrition in urologic cancer. This book is part of an international perspective in urology. Since this series will cover cancer of specific organs in future volumes, I have made an attempt to discuss only the general advances as applied to all organs of interest to the urologic surgeons.

NASSER JAVADPOUR, M.D.

Contributors

George G. Bosl, M.D.
Assistant Attending
Solid Tumor Service
Memorial Hospital
New York, N.Y.

David P. Byar, M.D.
Head, Clinical and Diagnostic
   Trials Section
Biometry Branch,
National Cancer Institute
Bethesda, MD

R. W. Casey, M.D.
Wellesly Hospital
Toronto, Canada

William J. Catalona, M.D.
Associate Professor of Surgery
   (Urology)
Washington University School
   of Medicine; Attending
Urologist, Barnes Hospital,
The Jewish Hospital of
St. Louis and St. Louis
Children's Hospital,
St. Louis, MO

Joseph N. Corriere, Jr., M.D.
Professor of Surgery (Urology)
The University of Texas
   Medical School at Houston
The Texas Medical Center
Houston, TX

Jean DeKernion, M.D.
Department of Urology
University of California at
   Los Angeles
Los Angeles, CA

N. Reed Dunnick, M.D.
Staff Radiologist
Chief, Special Procedures
Diagnostic Radiology
   Department
The Clinical Center,
   National Institutes of Health
Bethesda, MD

R. Ghanadian, Ph.D.
Senior Lecturer
Royal Postgraduate Medical
   School
Hammersmith Hospital and
   Institute of Urology
University of London,
United Kingdom

Nasser Javadpour, M.D.
Urologist In Charge and
   Senior Investigator
Surgery Branch,
National Cancer Institute
National Institutes of Health
Bethesda, MD

Michael Jewett, M.D.
Wellesly Hospital
Toronto, Canada

Nolan Karstaedt, M.B.,
  B.C.H.
Department of Radiology
Bowman Gray School of
  Medicine
Winston-Salem, NC

Robert E. McCool, Medical
  Student
Washington University School
  of Medicine
St. Louis, MO

David M. Ota, M.D.
Assistant Professor of Surgery
The University of Texas
  System Cancer Center
M. D. Anderson Hospital and
  Tumor Institute and
The University of Texas
  Medical School at Houston
The Texas Medical Center
Houston, TX

David Pistenma, M.D.
Chief of Radiotherapy
Development Branch
Cancer Therapy Evaluation
  Program
National Cancer Institute
Bethesda, MD

Martin I. Resnick, M.D.
Department of Surgery,
  Section of Urology
Bowman Gray School of
  Medicine
Winston-Salem, NC

Nicholas A. Romas
College of Physicians and
  Surgeons
Columbia University
New York, NY

John M. Russell, M.D.
Department of Surgery,
  Section of Urology
Bowman Gray School of
  Medicine
Winston-Salem, NC

Avery A. Sandberg, M.D.
Roswell Park Memorial
  Institute
Buffalo, NY

Howard Scher, M.D.
Fellow, Medical Oncology
Memorial Hospital
New York, NY

Myron Tannenbaum
College of Physicians and
  Surgeons
Columbia University
New York, NY

Sheila Tannenbaum
College of Physicians and
  Surgeons
Columbia University
New York, NY

Alan Yagoda, M.D.
Associate Attending
Solid Tumor Service
Memorial Hospital
New York, NY

Contents

CONTENTS   xiii

1

Statistical Procedures in Cancer

The attitudes of physicians toward the field of statistics vary widely, but seldom are physicians enthusiastic about the subject. Some feel that statistics are useless in medicine "since anything can be proved with statistics," while others admit that statistics may have some small role, particularly in specifying the sample size necessary for carrying out a study, or for evaluating the possible statistical significance of some finding. There seems to be little appreciation for what the whole field of statistics is about, what statisticians actually do, or how their activities may help us understand complex medical data.

Basically, statistics may be thought of as a discipline concerned with the study and application of methods for collecting, classifying, summarizing, and analyzing data, usually with the goal of making scientific inferences from such data. The discipline of statistics is particularly important in studying medical problems because the phenomena we wish to observe are usually obscured to some extent by chance effects, by errors of measurement, and possibly by various sorts of observation bias. Statistics helps us draw conclusions in the face of such uncertainty. For example, suppose we are comparing two treatments for the same cancer which are reported to have 5-year survival rates of 45% and 60%. Immediately, we would want to know if the two series were comparable, whether the data were collected in an appropriate manner, and how many patients were studied in each series. If the two series do seem appropriate for a comparison, then we might wonder whether the results reported could be due to chance alone if, in fact, the two treatments did not differ in their effectiveness. This is a statistical question since it involves an evaluation of the possible role of chance, and its answer will depend on the nature of the observations and the numbers of patients studied.

Biostatistics, the application of statistics to biologic problems, has become a specialty in itself in recent years. Keeping up with methodological progress in biostatistics is now a full time occupation requiring special training and experience. It is no more reasonable to expect a physician or laboratory researcher to design and analyze his own studies unaided than for an internist to perform thoracic surgery. Nevertheless, it is useful for physicians to have some general idea about what statisticians do and how statistics might be helpful to them in studying medical problems.

The purpose of this chapter will be to review some general statistical principles, to discuss some special topics which arise in the analysis of cancer data, to suggest some things to consider when reading articles, and make some comments about consulting with statisticians.

GENERAL PRINCIPLES

Before turning our attention to statistical procedures appropriate for the study of cancer, it will be useful to review some general principles of statistical thinking. Words denoting important concepts will be italicized.

Types of Questions

DESCRIPTIVE

The first kind of question is a *descriptive* one; for example, how many new cancers of a certain type occur every year, what is the average age of a group of patients, what proportion of patients are cured by a certain treatment, and what is the correlation between body weight and serum cholesterol? A statistician approaches such questions by imagining an abstract population governed by laws of chance which may be described by certain parameters. These laws of chance are referred to as statistical distributions and they determine the relative frequencies of different values. An example is the familiar bell-shaped normal distribution whose shape is governed by two parameters, the mean and the variance. The mean is just the average of the elements in this abstract population, sometimes referred to as a measure of central tendency, and the variance determines, roughly speaking, the degree of variation or dispersion of elements of the population from the average value.

One goal of descriptive statistics is to estimate such parameters. An example would be estimating the mean of a set of observations. Since these estimates are themselves random variables (subject to change variation) a measure of the variability is often supplied, for example, 95% *confidence limits.* These limits are constructed in such a way that the true parameter will lie somewhere between these limits 95% of the time.

Descriptive statistics can be thought of as summarizing important characteristics of a body of data. Often, experiments or surveys are conducted specifically for the purpose of obtaining such descriptive information. Examples include collection of data for determining incidence and mortality rates, estimation of response rates following certain forms of treatment, calculation of survival rates at various points in time, and estimation of the correlation between two variables. In studying a new drug, we may not be interested in comparing it with other drugs until we first determine that it has some anticancer activity. For this reason, many phase II clinical trials of new agents do not contain a control group; the main goal is simply to estimate the proportion of a group of patients in whom the new drug might produce objective responses.

COMPARATIVE

A second important kind of question is a comparative one, for example, whether one treatment is better than another in some respect. Such questions arise in a great variety of settings including the laboratory, the clinic, and in nature itself. Comparative questions lead to the statistical activity referred to as *hypothesis testing*. In the case of two groups to be compared, the familiar *null hypothesis* often states that there is no difference between the two groups (or there is some prestated difference). The statistician examines the data at hand to determine the probability that they could have arisen by chance if the null hypothesis were true. If this probability is small, for example less than 1 in 20 ($p = 0.05$), we may decide to reject the null hypothesis and conclude that a real difference (or a difference bigger than our prestated value) exists.

Types of Data

Data may occur in a variety of forms and both the design of studies and their analysis depend on the form the data take. Although there are several ways of classifying types of data, I would like first to distinguish between the *main end points* in a study and *ancillary data*. For example, in a study of survival following cancer treatment, the main end point would be the length of time the patient survived and ancillary data might include such things as the patient's age, sex, extent of tumor at diagnosis, and tumor cell type. Further, either the main end points or the ancillary data can occur in a variety of forms. Some of the most common of these are *counts*, *measurements*, and *times to response*.

COUNT DATA

Count data arise in situations where numbers of objects are the main end points of the study. Examples include the number of responders out of some total number of patients, the number of white cells seen within a 1-mm grid of a hemocytometer, the number of counts/minute emitted by a scintillation counter, the numbers of patients with various kinds of toxic reactions to a drug, and the number of new cases of cancer arising in a defined population in a year's time. If counts in more than one category are important, the data are often referred to as *categorical data*. Examples would be the numbers of patients in each of the four major blood groups or belonging to different racial or geographic groups. Such categorical data are often arranged in tables of two or more dimensions which statisticians refer to as *contingency tables*. Perhaps the most familiar of these is the simple *2 × 2 table*. Some of the most common distributions used for analyzing count data are the binomial, multinomial, and Poisson distributions.

MEASUREMENT DATA

Measurement data arise when the amount rather than the number of something is of interest. Measurements would include such things as weight, height, the amount of some substance in the blood, titers of an antibody, or the size of a tumor. The essential feature of measurement data is that it is quantitative in the sense of representing points on a continuous scale or representing naturally ordered values. Examples of the latter would include recording the extent of pedal edema, degree of toxicity, or severity of pain on a semiquantitative scale ranging from 1+ to 4+. Sometimes it would be appropriate to analyze such data as counts, that is the number of observations falling at each point on the ordered scale, but in other applications it may be appropriate to treat these as semiquantitative measurements.

The most important distribution used in analyzing measurement data is the familiar normal distribution. Even if the measurements themselves do not follow the normal distribution, the means (suitably standardized) of sets of observations may follow the normal distribution because of an important statistical concept called the *central limit theorem*. Roughly speaking, this theorem states that, for sufficiently large samples, the standardized means of observations from any distribution are distributed normally. In practice, the samples often need not be very large, sometimes as small as 5 or 10. Even without invoking the central limit theorem, it is often possible to perform some mathematical operation on the basic measurements, such as taking logarithms or square roots, so that the resulting quantities follow the normal distribution reasonably well. This process is referred to as *transformation* of the data.

TIMES TO RESPONSE

Times to response comprise another type of data which usually require completely different analyses from those appropriate for count or measurement data. The main reason for this is that not all patients may have achieved the response under study (for example, recurrence of tumor or death) before the end of the study, but we will know that they have not yet responded at the time last seen. Statisticians refer to such observations as *censored*, indicating that we do not know the actual response time but we do know that it was greater than the censoring time. The important point is that these censored observations do provide some information, albeit incomplete, and therefore must be accounted for in the analysis. Statistical distributions used for analyzing response time data, sometimes called *survival models*, include the log-normal, exponential, and Weibull distributions.

ANCILLARY DATA

Ancillary data, often referred to as *covariates* or *concomitant information*, may be of any of these types. The important questions for the medical researcher and statistician are how much of this kind of data to collect and what to do with it in the analysis. In formal clinical trials, there is a tendency to collect much more ancillary information than is really needed. The result is unnecessarily, complex data forms which are tedious to complete. In addition, there is an informal law stating that the quality of data collection is inversely proportional to the amount collected. These considerations suggest that careful attention should be paid to what ancillary data are really essential and one should resist the temptation to include every variable known or suspected to influence the outcome in clinical studies.

Comments on Analysis

The type of analysis appropriate in any study must be tailored to the kind of question being asked and the form the data take. For example, if one wished to compare survival experience in two groups of patients where some of the data are censored, it would not be appropriate simply to compare the average follow-up times for the two groups using the familiar t-test (see below). Nevertheless, such incorrect analyses appear in published papers.

PARAMETRIC VERSUS NONPARAMETRIC

Two major classes of statistical analyses are parametric and nonparametric analyses. *Parametric analyses* rely on theoretical statistical distributions which describe the actual data and the extent of their variation, sometimes with a remarkable accuracy, particularly when there are large amounts of data. When appropriate, these analyses permit us to summarize large amounts of often complex data with a few meaningful numbers (the parameters), facilitating comparisons and communication, and sometimes providing useful insights into the behavior of the data. When employing a parametric method of analysis, the statistician must check to see that the assumed statistical distribution fits the data at hand; this is usually done by graphical methods and *"goodness of fit"* tests (see below). If there is substantial evidence that the data do not fit the statistical distribution, then a parametric analysis can be quite misleading. *Nonparametric methods*, on the other hand, require fewer theoretical assumptions, and rely instead only on such things as the ordering of measurements or times. These methods are therefore less likely to be misleading, but they are generally less useful in summarizing data. Nonparametric analyses are particularly useful when there are small amounts of data, since then it is very difficult to carry out meaningful goodness of fit tests.

INTERPRETING p-VALUES

The results of statistical tests are often reported as p-values which refer to the probability of obtaining the observed or more extreme results by chance if a prespecified null hypothesis were true. In general, the smaller the p-value, the less likely it is that our results just arose by chance. Instead we reason that since our data would have been so unlikely under the null hypothesis, it is more reasonable to believe that a true difference exists. However, since the null hypothesis is usually formulated in terms of two quantities, A and B, being equal (or differing by some fixed amount), there are two ways it can be untrue: A may be larger than B, or B may be larger than A. These possibilities give rise to two kinds of p-values, *one-tailed* and *two-tailed*. One-tailed p-values put all the probability in one tail of the distribution, but two-tailed p-values split the probability (often equally) between the two tails. One-tailed values may be used only when we are able to specify the anticipated direction of the findings before doing the study, or are only interested in results in one direction. In treatment studies, this is seldom the case because new therapies that we hope may be better than the control treatment may have unanticipated toxicity. In this situation, one should use two-tailed p-values. For symmetrical distributions like the normal and t-distributions the two-tailed values are just twice the one-tailed p-values, so we can convert one-tailed p-values to two-tailed ones by simple multiplication. Sometimes, investigators who are aware of this fact choose to report one-tailed p-values simply because they appear to be more significant, even when they are not entitled to use them. Even more often, articles do not state whether the p-values are one- or two-tailed. The methods section of a well written paper should state which choice was made and why.

MULTIPLE COMPARISON PROBLEM

Since, in most studies, it is possible to break down the whole study into a potentially great number of possibly meaningful subsets, there is always a temptation to perform many significance tests. This is a perfectly valid activity if motivated by a desire to explore the data, but it should not be confused with testing the hypothesis that gave rise to the study. The reason for this is that the more things we look at, the more likely we are to find "significant" differences due to chance alone. For example, if we performed two independent statistical tests at the 0.05 level, then under the null hypothesis we would expect to find a significant result about 1 in 10 times rather than 1 in 20. If we performed five such tests, then under the null hypothesis we would expect to find a significant result about 1 out of 4 times. Clearly, we should not believe these results since they occur so frequently by chance alone, even though in isolation they appear to be significant. The same principle applies when the tests are not independent, although then it is more difficult to state the true probability. This principle also applies to monitoring clinical trial results over time. If we just wait until the comparison of treatments is first significant at the usual level and then report that p-value, we will exaggerate the significance of our findings, deluding ourselves and others. The lesson in all of this is that we should be careful to distinguish hypothesis testing from exploratory data analyses in reporting our results. The interesting things we find by exploring the data may in fact be true, but they can best be thought of as hypotheses to be tested in the future or looked for in other studies.

Some Common Statistical Tests and Techniques

Although space does not permit review of the great variety of types of analysis appropriate for biomedical data, some of the more common tests and techniques one sees mentioned in the literature are described below along with their main uses.

THE χ^2 TEST

Statisticians use χ^2 tests in a great variety of situations, but those most likely to be encountered in medical articles are concerned with analyzing cross-classified or contingency-table data and for testing goodness of fit of the data to some assumed theoretical distribution by comparing the observed data with theoretical predictions. An example of the former use would be the test of independence between row and column variables in a cross-classification of counts. In the familiar 2×2 contingency table, a test of independence of rows and columns is equivalent to comparing two proportions. For example, if we wish to compare the response rates of males and females to some drug, we might construct a table with two rows representing the sexes and two columns representing response or nonresponse. The χ^2 tests allow us to determine whether the classification by sex is independent of the classification by response, but this is equivalent to asking whether the response rates in males and females are the same. An example of a χ^2 goodness of fit test might arise if one wished to compare observed frequencies of phenotypes with those predicted theoretically by Mendel's laws.

t-TEST

The t-test is used for comparing the means of two independent sets of measurements. It is based on the assumption that both sets of measurements follow normal distributions with the same variance but, in practice, these two requirements can be relaxed somewhat. Roughly speaking, it is usually sufficient that the two frequency distributions of the observations have a single large hump in the middle, not be badly skewed in either direction, and that sample variances do not differ by more than a factor of 4. If there is serious doubt about the assumptions, statisticians usually prefer to use a nonparametric test which only takes into account the ordering of the observations in each group, rather than the actual measurements. A common test of this type is the *Wilcoxon test*.

PAIRED ANALYSIS

A method often appropriate in medical studies, but frequently overlooked, is that of paired analyses. This technique may be used when the observations are naturally paired in some way, such as blood sugar measured before and after treatment for each of a group of individuals. An example will make this concept clear. In his textbook, *Statistics in Biology*, Bliss[1] describes an experiment in which the length in millimeters of the left and right external ears of each of 477 young men were measured to determine whether one ear was longer than the other. If one disregarded the paired nature of the data, the difference between the two ears (0.449 mm) was not significant, $p = 0.08$, despite the large number of measurements. In fact, such an analysis would be incorrect since the ear measurements are correlated and the unpaired t-test assumes independence. However, when an appropriate paired analysis was performed, the difference was significant at $p < 0.0000001$. The reason for this discrepancy is that big people generally have big ears and little people have little ears so that the variation in ear lengths related to body size obscured a highly significant difference between the average lengths of left and right ears. The effect of body size disappears when a paired analysis is performed. Usually the gain in statistical significance is not so striking, but paired analysis should definitely be used when appropriate. It is very closely related to the concept of adjusting for covariate information.

ANALYSIS OF VARIANCE

The analysis of variance is an important technique for analyzing designed experiments where the goal is to compare averages of measurement data cross-classified in sometimes rather complex ways. In its simplest form, it is identical to the t-test described above and, like that test, assumes that the averages of observations in the groups being compared follow normal distributions with equal variances, at least after appropriate transformation of the data. This form of analysis grew out of agricultural research concerned with fertilizers, pesticides and the like, but it sometimes appears in the medical literature, particularly in the analyses of laboratory experiments. The fundamental concept underlying the analysis of variance is that of comparing the *variation within* the groups to the *variation between* the groups. If the variation between groups is much greater than the variation within groups, we reason that the groups must be different.

MULTIPLE REGRESSION

Multiple regression refers to a group of techniques designed to estimate the effects of a number of variables acting simultaneously on a single outcome variable. For example, we might want to know how the level of some biological marker for cancer is related to the age and sex of the patient, and the stage and cell type of his tumor. Of course we could examine the relationship separately for each of these variables, but since the variables themselves are likely to be correlated, we may be more interested in some meaningful summary of how they all act together since that is obviously the way they behave in the patient. The most common types of multiple regression are *multiple linear regression* (linear refers to the assumed statistical model relating the several variables to a *quantitative* outcome) and *logistic regression*, a form of analysis appropriate when the outcome variable is an all-or-nothing or a so-called *qualitative* or *binary response*. When the outcome variable is a count in a cross-classified table, then a closely related methodology based on a *log-linear model* may be used to determine how the counts depend on the variables used to cross-classify them.

LIFE TABLES AND SURVIVAL CURVES

A life table is a set of calculations defining the probability of survival at various points in time after entry into a study. The survival curve is a plot of these probabilities versus time. These techniques were originally used by actuaries in determining insurance rates for defined groups of people. They are familiar to almost all physicians and medical researchers and play an important role in comparing treatments of cancer patients. A more detailed, but still nontechnical discussion of these techniques appears in Ref. 2. The aspect of survival analysis that most often seems to confuse medical audiences is the method of using censored data. For example, many people seem to feel that a 5-year survival rate cannot be calculated unless all patients could have been followed for 5 years, but these statistical procedures use the censored data and thereby gain greater precision. Cutler and Ederer[3] have a readable explanation of the principles involved.

SURVIVAL MODELS WITH COVARIATES

Although survival curves such as those described in the last section can be constructed to show the importance of a factor such as sex, age, cell type, menopausal status, or type of treatment, such a profusion of survival curves scarcely satisifies our desire for a simple summary of a complex set of data. In the past decade and a half, a great deal of both theoretical and applied statistical work has been directed toward developing statistical models for survival which may incorporate the effects produced by several variables acting together. Most of these methods can be viewed as special cases of *multiple regression*, specially adapted for dealing with censored survival data. Some of these methods are based on theoretical distributions such as the *Weibull model*. This model is capable of fitting sets of data in which the death rate either increases or decreases with the passage of time. When the death rate remains constant over time, the Weibull distribution reduces to the *exponential distribution* familiar to many laboratory researchers as the statistical law describing the times between decay events of radioactive elements. Some of the most important recent work concerning survival analysis with covariate information has been based on a model proposed by Cox[4] in 1972. The *Cox model* does not require any assumptions about the nature of the death rate. The effects of covariates are introduced by assuming that they increase or decrease the underlying death rate (whatever it may be) in a multiplicative fashion. The techniques based on this approach are referred to as *proportional hazard models* since in statistical language the term "hazard" refers to a death rate. All of these survival models incorporating covariates have been extremely useful in identifying prognostic variables and in performing adjusted survival analyses in cases where it is feared that unequal distributions of important prognostic variables may have confused any simple unadjusted treatment comparisons.

Design of Studies

Design issues have been saved until last because a study cannot be designed until the nature of the questions to be asked, the kind of data, and the type of analysis to be undertaken have been specified. One might argue that these are all aspects of the design (and I would not seriously disagree), but there are a number of other important matters to consider.

SAMPLE SIZE, ERROR RATES, AND POWER

One of the most fundamental questions is how many experimental subjects will be required. If the main question being asked in the study is of a descriptive nature, then the number of subjects will be directly related to the precision of the estimates to be obtained. For example, we may wish to estimate the percent response to a new treatment with 95% confidence limits for this estimate ranging only to ±10%. Once this degree of precision has been specified, it will ordinarily be possible to state the sample size required to guarantee that degree of precision.

If the main question is of the comparative type, statisticians determine sample size by calculating probabilities that the wrong conclusion may be derived from the study. These probabilities are referred to as *error probabilities* and they are of two types usually designated type I and type II. A *type I error* refers to rejecting the null hypothesis when it is in fact true, while a *type II error* refers to failing to reject (accepting) the null hypothesis when it is in fact untrue. For example, if we compared two treatments which in fact had identical response rates, but by chance we observed and reported a significant difference, then we would have made a type I error. On the other hand, if two treatments really had a true difference in response rates, but because of chance fluctuations we failed to find it, then we would have made a type II error. In designing comparative studies, the probability of a type I error is often set at the familiar p value of 0.05 or less on the grounds that we are willing to make a type I error in 1 out of every 20 or more experiments. Reducing the probability of a type I error even further may require the study of an inordinately large number of subjects and we may feel that such further effort is unwarranted since 1 in 20 is usually an acceptable probability for making an error of this type. Larger probabilities are generally accepted for type II errors, often as high as $p = 0.10$ or even 0.20 (1 out of 10 or 1 out of 5). If we subtract the probability of a type II error from 1.0; we obtain what is referred to as the *power of the statistical test*.

The probability of a type II error (or equivalently the power of the statistical test) depends on how different the *alternative hypothesis* (some postulated true difference) is from the null hypothesis. For example, for any given sample size, it may be easy to detect a difference between two response rates as great as 50%, but we would be much more likely to miss a difference as small as 5%. The power of the test refers to the probability that we will detect a significant difference between two sets of observations (reject the null hypothesis) if the true difference is of some specified magnitude. Thus, in calculating the needed sample size, we must first identify differences of sufficient magnitude and importance that we would want an acceptably low probability of failing to find such differences in our study. We would almost never want the power of our statistical test to be less than 0.5 because that would mean we were more likely to fail to find a significant difference than to find one, even when such a true difference exists.

It is a sad fact that many comparative studies of treatment are conducted with so few subjects that the power to detect modest but medically important differences is in fact less than 0.5. For example, if the control response rate was about 50% and we were interested in detecting a difference as small as 10% (a response rate of 60% with the new treatment), then 306 patients would be required in each group if we want 8 chances out of 10 of detecting the difference (power $-$ 0.80) at a one-tailed significance level of $p = 0.05$. For a power of 0.5 (even chances of missing the difference), we would still require 134 patients in each group.

OTHER DESIGN ISSUES

Another design question concerns the allocation of patients to two or more treatment groups, that is, what proportion of the total number of subjects should be assigned to each group. Unless there are markedly different costs associated with the different treatment groups, it is usually best to put equal numbers of subjects in all groups since, in most situations, fewer total patients will then be required.

If the purpose of the study is to obtain descriptive information which is meant to be applied to a larger population, then formal sampling techniques may be required to permit such generalization of the results. In many situations, a formal random sample may be a sensible solution. In comparative studies, on the other hand, randomization may be needed to assure comparability of groups. A further assurance of comparability may be obtained by adding stratification on important prognostic factors to the randomization scheme, a feature which will be particularly important in small studies. Whether or not stratification is a part of the design, a stratified analysis is usually desirable.

In the final stages of planning, we must decide how much covariate information to record. However tempting it may be, it is usually unwise to expect any single study to answer too many questions. Indeed, it is often difficult to design a study with sufficient care to provide a clear answer to even a single question.

RESOURCES AND USING COMPUTERS

A final consideration in design which influences decisions on every other aspect of the study concerns the resources available for carrying it out. These resources include money, time, and the availability of interested, well trained and dedicated personnel as well as the availability of subjects for study. Another consideration is whether or not computers will be available to help us collect, store, edit, and analyze the data.

Computers are by no means essential, but when properly used they can be extremely helpful, mainly because they can store large amounts of data conveniently and perform extremely rapid calculations. Indeed, they have made many statistical analyses possible that in previous years would have been unthinkable simply because of the enormous amounts of calculation involved. Great care must be taken in deciding how to enter data into the computer. For example, it is important to distinguish carefully between negative, missing, and unknown data. Occasionally, one sees forms where there are check lists for symptoms or positive physical findings. If the physician just checks off those items that apply, then when it comes time to enter the data into the computer, it is impossible to distinguish between the absence of findings, missing values, and unknown values. This problem arises more frequently than one might imagine. It is important to realize that computers do not think, and that having the data in a computer in no way sanctifies them or endows them with any special characteristics which should cause us to believe that they are somehow better or more reliable than information written on sheets of paper.

SPECIAL TOPICS IN CANCER

Population Rates

Incidence and *mortality rates* for cancer are descriptive statistics collected to give us some general ideas about how many new cases of cancer occur each year and how many patients die each year. These statistics are usually compiled from very large populations so that it is possible to present specific rates for separate age categories, sexes, races, and geographical locations. Mortality statistics are available for the entire United States and are obtained from death certificates which are required by law in all states. Data on incidence are much more difficult to obtain. National studies of cancer incidence were conducted in 1937, 1947, and in the 3-year period 1969–1971 overlapping the 1970 census. In the last of these, a population of some 20 million people, or roughly 1/10 of the United States population, was studied. Cancer registries for selected geographical regions of the country have supplied annual incidence figures since 1973. *Survival rates* from the time of diagnosis for specific types of cancer also have been compiled from these and other cancer registries. *Prevalence rates* estimate the number of people who have cancer at any one time and are less commonly available, although they may be estimated crudely from the incidence and survival rates. These rates are useful for giving us an idea of the magnitude and variation of the cancer problem and for deciding which cancers are more common or more lethal. Incidence rates are particularly useful to epidemiologists because variations in these rates in different segments of the population suggest epidemiologic hypotheses which may be tested by a more detailed study. Despite their general usefulness, population rates are often over interpreted and misinterpreted, especially when comparisons are made of rates determined at different points in time. For example, an apparent increase in incidence of cancer may simply reflect more careful efforts at diagnosis, better record keeping, or changes in the definitions of diagnostic entities. When interpreting national death rates, it is important to realize that the information is based on diagnoses listed on death certificates and is therefore somewhat crude and inaccurate. More detailed data on stage of disease at diagnosis and histological type are generally supplied by cancer registries, but data on certain other important variables are almost never available except in special studies. Population survival rates are also subject to misinterpretation. For example, early diagnosis, such as that brought about by mass screening programs, will make the survival of patients appear longer even though no progress has been made in treatment. The role of these programs should be evaluated by controlled scientific experiments. So far only a few such controlled studies have been carried out.

Epidemiologic Studies

Epidemiologic studies in cancer are usually designed to investigate possible causes of cancer or the role of factors which may affect the risk of cancer. Since we know the etiology of very few cancers, the list of possible causes is quite long and includes such things as genetics, diet, personal habits such as smoking and drinking, x-rays, chemicals, and viruses. Factors which may affect risk include such things as race, national origin, age at first pregnancy, obesity, or a history of cancer in the family. For simplicity in the ensuing discussion, we may lump all these things together and refer to them as exposure.

TYPES OF STUDIES

There are two general types of epidemiologic studies, prospective and retrospective. *Prospective studies* (also called *cohort studies*) generally require large numbers of subjects and long periods of observation. They proceed by first identifying a group of exposed subjects and then choosing an appropriate group of unexposed control subjects, usually matched on such factors as age, sex or other variables likely to influence the later development of cancer. These two groups are followed in time to determine whether cancer develops more frequently in one group than the other. *Retrospective studies* (often called *case-control studies*) are much more common than prospective ones, possibly because they generally require fewer subjects and much less time to complete. These studies begin by identifying a group of patients with cancer or some other disease and then identifying an appropriate control group, usually matched on important variables which are not under study, just as in prospective studies. After these two groups are identified, past exposure to some factor of interest is determined by questioning the subjects if they are still alive or by studying medical records. Mantel and Haenszel provide a good discussion of retrospective studies.[5]

The goal of the analysis in both kinds of epidemiologic studies is to determine if there is a significant association between the exposure, or factor under study, and the presence of the disease. The degree of association is usually measured by the *relative risk* in prospective studies and the *odds ratio* in retrospective studies. When there is no association between disease and exposure, these two measures take on the value 1.0. A value of 2.0 for the relative risk would mean that the disease was twice as likely among the exposed.

INTERPRETATION

Epidemiologic studies are observational in nature rather than experimental since we can not try deliberately to cause cancer in humans. For this reason, unusual caution is required in their interpretation. First, we must ask if the study was conducted and analyzed correctly because there are many pitfalls in this kind of research. Determining the answer to this question is even difficult for professional biostatisticians. A second point is the strength of the association reported. The higher the relative risk, the more convincing the evidence—other things being equal. Relative risks less than 2.0, even when statistically significant, are not very convincing because all kinds of subtle biases can produce effects of that magnitude. If the exposure under study can be characterized as occurring at different levels of intensity, then evidence of a dose-response relationship provides more convincing evidence. Another feature useful to consider is biological plausibility. Since it is known that many cancers take years to develop, epidemiologic studies reporting significant positive association for recent short-term exposures are unconvincing to many scientists, while others may regard them as evidence for late promotion of a carcinogenic process which was already underway. One cannot rely too much on the criteria of biologic plausibility since this would prevent us from finding new biologic principles. Nevertheless, it is usually comforting when the finding in human epidemiologic studies agree with the findings in experimental animals. A final point to consider is the consistency of findings across different epidemiologic studies. When several studies carried out by competent investigators produce contradictory results, it is difficult to know what to conclude.

Evaluation of Diagnostic Tests

When a new diagnostic test is proposed, it is usually evaluated in both diseased and control subjects. The results are often displayed in a 2 × 2 table containing numbers of subjects with and without the disease cross-classified by the results of the new diagnostic test. Here it is not enough to see if the results of a new test are significantly associated with the presence of disease or, equivalently, that the average value of the diagnostic test differs between cases and controls. We must also concern ourselves with the concepts of sensitivity and specificity.

Sensitivity is the percentage of subjects known to have the disease who are identified by the new test, while *specificity* is the percentage of control subjects classified by the new test as negative. A perfect test would have both sensitivity and specificity of 100%. These two measures are more informative than simply quoting the percent agreement between the true state of the patient and the results of the test or quoting the numbers of false negatives and false positives. This point may be clarified by an example. Suppose we were studying a group of 100 subjects encountered on the street corner and only one of them turned out to have cancer. Our new test consists in simply saying that no one has cancer. Using this ridiculous test, we would find that there was 99% agreement between the results of our test and the truth, no false positives, and only one false negative. However, it is clear that the test is useless and in fact the sensitivity of the test would be 0% even though the specificity is 100%±.

Even if we have a test with high sensitivity and specificity, that still does not mean that the test is useful since we must consider its cost and how much it adds to whatever diagnostic information may already be available. These last points are frequently overlooked in articles describing new diagnostic tests. If the result of the diagnostic test is a measurement (such as the amount of some substance in the serum) then a frequent error of analysis is choosing that value of the test which best separates the cases from the controls and using this as a cutoff value for constructing and analyzing the 2 × 2 table. This procedure is statistically improper and will result in overestimating the statistical significance of the test. In effect, what we have done is peek at the data before deciding on the form of analysis. Of course, this may be useful in suggesting a cutoff value to be used in future studies.

Treatment Comparisons

CASE REPORTS AND PERSONAL SERIES

The publication of case reports and personal series have been important in the history of medicine. However, unless one succeeds in curing a previously incurable disease, case reports generally provide little information about the efficacy of treatment, although they may provide useful information about pathophysiology, unusual features of a disease, or toxicity of treatments. The publication of personal series, results for a group of patients treated by a single physician or at a single center, began in Europe in the late 19th century. These reports were a definite step forward since before that time physicians seldom made serious efforts to obtain follow-up information on their patients to evaluate carefully the results of their therapeutic actions and possible undesirable sequelae. This practice has continued to the present and much effort is spent in informal comparisons of series, usually accompanied by excessive rhetoric, for the purpose of determining which treatments appear to be the most effective. Even now, these publications have a certain limited usefulness, but they occupy far too much space in medical journals in comparison to what can be learned from reading them.

SERIES WITH HISTORICAL CONTROLS

An improvement over reporting results of treatment in series of patients without any control group, other than references to the summary results obtained in other similar series, is the use of historical control groups. This term is meant to imply that complete data for individual patients treated by another method are used for comparison with the reported series. Often, this control group consists of patients treated previously by the same investigator or at the same institution just before some new therapy was introduced. Reports of this kind usually contain fairly elaborate adjusted analyses designed to correct for the effects of important prognostic variables which might not have been well balanced across the two treatment groups. In situations where it is not possible to do a randomized clinical trial, this is a reasonable procedure if sufficient care is taken to assure that patients were comparable in all regards except the treatments administered and that sufficient data are available to perform convincing adjusted analyses.

Comparability of patients includes such things as the precise criteria for eligibility in the studies, identical methods for diagnosing and staging the disease, the same kind and extent of supportive care, and identical follow-up procedures. Comparability can be destroyed by subtle changes in time concerning the nature of the patient population, diagnostic methods, details of treatment, or supportive care. Other problems include the absence of information needed for adjusted analyses and the necessity of relying on a mathematical model even when information is available. The effects of unmeasured or unknown prognostic factors may play a decisive role, but cannot be assessed.

For these reasons, there is often considerable uncertainty concerning whether any improvement claimed for a new treatment should be believed since the differences found in most treatment comparisons, though medically important, are relatively small compared to the possible effects of systematic bias or unnoticed selection of patients. Three articles[6-8] written for medical readers discuss in more detail the difficulties with historically controlled studies and argue in favor of the use of randomized clinical trials whenever possible.

RANDOMIZED CLINICAL TRIALS

Randomized clinical trials are a fairly recent development in medical research. The first such trials were carried out in England in the 1940s in evaluating streptomycin as a treatment for tuberculosis. Their use in evaluating cancer therapies began in the early 1960s and has increased rapidly since that time. These studies may be regarded as proper scientific experiments which need suffer from none of the objections made to historically controlled studies. The main purpose of randomizing patients is to eliminate bias, whether conscious or unconscious, from the treatment comparisons. Patients are admitted to the study, then treated and followed according to carefully written protocols which attempt to standardize all aspects of the patient's care so that sound conclusions can be drawn from the eventual results. Since randomized trials are often rather complicated experiments, I will not attempt to discuss the principles of their design, conduct, and analysis, but instead refer the reader to an excellent two-part article appearing in the *British Journal of Cancer*[9, 10] which contains an up-to-date, thorough, and readable account of these matters. It is important to understand and participate in randomized clinical trials since, when properly conducted, they provide the most reliable information available about treatment comparisons.

THINGS TO CONSIDER IN READING ARTICLES

The general statistical principles presented under "General Principles" provide a convenient framework for evaluating scientific articles. For example, we should determine whether the question addressed by the paper was descriptive or comparative. We should ask ourselves what kind of data were studied and how they were obtained. If the data were measurements, what do we know about their accuracy? If times to response were studied, were any of the observations censored, and how did this censoring come about? What kind of analysis was performed and was it appropriate for the kind of questions asked and the type of data? What was the source of the p-values cited in the article, and were these one- or two-tailed? Could paired analysis have been used and have the authors taken into account the problem of multiple comparisons when quoting p-values?

Concerning the design, we should first check to see what sample sizes were involved and then check to see if all these subjects are accounted for in all tables and graphs, or whether some have been purposely or unwittingly omitted. It is remarkable how often this simple requirement is not met. Even in well designed studies, there is often a temptation to leave out certain patients for one reason or another. For instance, in analyzing randomized clinical trials, investigators often decide to compare only those patients receiving, for example, adequate doses of radiation or chemotherapy. Unfortunately, this may lead to an improper comparison because marked selection biases may result due to such things as elimination of patients who died before they could complete the course of therapy. A good example of this in urology has to do with reporting survival figures for patients with stage B prostatic cancer treated by radical prostatectomy. A frequent practice is to exclude patients who are found at operation to have had more extensive disease. Since these patients have worse chances of survival, it should be obvious that this practice gives too high an estimate of survival if the results are to be compared to unoperated series. The general rule about dropping patients from an analysis in comparative studies is that only things which could have been known before the study began may be used as reasons, and patients should never be dropped because of things occurring during the course of the study.

Other important design questions are: was the study controlled, and if so what was the nature of the control group; are we convinced that it was comparable; and was stratification needed or done? Finally, we must consider the report of conclusions: do we believe them, how general are they, and can they be applied to other groups of patients? Were the investigators really testing a previously specified hypothesis, or is there some suspicion that they may just be reporting chance findings which happened to appear in their data? What should we conclude if the results of the study were negative? Was the sample size large enough that the investigators had a reasonable chance of finding significant differences if they, in fact, existed? Are confidence limits cited which allow us to determine what magnitude of differences are consistent with the data?

CONSULTING WITH STATISTICIANS

It should be obvious from the foregoing that statistical considerations can affect every aspect of a scientific study. For this reason, when planning a new study, it is usually desirable to consult a statistician in the early stages after some preliminary plan has been developed. All too often, statisticians are consulted only after the study is completed and some kind of analysis is required. This is unfortunate because sometimes even the most ingenious analytic techniques are incapable of producing meaningful results from poorly designed or conducted studies. When consulting with a statistician, the physician should assure himself that the statistician understands the scientific background of the problem as completely as possible, the nature of the questions asked, and the kind of data that can be obtained. Only then will he be able to consider possible types of analyses and help devise an appropriate design. It is almost never appropriate simply to call the statistician on the telephone and ask if he happens to have a computer program for performing the analysis of variance or for constructing survival curves.

Proper collaboration requires a thorough exchange of ideas between the statistical and medical specialists, each bringing information from his specialty to bear on the problem. The medical researcher should require that the statistician explain the reasons for the design he proposes and the nature of the analyses he intends to perform. This effort will help them both avoid what is sometimes referred to as type III error—obtaining the right answer to the wrong question. Since both the medical researcher and the statistician are responsible for the published results, it is usually desirable to include the statistician as a coauthor. In the past, statisticians often played a less important role, simply computing p-values from time to time, without really becoming involved in the study. This practice doubtless led to many foolish errors. Today there are many statisticians with considerable knowledge of biology and medicine who are experienced in collaborating with medical researchers. It is important to try and find such individuals if one wants to obtain the most that statistics has to offer.

REFERENCES

1. Bliss, C. I. *Statistics in Biology*. McGraw Hill, New York, 1967.
2. Byar, D. P. Analysis of survival data. *Proceedings of the 2nd Veterans Administration Cooperative Studies Program Symposium*, Chicago, Sept. 21–22, 1978.
3. Cutler, S. J., and Ederer, F. Maximuim utilization of the life table method in analyzing survival. *J. Chronic Dis. 8:*699, 1958.
4. Cox, D. R. Regression models and life tables. *J. R. Stat. Soc. B 34:*187, 1972.
5. Mantel, N., and Haenszel, W. Statistical aspects of the analysis of data from retrospective studies of disease. *J. Nat. Cancer Inst. 22:*719, 1959.
6. Byar, D. P. The necessity and justification of randomized clinical trials. In *Controversies in Cancer: design of trials and treatment.* Edited by H. J. Tagnon and M. J. Staquet. Masson Publishing Company, New York, 1979.
7. Byar, D. P. Why data bases should not replace randomized clinical trials. *Biometrics 36:* 337, 1980.
8. Byar, D. P., Simon, R. M., Friedewald, W. T., Schlesselman, J. J., DeMets, D. L., Ellenberg, J. H., Gail, M. H., and Ware, J. H. Randomized clinical trials: perspectives on some recent ideas. *N. Engl. J. Med. 295:*74, 1976.
9. Peto, R., Pike, M. C., Armitage, P., Breslow, N. E., Cox, D. R., Howard, S. V., Mantel, N., McPherson, K., Peto, J., and Smith, P. G. Design and analysis of randomized

clinical trials requiring prolonged observations of each patient. I. Introduction and design. *B. J. Cancer 34:*585, 1976.

10. Peto, R., Pike, M. C., Armitage, P., Breslow, N. E., Cox, D. R., Howard, S. V., Mantel, N., McPherson, K., Peto, J., and Smith, P. G. Design and analysis of randomized clinical trials requiring prolonged observations of each patient. II. Analysis and examples. *Br. J. Cancer 35:*1, 1977.

2

Chromosomes in Urologic Cancers*

CHROMOSOME ANALYSIS IN SOLID TUMORS

The present review will attempt to draw attention to the salient accomplishments to date in the cytogenetics of urologic cancers and will deal primarily with the chromosomal findings and their possible clinical application in those conditions of direct interest to the urologist. Progress in this area has been relatively slow as compared, for example, to the voluminous amount of karyotypic‡ data available in hematologic conditions (*e.g.* leukemia and lymphoma).[1] This discrepancy has been due almost entirely to methodologic factors which have made chromosome analysis in solid tumors, particularly those of the prostate and bladder, difficult, inefficient, and less than optimal. However, recent developments in cytologic and cytogenetic techniques as applied to solid tumors,[2-4] and undoubtedly those which will be developed in the future, will greatly expand the amount and quality of the karyotypic data in urologic cancers.

For more details regarding the terminology, classification and nomenclature of chromosomes and methods for karyotypic analysis, the background to the cytogenetics of urologic cancers, presentation of karyotypic data obtained in such cancers,and a comprehensive discussion of their significance and meaning and for a complete listing of the references, the reader is referred to the book, *The Chromosomes in Human Cancer and Leukemia*,[1] recently published by the author.

* The author's studies reported in this paper have been supported in part by Grant CA-14555 from the National Cancer Institute.

‡ The terms "chromosomal," "karyotypic," and "cytogenetic" will be used interchangeably and will carry the same meaning.

CHROMOSOMES IN ESTABLISHED CANCER CELL LINES

The shortcomings of chromosomal data based on material obtained on long-term cell lines have been stressed by the present author,[1] *e.g.* selection of a karyotype *in vitro* which may not be representative of the *in vivo* status of the tumor, not infrequent overgrowth of the neoplastic cells by normal (diploid) cellular elements present in the cancer, the rather long time necessary for the cell line to be established before chromosome analysis can be performed and, most importantly, the failure to establish a viable cell line in the preponderant percentage of urologic tumors. Nevertheless, keeping these shortcomings in mind, I shall refer to cytogenetic data obtained on long-term cultures of urologic cancers when these appear to be appropriate to the presentation.

DNA MEASUREMENTS IN TUMORS

The determination of ploidy (chromosome number) by measuring nuclear DNA content by one spectrophotometric technique or another also will be mentioned in this review, even though the shortcomings are just as putative as those of long-term cultures, *e.g.* failure to detect minor chromosomal changes (loss or gain of a whole or part of a small chromosome) or recognize pseudodiploidy (presence of 46 chromosomes, but of abnormal distribution and/or morphology).

NORMAL AND ABNORMAL KARYOTYPES

The correct number of chromosomes in human cells was established only about 25 years ago[5] (Fig. 2.1). This number was shown to be 46, consisting of 22 pairs of autosomes (nonsex chromosomes) and one set of sex chromosomes (gonosomes), *i.e.* XX in the female and XY in the male (Figs. 2.2–2.4). Each somatic cell in the human obtains 23 chromosomes from the father through the sperm and 23 chromosomes from the mother through the ovum. Any deviation from the normal (diploid) number of 46 chromosomes is considered aneuploidy, *i.e.* hypodiploidy is less than 46 and hyperdiploidy is more than 46 chromosomes. Triploidy and tetraploidy refer to cells with 69 and 92 chromosomes, respectively. It is possible for a cell to be abnormal and still contain 46 chromosomes, so called pseudodiploidy, if the distribution of the chromosomes among the 23 pairs is deviant and/or if morphologically abnormal chromosomes (markers) are present. The latter may be due to simple or complex (reciprocal or not), balanced or unbalanced translocations among chromosomes to deletion of part of a chromosome, or to the presence of extra material on a chromosome. The data on urologic cancers to be discussed below will essentially be considered in terms of changed chromosome numbers and/or the presence of marker chromosomes. For all practical purposes, when a tumor contains several cells with an identical karyotype

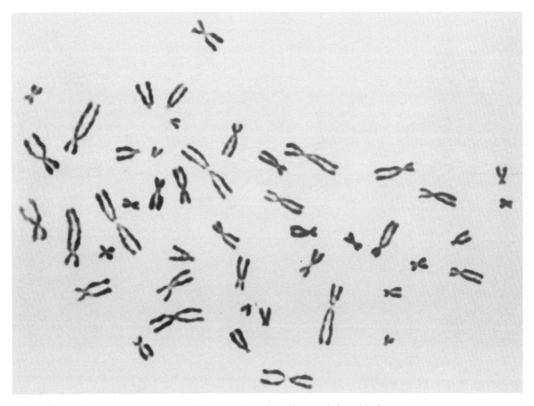

Figure 2.1. Metaphase of a normal human female cell containing 46 chromosomes. The chromosomes vary in length and location of the centromere; some of them contain satellites (the acrocentric chromosomes). These characteristics allow the identification and classification of the various chromosomes.

which is shown to contain a marker and/or numerical abnormalities of the chromosomes, such cells can be considered to be cancerous. In some cases, a possible congenital cytogenetic anomaly affecting the individual may have to be ruled out and the best way to do so is to determine the chromosome constitution of the individual in cultured blood lymphocytes. The constitution of the cancer cells can only be established on the cancer *per se*. In my opinion, when cells of a tumor are shown to be exclusively diploid in nature, the tumor is either benign (*e.g.* adenoma) or the metaphases observed may belong to normal cells present in the tumor without the tumor contributing any mitotic cells.

The identification of the various human chromosomes is based on the following: length of the chromosome relative to the others in the set, location of the centromere (kinetochore) dividing the chromosome into two arms (the arm above the centromere is labeled p, below q; often p is the *short* arm and q the *long* arm), presence of satellites and, most importantly, the distribution of the bands within a chromosome. The introduction of various banding techniques allowed the rigorous identification of all the chromosomes in the human set[6] (Figs. 2.2–2.5) and, in relation to cancer cells, the identification of abnormal (marker) chromo-

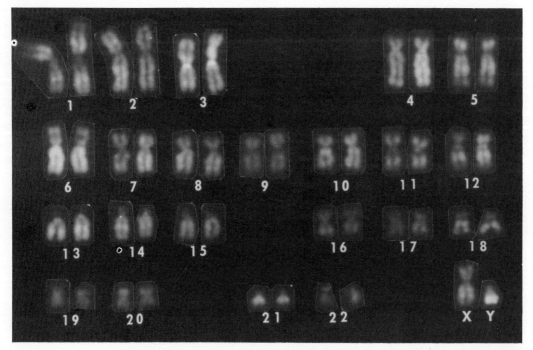

Figure 2.2. Arrangement of the chromosomes of a normal male cell into 22 pairs of autosomes and 1 pair of sex chromosomes (gonosomes). Each of the 22 pairs of autosomes consists of 1 paternal and 1 maternal chromosome. The sex chromosomes are *X* and *Y*, the former obtained from the mother and the latter from the father. This karyotype has been stained with quinacrine, thus yielding Q bands. These bands afford the opportunity to identify each chromosome with considerable certainty. Note the high fluorescence of the long arms of the Y chromosome. Q-banding was the first banding technique introduced into human cytogenetics in 1970 and initiated an era in which not only normal but also abnormal chromosomes could be identified as to their identity and origin.

somes and the derivation of the markers and various translocations (Fig. 2.6). In the discussion below, reference will be made to findings obtained prior to banding (before 1970); it should be realized that without banding, markers may spuriously be labeled as normal chromosomes. Thus, the results obtained prior to banding must be interpreted with this reservation in mind. In other words, it is possible for a chromosome to morphologically resemble a normal one and at the same time be quite abnormal when analyzed with banding, the banding pattern revealing the abnormal origin or constitution of such a chromosome (Fig. 2.7).

CANCERS OF URINARY SYSTEM

Tumors of Kidney

Chromosome analysis is available only on about 12 cases of kidney tumors.[1] Most of these were done prior to banding. Thus, Cox[7] in 1966 reported studies on seven nephroblastomas. Except for one case in which the modal chromosome number was 55–58, in all others it was at, or near, 46. In fact, three patients, including the two youngest (age 11 and 18 months), yielded diploid karyotypes only. Two additional tumors had some hyperdiploid cells with extra C or ≠1 chromosomes, whereas the tumor in the oldest patient (13 years) had a consistent karyotype of 46 chromosomes in which a chromosome ≠1 was missing and an extra C-like chromosome, which might have been derived from the chromosome ≠1, was seen.

In other unbanded studies, three renal carcinomas and two of the renal pelvis were studied. Four were found to be hypodiploid and one hyperdiploid. The range of chromosome numbers was 23–85.[8] A carcinoma of the kidney was found to have 50–51 chromosomes with similar karyotypes on two occasions.[9]

A biopsy specimen of a liver metastasis from a rapidly progressing renal adenocarcinoma was investigated with banding.[10] Of the metaphases studied, 40% had a chromosome number in the triploid range. A characteristic set of markers was consistently present in these metaphases. The main part of the metaphases studied, however, had a normal diploid karyotype and the authors[10] postulated that these cells apparently repre-

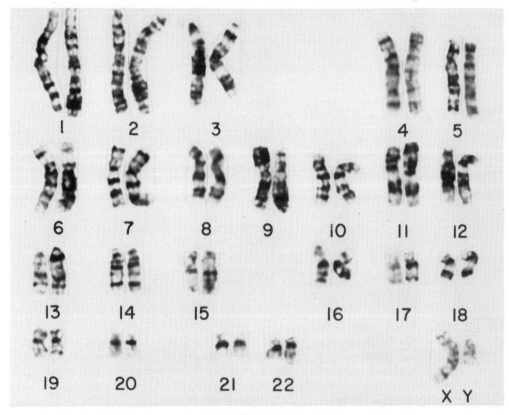

Figure 2.3. G-banded (stained with Giemsa) karyotype of a normal male cell showing bands of varying intensity and in each case affording the opportunity to identify the chromosomes of each pair.

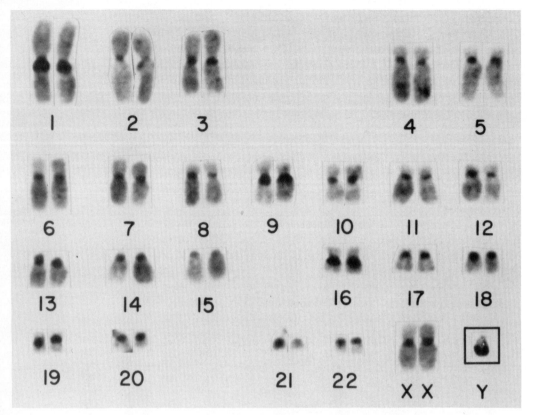

Figure 2.4. C-banded karyotype of a normal female cell, a procedure which tends to stain the paracentric areas and with particular intensity those of chromosomes *1, 9* and *16*. It can be noted that there is some variation in the size and shape of the C-chromatin, this being a characteristic related to whether the chromosome is of paternal or maternal origin. The *inset* shows a Y chromosome from another cell, to indicate the heavy staining of its long arms with C-banding.

sent normal host cells stimulated to mitotic activity by the presence of the neoplasm.

Banding analysis was performed on three clonal cell lines derived from a human renal carcinoma and its lymph node metastasis.[11] Banding revealed a rather variable chromosome number depending on the manipulations performed with these cell lines. However, most of the marker chromosomes could be identified and were derived by deletion, inversion, translocation, or isochromosome formation of chromosomes ≸1, ≸3, ≸4, ≸5, ≸8, ≸9 and ≸17. Three marker chromosomes were shown to be shared by the three cell lines which, according to the authors,[11] confirmed the common origin of these lines. Other established cell lines from human renal cell cancers have revealed various karyotypic pictures ranging from hypodiploidy with nonrandom loss of chromosomes and without the presence of markers to hypertetraploidy and the presence of definite marker chromosomes.[12-14] Thus, to date, the cytogenetic findings in renal cell carcinoma reveal no consistent karyotypic change which characterizes this tumor, although it is hoped that the application of banding techniques

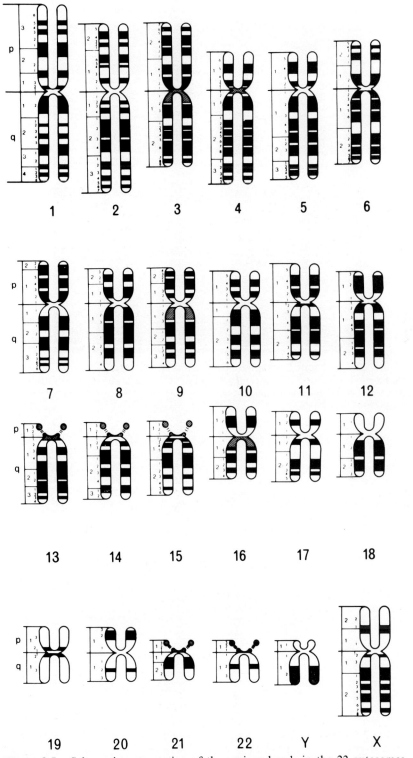

Figure 2.5. Schematic presentation of the various bands in the 22 autosomes and sex chromosomes of normal human cells according to the 1971 Paris Conference.[6]

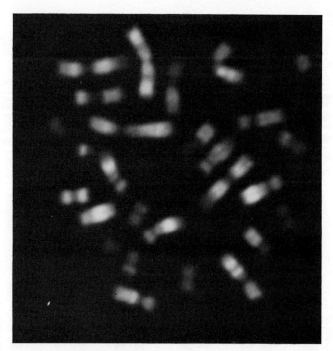

Figure 2.6. Q-banded metaphase from a tumor cell containing much less than the normal number of 46 chromosomes but showing a rather large number of abnormal chromosomes (markers), either due to translocation between chromosomes or to the formation of so-called isochromosomes.

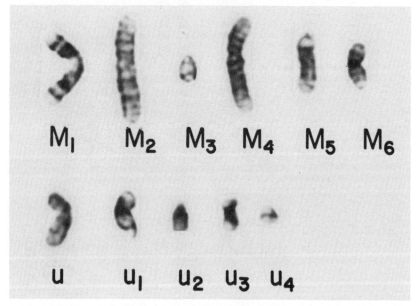

Figure 2.7. Marker chromosomes from a tumor cell in which six of the markers (M_1–M_6) could be identified as to their origin, whereas the five (U–U_4) remain unidentified. It is not uncommon in human cancers for one to be able to identify some of the markers and not others. Marker chromosomes by definition are those which deviate morphologically from any chromosomes of the normal set.

to a much larger number of such tumors will ultimately reveal some nonrandom changes akin to those described for other tumors, e.g. meningioma (−22),[15] ovarian cystadenocarcinoma [t(6;14)][16] and mixed tumor of the parotid [t(3;8)].[17]

HEREDITARY RENAL CELL CARCINOMA

An interesting family with renal-cell carcinoma associated with a chromosomal translocation, t(3;8)(p21;q24), has been described by Cohen et al.[18] This family contained members with an inherited chromosomal translocation which predisposed to renal cancer. The balanced reciprocal translocation between chromosomes #3 and #8 was found in 8 of the 10 patients with renal cancer whose karyotype was known and no family member with a normal karyotype had renal cancer. An unbalanced chromosomal translocation was not detected in the family and may well be lethal; early spontaneous abortions may have gone unnoticed. The balanced translocation was transmitted to approximately one half of the living male and female progeny in three consecutive generations. Development of renal cancer in such heterozygous persons with the translocation appeared to follow an autosomal dominant pattern of inheritance. The chromosomal abnormality is prezygotic, detected in somatic cells and distinct from postzygotic chromosomal lesions reported in malignant cell lines of other cancers.

The family discussed above should spur urologists to undertake similar studies in other families in whom kidney and other urologic tumors appear to occur with a higher frequency than expected. Only through further cytogenetic studies will the significance of the t(3;8), in relation to the development of renal cell cancer and the exact mechanism by which such cytogenetic changes lead to neoplasia, be established. Unfortunately, the tumors in this case were not studied so that we do not have an exact karyotypic picture of the renal cell cancers, i.e. whether they contain the translocation and/or other chromosomal changes which would differentiate these tumors from others.

WILMS' TUMOR ASSOCIATED WITH ABNORMALITY OF CHROMOSOME #11

The association of Wilms' tumor with mental retardation, microcephaly, bilateral aniridia, ambiguous genitalia in males, and other congenital anomalies has been reported in more than 50 cases, selected primarily on the basis of the unusual association of aniridia and Wilms' tumor.[1] The occurrence of this syndrome is usually sporadic and has been found to be due to an interstitial deletion of the short arm of chromosome #11.[19-22] The data to date would seem to indicate that a specific deletion at 11p13 appears to cause aniridia with a one-to-three risk for the development of Wilms' tumor and an even greater risk for mental retardation (Fig. 2.8). Aside from an increased frequency of genitourinary abnormalities (from mild hypospadias to ambiguous genitalia) in males, there is no clear-cut dysmorphic syndrome associated with the deletion. High resolution banding studies of patients with partial manifestations of the syndrome may

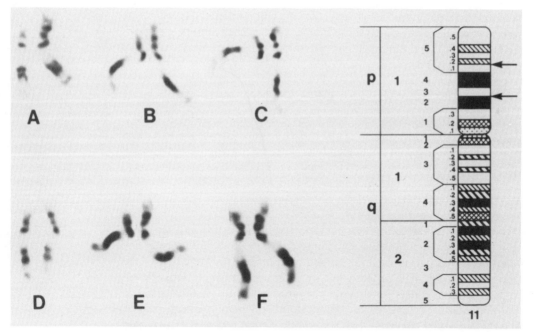

Figure 2.8. Partial trypsin C-banded prometaphase karyotypes from a case with aniridia and Wilms' tumor with abnormalities of chromosome #11. The breakpoints are depicted by the *arrows* at the edge of the *schematic chromosome #11*. (Reproduced by permission from U. Franke *et al., Cytogenet. Cell Genetics 24:* 185, 1979.[20])

allow further dissection of the responsible chromosome region,[21] while elucidation of the number and nature of genes involved will require investigation at the molecular level. Thus, the 11p− story in Wilms' tumor again points to the necessity of performing cytogenetic studies in patients with urologic tumors with the hope that knowledge regarding these tumors and their possible transmission and genesis can be gained through such approaches. Unfortunately, very few Wilms' tumors have been studied cytogenetically, so that the exact karyotypic picture in these tumors has not been established with certainty. In some cases, it has been shown that the amount of the short arm of chromosome #11 deleted (11p13−4.1) is very small indeed[21] and illustrates the need to use refined chromosome analysis for more accurate assessment of chromosomal defects.

Tumors of Urinary Bladder

Of all urologic cancers more cytogenetic studies have been done in bladder cancer than in any other condition.[1, 23] The results prior to banding were primarily obtained in transitional cell carcinomas and showed modal chromosome numbers in the diploid, triploid, and tetraploid ranges with some correlation between the number and the behavior of the tumor, both biologically and therapeutically. However, the correlation was not a very reproducible one and it still remains to be determined as to whether the chromosome number in advanced bladder cancer correlates with the parameters mentioned.

The examination of noninvasive or only submucosally invasive bladder cancer has revealed a very interesting cytogenetic correlation[23-26] (Figs. 2.9, and 2.10). Most of these tumors have been shown to have chromosome numbers in the diploid range, with the presence of marker chromosomes apparently having an important prognostic implication (Figs. 2.11, and 2.12). Thus, studies have shown that those papillary (noninvasive) tumors which contain marker chromosomes stand a 95% chance of recurrence, whereas those tumors not containing markers have less than a 5% chance of recurrence. A number of other interesting observations related to such tumors have been obtained: multiple tumors appear to have the same karyotypic picture, possibly indicative of seeding of the original tumor onto the bladder mucosa; when tumors recur, the karyotype is usually of the same nature as that observed in the original tumor; and that the triad of tetraploidy, markers, and submucosal invasiveness in moderately well differentiated cancers appear to carry such a poor prognosis as to point to early radical resection.

Because of the significance of marker chromosomes in noninvasive bladder cancer, it may be worthwhile to mention the occurrence of nuclear protrusions in cancer cells. These have been observed by several investigators in the past and the interpretation advanced has been that these

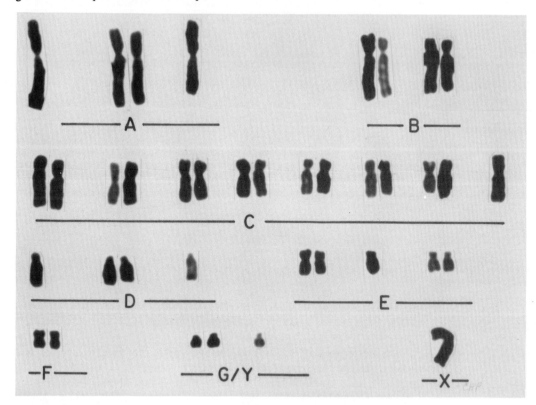

Figure 2.9. Unbanded karyotype from a papillary carcinoma of the bladder having a hypodiploid chromosome number, *i.e.* chromosomes missing in groups *A*, *D*, *E*, and *G/Y*. No definite marker chromosomes could be identified in this unbanded preparation.

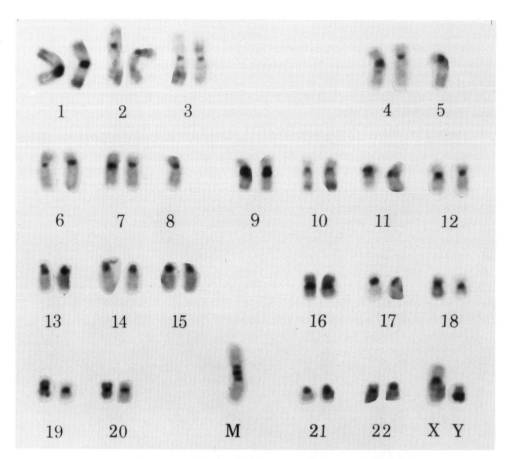

Figure 2.10. C-banded hypodiploid (45 chromosomes) karyotype from a papillary carcinoma of the bladder showing loss of chromosomes in groups *5* and *8* and, more importantly, a marker chromosome (*M*) with dicentric morphology, possibly consisting of the two missing chromosomes. The presence of such a marker in papillary cancer carries with it a very high risk of recurrence, whereas those tumors without markers carry very little risk of recurrence.

represent large marker chromosomes present in such cells.[9, 27] If that is true, examination of isolated bladder cancer cells for the presence of protrusions should be undertaken, particularly in cases in which there are very few metaphases for examination, for apparently their significance is the same as that of markers. Thus, the presence of nuclear protrusions in such cancers would carry the same prognostic implications as does the presence of marker chromosomes.

A correlation of chromosomal changes with the 5-year survival in invasive bladder tumors reveals an interesting correlation, although more cases will have to be studied in order to understand and expand the implications (Fig. 2.13). Thus, when the invasive tumors are in the near diploid range, bout 40% of the patients survive 5 years; this decreases to only 20% when the tumors are near triploid and only to about 5% when the tumors are near tetraploid. Thus, there does appear to be some correlation between the modal chromosome number and either the progression of the tumor and/or the biologic behavior of the cancer.

The karyotypic changes obtained on bladder cancer cells in culture have varied considerably.[28-32] Most of the established cultures have originated from rather well advanced cancers and, thus, one would expect the chromosomal picture to be complicated and to be accompanied by hyperdiploidy in most cases.

Where banding studies have been performed in established cell lines, they have revealed some interesting findings. For example, a mode of 58 chromosomes with retention of the X and Y was found in an established cell line from a transitional cell cancer and, in addition, the origin of 10 markers was established, including abnormalities of chromosome #1, deletion of chromosome #3, and a dicentric and several isochromosomes.[32] However, a number of other markers remain unidentified.

As mentioned previously, the results obtained with established cell lines have generally consisted of reports on the chromosome number and the presence or absence of markers, with very few of the papers actually presenting detailed banded karyotypes. Again, it must be stressed that these changes may not represent those of the *in vivo* tumor, since these cell lines had existed *in vitro* for a rather lengthy period of time during which selection of one karyotype over another may have occurred.

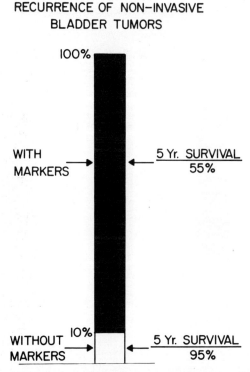

RECURRENCE OF NON—INVASIVE
BLADDER TUMORS

100%

WITH MARKERS → ← 5 Yr. SURVIVAL 55%

WITHOUT MARKERS 10% → ← 5 Yr. SURVIVAL 95%

Figure 2.11. Recurrence rate and 5-year survival rate in bladder cancer of noninvasive nature as related to the presence or absence of marker chromosomes.

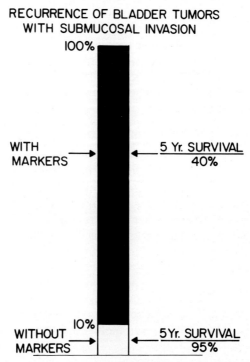

RECURRENCE OF BLADDER TUMORS
WITH SUBMUCOSAL INVASION

100%

WITH
MARKERS →   ← 5 Yr. SURVIVAL
                                40%

10%
WITHOUT →   ← 5 Yr. SURVIVAL
MARKERS   95%

Figure 2.12. Recurrence and 5-year survival rate in bladder cancers with submucosal invasion only as related to the presence of marker chromosomes in such tumors.

5-YEAR SURVIVAL IN INVASIVE BLADDER TUMORS

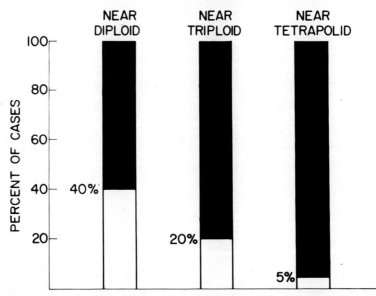

NEAR   NEAR   NEAR
DIPLOID   TRIPLOID   TETRAPOLID

100

80

60

PERCENT OF CASES

40   40%

20   20%

                              5%

Figure 2.13. The 5-year survival rate in invasive (transitional) bladder cancer as related to the modal chromosome number. Tumors with near diploid chromosome number appear to carry a better prognosis than those with higher ploidies.

34   RECENT ADVANCES IN UROLOGIC CANCER

The utilization of spectrophotometric DNA measurements in bladder cancer has been studied by a number of clinics[33-37] and appears to have some utility in the management of bladder cancer. Even though the method is not acceptable as a screening procedure and does not appear to offer a reliable correlation between the degree of malignancy and ploidy, DNA measurement of the cells may be significant in the management of bladder cancer.

Newly developed techniques[2-4] for examining cancer cells cytogenetically (Figs. 2.14 and 2.15) should spur urologists to undertake studies not only in early tumors, already discussed above, but also in *carcinoma in situ* on which cytogenetic data, for all practical purposes, do not exist. If a sufficient number of cells can be obtained through bladder washings, the application of cytogenetic analysis should aid greatly in the diagnosis and differentiation of these perplexing lesions, for the presence of any chromosomal deviation from diploidy, even in a small number of cells, if consistent, would definitely indicate a neoplastic condition.

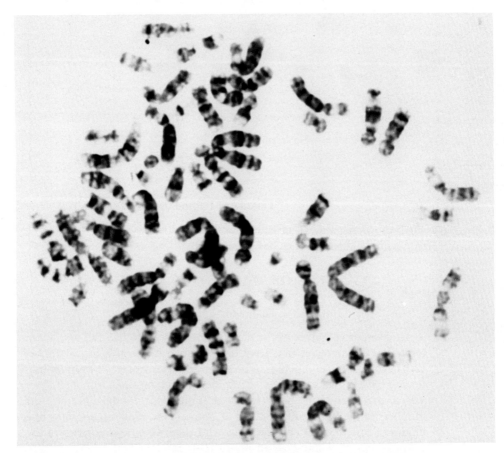

Figures 2.14 and 2.15. Two metaphases from bladder cancers demonstrating chromosome banding as ascertained with a G-banding technique. The number of chromosomes is definitely increased and the presence of abnormal chromosomes was readily established with the banding pattern.

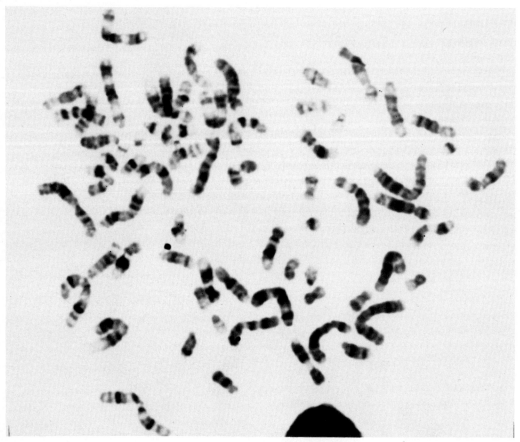

Figure 2.15

Tumors of Uretha

Chromosome studies in cancer of the urethra have been scarce. One case with 48 chromosomes has been reported.[38]

CANCERS OF MALE GENITAL SYSTEM

Testicular Tumors

An interesting feature of the more than 100 seminomas and malignant teratomas of the testes that have been studied is the absence of tumors with chromosome numbers at or below the diploid range.[1] The seminomas tend to have higher chromosome numbers than teratomas, although there was a predilection in both types of tumors for modal chromosome numbers in the hypotriploid range or above. Few of the seminomas had modes of less than 60 chromosomes and they were concentrated in the range of 60–69. There was an appreciable number with higher modes. Malignant teratomas, however, had modes of 50–59 and less frequently 60–69 and only a few tumors had higher modes. A nonrandom distribution of chromosomes in both malignant teratomas and seminomas and particular deficiency of group B and excessive group C chromosomes have been noted,[1] but since most of these studies were based on unbanded preparations it is difficult to decide with certainty the exact significance of these changes.

Nearly all malignant testicular tumors have at least one large or medium sized marker; however, a seminoma without any obvious marker has been observed.[39] Testicular teratomas are frequently X-chromatin positive; seminomas lack this feature. The reason for this is unknown, but it is clear that studies of the sex chromosomes are of special interest in teratomas. How this is related to the androgenetic origin of ovarian teratomas and hydatidiform moles in females is an intriguing question and hopefully data regarding the exact genetic origin of these teratomas will be forthcoming in the near future. Quinacrine fluorescence observations of metaphases and interphases have confirmed, or at least suggested, the presence of a Y in most seminomas and malignant teratomas, including among the latter some that were X chromatin positive and some in the form of double Y bodies.[40, 41]

MARKER CHROMOSOME IN TESTICULAR TUMORS

Much has been written in the past regarding a somewhat specific marker chromosome in testicular tumors.[42] Without banding, it was difficult to decide on the exact nature of such a marker and, in fact, controversy existed as to whether such a marker was observed in all tumors.[43] It is hoped that, as banding techniques are applied to testicular tumors, the nature and/or existence of such a marker will be settled. Of interest in this connection is the paper by Wang et al.[44] in which G-banding was performed on metaphase chromosomes from fourteen cell lines derived from primary tumors or metastases of eleven patients with testicular cancer. Break points in chromosome #1 were nonrandom being concentrated in the regions of p12, q12, p36 and p22 which resulted in morphologically identical marker chromosomes in different cases. In one instance, three lines derived from the same patient, one from tissue removed at operation and two from separate metastases removed at autopsy nearly 3 years later after successful radiotherapy and chemotherapy, had an identical chromosome composition. In another case, lines derived from a primary tumor and a metastasis from the same patient also had identical marker chromosomes. The authors indicated that the consistent involvement of chromosome #1 in aberrations may be associated with the highly malignant nature of testicular cancers. It is also possible that the abnormal chromosome #1 present in these cell lines may be related to the marker chromosome described in the past and based on nonbanded preparations. This is particularly cogent since Wang et al.[44] had indicated that all their lines had numerical and structural changes involving chromosome #1 with trisomy of the long arm being the most common aberration. Obviously, more studies are needed on primary and metastatic tumors of the testes examined directly without any long term culture in order to establish with certainty the exact nature of the marker referred to above.

In another study,[45] 10 testicular tumors were analyzed, and the karyo-types of all cells were diverse. Extra chromosomes were distributed irregularly among all groups, with the most prominent increase being in group C. An outstanding feature of the tumors was the presence of markers. A chromosome with a subterminal centromere was present in every tumor and in 35%–95% of the cells. A long marker with a secondary centromere or constriction was found in at least 50% of the cells of four cases.

Referring back to the long marker in testicular tumors, if there is specificity to this marker it would be site specific, because this long chromosome has been observed in testicular tumors of different histology and pathology, *e.g.* seminoma and malignant teratoma. The morphology of the marker is similar but not identical in different reported specimens. The proportion of the long and short arms, as well as the relative length of the chromosome varied. On the other hand, the marker has not been seen in duplicate in any cell and appears to be quite characteristic for stem line cells in the tumors described. In one case, it occurred in seminomas of both testes.[45]

FURTHER COMMENTS ON TUMORS OF TESTES

There is uncertainty about the histogenesis of testicular tumors and, hence, there is no universally accepted classification. Most tumors, how-ever, can be broadly classified as either teratomas or seminomas, even though mixed forms occur. Two main cytogenetic features of testicular tumors are the frequent occurrence of Barr bodies in teratomas[46] and the apparent universally high chromosome numbers (*i.e.* over 50) in both teratomas and seminomas.[40, 41]

Unlike the common teratomas (dermoid cysts) of the ovary, which are benign tumors, teratomas of the testis are rather uncommon and usually malignant tumors. In the more differentiated examples, elements of all three embryonic germ layers are usually present; in the undifferentiated tumors there may only be cells of carcinomatous appearance. Even though there have been several theories as to the origin of testicular teratomas, perhaps the most generally accepted one is that they arise from pluripo-tential cells that have escaped the influence of organizers.

Seminomas have a uniform histological appearance and may arise from the germinal (seminiferous) epithelium of the mature or maturing testis. They are malignant tumors, however, that are radiosensitive and carry a better prognosis than teratomas. Barr bodies have not been described in seminomas.

It is interesting to note that Atkin[40] in discussing two seminomas that had modal DNA values equivalent to 52 and 80 chromosomes, respec-tively, and were histologically of the spermatocytic variety, raised the possibility that this type of seminoma may arise from spermatocytes.

On the basis of enzyme and chromosome studies, Linder *et al.*[47] examined a number of extragonadal teratomas and endodermal sinus tumors and came to the conclusion that these tumors develop from mitotic cells; and that the cell origin could be either a somatic cell or a misplaced germ cell that failed to undergo meiosis and had proceeded directly into mitosis. Reports have appeared on the role of chromosome breakage in teratology, on the distribution of chromosome spiralization in testicular tumors, and on extragonadal teratomas.[1]

Barr bodies in teratomas were first described in 1954[48] and subsequently by other authors. In a review,[49] Barr bodies had been found in 110 out of 240 male teratomas (including some arising at extragenital sites). Sometimes they were present in some regions of the tumor but not in others; or they were confined to certain cellular components. Even though Barr bodies can occasionally be explained on other bases, *e.g.* in a case of Klinefelter's syndrome with a pineal teratoma,[48] this is exceptional in the great majority of cases, and almost all patients with testicular teratomas appear to be chromosomally normal. Various theories have been put forward to account for the appearance of Barr bodies in teratomas of males; some light recently has been shed by the demonstration that most chromatin-positive teratomas, as well as chromatin-negative teratomas and seminomas, contain Y chromosomes, either as seen in metaphases, where they are particularly easy to identify with Q- and C-banding, or revealed in interphase nuclei where in Q-stained preparations they are represented by Y-chromatin bodies.[40] The presence of both X and Y chromosomes in chromatin-positive teratomas is not in accord with theories that postulate their development from haploid cells containing an X, with subsequent conjugation of two cells, or chromosome duplication in a single cell to give XX diploid cells. Aneuploidy *per se* would not appear to explain the occurrence of Barr bodies in teratomas because, with extremely rare exceptions, other types of malignant tumors in males are chromatin negative. If, however, the aneuploidy first occurred in developing teratomas in cells where, like those in the early stages of fetal development, differentiation of X chromosomes to allocyclic behavior (formation of Barr body) had not yet occurred, the subsequent development of the latter properties might result in the appearance of Barr bodies, as it does in patients with Klinefelter's syndrome. One possibility is that the precursor cells are triploid; it is known that triploid embryos with both XXX and XXY sex chromosomes may have Barr bodies. Whether teratomas originate from diploid or triploid cells, secondary chromosome changes may, of course, involve the sex chromosomes and could account for the duplication of the Y seen in some teratomas.[40] An origin from triploid cells might also explain the consistently high chromosome numbers of both teratomas and seminomas. Kaiser-McCaw and Latt[50] showed that in ovarian tumors the pattern of duplication of the late-replicating X is identical to that of normal fibroblasts, but different from that usually observed in peripheral lymphocytes. Thus, if late replication is an accurate gauge of X inactivation, the data confirmed that such an activation can occur without fertilization.

A distinction between benign and well differentiated malignant teratomas cannot always readily be made on histologic criteria, especially in young adults. In infants and young children, however, a polycystic tumor with completely differentiated elements occurs and carries a good prognosis. According to a report on eight of these tumors,[46] there was a lack or a very low incidence of Barr bodies; more cases should be studied in order to confirm whether these tumors are generally chromatin negative. Chromosome studies on benign teratomas have not been reported, but the modal DNA value of a presumably benign well differentiated teratoma was compatible with a diploid complement.[40, 51]

Choriocarcinomas of the testes are highly malignant tumors generally considered to be a variety of teratoma. Barr bodies have been described in one tumor.[52]

Cancer of Prostate

Detailed chromosome analyses of human prostatic cancer, either primary or metastatic, are lacking. Studies on cellular DNA content of cancer of the prostate have been published and correlated with prognosis,[53] however, these methodologies lack the specificity and morphologic detail of chromosome analysis, particularly regarding the possibility of a specific karyotypic change characterizing all or some cancers of the prostate.

We reported[54] the presence of an isochromosome 17 [i(17q)], established with Q- and G-banding, in the metastatic cells (in the bone marrow) of a prostatic cancer (Fig. 2.16). Direct marrow chromosome preparations showed a mode of 70 with considerable scatter in counts and the presence (about 15%) of normal diploid metaphases with 46 chromosomes. The latter were undoubtedly of normal origin.

A prostatic cancer with hypodiploidy and no markers was described by Sekine.[8]

Chromosome studies have been performed in several human prostatic carcinoma cell lines established in long term culture[55-62] (Figs. 2.17 and 2.18). Thus, in one, the investigators[55, 56] utilized Q-banding which revealed the cells to be completely aneuploid with a modal chromosome number in the hypertriploid range. At least 10 distinctive marker chromosomes were identified. However, the modal chromosome number shifted from 62 to 55 between the 5th and 50th passage and certain karyotypic variability occurred. In another cell line originating from a primary prostatic adenocarcinoma, 28% of the cells were found to be pseudodiploid and 72% pseudotetraploid.[55] All metaphases examined were partially trisomic for chromosome #9 and lacked a demonstrable Y chromosome. The overall karyotypic patterns of the cell lines studied, as well as their marker chromosomes, clearly distinguish these lines from other cancer lines including HeLa. The latter is of importance since the authenticity of other putative prostatic cancer lines has been disputed.

Studies based on spectrophotometric DNA measurements in prostatic cancer[53, 63, 64] have indicated that the results obtained with this method could serve as a useful approach in following cancers with a hyperdiploid chromosome number as well as serve under appropriate conditions as a guide in therapy particularly in those cases in which the DNA content decreases to levels usually found in normal or benign tumors. Taken in total, however, neither the DNA studies nor those based on established cell lines have shed much light on any specific or nonrandom changes in

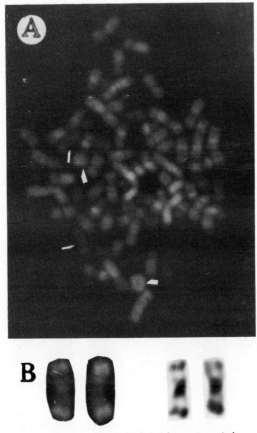

Figure 2.16. Isochromosomes of 17, i(17q) (*thin pointers*), in an invasive cancer of the prostate. The metaphase (*A*), in addition, shows the presence of ring chromosomes (*thick pointers*), a finding not uncommon in cancer cells. In *part B* are shown Q- and G-banded partial karyotypes of the iso-17 chromosome. (Reproduced by permission from M. Oshimura and A. A. Sandberg. *Journal of Urology 114:*249, 1975.[54])

prostatic cancer. To accomplish this, it will be necessary to utilize some of the newer techniques and to examine the tumors directly without resort to long-term culture. Only on the basis of such analysis will it be possible to ascertain whether cancer of the prostate is characterized by unusual changes.

Because studies[53] based on DNA content in prostatic carcinoma have indicated that ploidy may have some relationship in response to estrogens, *i.e.* all but 1 of the 9 triploid and hexaploid tumors did not respond to estrogen therapy, sharply contrasting with 22 or 24 diploid and tetraploid tumors that did respond, it becomes important to ascertain with chromosomal studies whether this particular relationship holds up.

Cancer of Penis

Very few studies have appeared on tumors or on neoplasms of the penis and as far as I know only two cases of squamous cell carcinoma of the

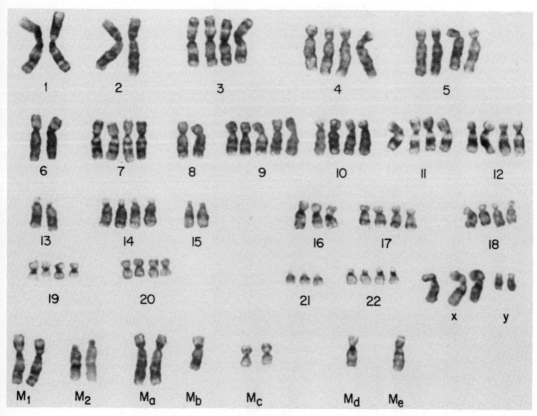

Figure 2.17. A G-banded karyotype of a cell from the LNCaP line of a human prostatic carcinoma carried in cell culture. The chromosome number is greatly increased with many of the groups containing two to three extra chromosomes. At the *bottom* are shown marker chromosomes, two of which could be identified with certainty as to their origin. The origin of the other five markers could not be ascertained.

penis, both with a stem line in the range of 71–80 chromosomes with no markers, have been examined.[65, 66]

CONCLUSION

Even though at present the chromosome changes in urologic cancers have not shed much light on the causation of these diseases or the etiologic factors associated with these conditions, urologists have not taken advantage of the possibly important potential information that cytogenetic analysis of urological cancers may yield. Such information may have a direct relevance to the success of therapeutic approaches, the chances of tumor recurrence, sensitivity of the cancers to radiation and/or chemotherapy, more concise classification of the cancers, and biologic behavior of the tumors, to mention only a few parameters. It is hoped that the situation will be ameliorated by urologists taking advantage of cytogenetic data obtained on cancers, for only through adequate application of these

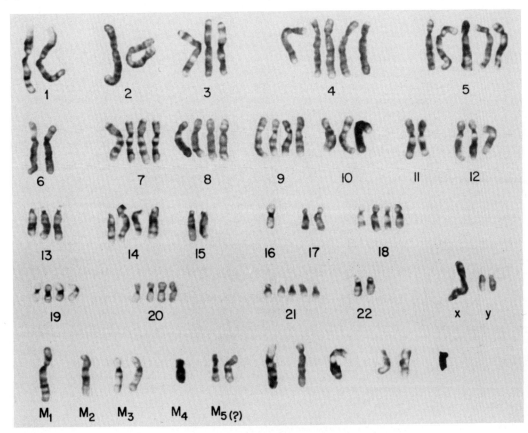

Figure 2.18. A G-banded karyotype of a LNCaP cell from a tumor grown in a nude mouse. The karyotype resembles very much that seen in cell culture (*see* Fig. 2.17) although, in this case, the origin of three of the markers could be identified, but not that of six other markers.

data and experience will it be possible to establish the significance of karyotypic analysis in urological neoplasia.

REFERENCES

1. Sandberg, A. A. *Chromosomes in Human Cancer and Leukemia.* Elsevier North-Holland, New York, 1980.
2. Wake, N., Slocum, H. K., Rustum, Y. M., Matsui, S.-I., and Sandberg, A. A. Chromosomes and causation of human cancer and leukemia. XLIV. A method for chromosome analysis of solid tumors. *Cancer Genet. Cytogenet. 3:*1, 1981.
3. Kusyk, C., Edwards, C., Arrighi, F., and Romsdahl, M. Improved method for cytogenetic studies of solid tumors. *J. Natl. Cancer Inst. 63:*1199, 1979.
4. Trent, J., and Salmon, S. E. Potential applications of a human tumor stem cell bioassay to the cytogenetic assessment of human cancer. *Cancer Genet. Cytogenet. 1:*291, 1980.
5. Tjio, J. H. and Levan, A. The chromosome number of man. *Hereditas 42:*1, 1956.
6. Paris Conference (1971). Standardization in human cytogenetics. Birth Defects: Orig. Art. Ser., Vol. VIII, No. 7. The National Foundation, New York, 1972.
7. Cox, D. Chromosome constitution of nephroblastomas. *Cancer 19:*1217, 1966.
8. Sekine, S. Cytogenetic observations in tumours of the urinary tract and male genitals. *Jpn. J. Urol. 67:*452, 1976.
9. Atkin, N. B. Cytogenetic aspects of malignant transformations. S. Karger, Basel, 1976.

10. Gripenberg, U., Ahlquist, S., Stenstrom, R., and Gripenberg, L. Two chromosomally different cell populations in a human neoplasm. *Hereditas 87:*51, 1977.
11. Hagemeijer, A., Hoehn, W., and Smit, E. M. E. Cytogenetic analysis of human renal carcinoma cell lines of common origin (NC 65). *Cancer Res. 39:*4662, 1979.
12. Komatsuhara, S. Establishment and characterization of a new cell line (NRC-12) derived from a human renal cell carcinoma. *Jpn. J. Urol. 69:*1535, 1978.
13. Williams, R. D., Elliott, A. Y., Stein, N., and Fraley, E. E. In vitro cultivation of human renal cell cancer. II. Characterization of cell lines. *In Vitro 14:*779, 1978.
14. Matsuda, M., Osafune, M., Nakano, E., Kotake, T., Sonoda, T., Watanabe, S., Hada, T., Okochi, T., Higashino, K., Yamamura, Y., and Abe, T. Characterization of an established cell line from human renal carcinoma. *Cancer Res. 39:*4694, 1979.
15. Zankl, H., and Zang, K. D. Correlations between clinical and cytogenetical data in 180 human meningiomas. *Cancer Genet. Cytogenet. 1:*351, 1980.
16. Wake, N., Hreshchyshyn, M. M., Piver, S. M., Matsui, S., and Sandberg, A. A. Specific chromosome change in ovarian cancer. *Cancer Genet. Cytogenet. 2:*87, 1980.
17. Mark, J., Dahlenfors, R., Ekedahl, C., and Stenman, G. The mixed salivary gland tumor—a usually benign human neoplasm frequently showing specific chromosomal abnormalities. *Cancer Genet. Cytogenet. 2:*231, 1980.
18. Cohen, A. J., Li, F. P., Berg, S., Marchetto, D. J., Tsai, S., Jacobs, S. C., and Brown, R. S. Hereditary renal-cell carcinoma associated with a chromosomal translocation. *N. Engl. J. Med. 301:*592, 1979.
19. Riccardi, V. M., Sujanski, E., Smith, A. C., and Francke, U. Chromosomal imbalance in the aniridia-Wilms' tumor association: 11p interstitial deletion. *Pediatrics 61:*604, 1978.
20. Francke U., Holmes, L. B., Atkins, L., and Riccardi, V. M. Aniridia-Wilms' tumor association: evidence for specific deletion of 11p13. *Cytogenet. Cell Genet. 24:*185, 1979.
21. Yunis, J. J., and Ramsay, N. K. C. Familial occurrence of the aniridia-Wilms' tumor syndrome with deletion 11p13−14.1. *J. Pediatr. 96:*1027, 1980.
22. Kolata, G. B. Genes and cancer: the story of Wilms' tumor. *Science 207:*970, 1980.
23. Sandberg, A. A. Chromosome markers and progression in bladder cancer. *Cancer Res. 37:*222, 1977.
24. Falor, W. H., and Ward, R. M. Cytogenetic analysis. A potential index for recurrence of early carcinoma of the bladder. *J. Urol. 115:*49, 1976.
25. Falor, W. H., and Ward, R. M. Fifty-three month persistence of ring chromosome in noninvasive bladder carcinoma. *Acta Cytol. 20:*270, 1976.
26. Falor, W. H., and Ward, R. M. Prognosis in early carcinoma of the bladder based on chromosomal analysis. *J. Urol. 119:*44, 1978.
27. Atkin, N. B. and Baker, M. C. Nuclear protrusions in malignant tumours with large abnormal chromosomes: Observations on C-banded preparations. *Experientia 35:*899, 1979.
28. Sanford, E. J., Geder, L., Dagen, J. E., Laychock, A. M., Ladda, R., and Rohner, T., Jr. Establishment and characterization of a new human urinary bladder carcinoma cell line (PS-1). *Invest. Urol. 16:*246, 1978.
29. O'Toole, C., Price, Z. H., Ohnuki, Y., and Unsgaard, B. Ultrastructure, karyology and immunology of a cell line originated from a human transitional-cell carcinoma. *Br. J. Cancer 38:*64, 1978.
30. Yamamoto, T. Establishment of a new cell line (NBT-2) derived from a human urinary bladder carcinoma and its characteristics. *Jpn. J. Urol. 70:*351, 1979.
31. Hisazumi, H., Kanakogi, M., Nakajima, K., Kobayashi, T., Tsukahara, K., Naito, K., Kuroda, K., and Matsubara, F. A cell line derived from urinary bladder carcinoma (KK-47): growth, heterotransplantation, microscopic structure and chromosome pattern. *Nippon Hinyokika Gakkai Zasshi 70:*485, 1979.
32. Moore, G. E., Morgan, R. T., Quinn, L. A., and Woods, L. K. A transitional cell carcinoma cell line. *In Vitro 14:*301, 1978.
33. Melamed, M. R., Darzynkiewicz, Z., Traganos, F., and Sharpless, T. K. Nuclear-chromatin structure of human bladder cell culture lines as studied by flow cytofluorometry. *Cancer Res. 37:*1227, 1977.
34. Pedersen, T., and Larsen, J. K. Flow-cytometry in bladder washings. *Ugeskr. Laeger 140:*161, 1978.

35. Peikov, Ts., and Khristov, K. Cytophotometrical determination of DNA content in transitional cell carcinoma of the urinary bladder. *Onkologie 15:*74, 1978.

36. Tribukait, B., Gustafson, H., and Esposti, P. Ploidy and proliferation in human bladder tumors as measured by flow-cytofluorometric DNA-analysis and its relations to histopathology and cytology. *Cancer 43:*1742, 1979.

37. Atkin, N. B., and Kay, R. Prognostic significance of modal DNA value and other factors in malignant tumours, based on 1465 cases. *Br. J. Cancer 40:*210, 1979.

38. Makino, S., Tonumura, A., and Ishihara, T. Studies on the chromosomes of some types of human cancer cells. *Dōbutsugaku Zasshi* (Tokyo) *68:*142, 1959.

39. Atkin, N. B. Y bodies and similar fluorescent chromocentres in human tumours including teratomata. *Br. J. Cancer 27:*183, 1973.

40. Atkin, N. B. High chromosome numbers of seminomata and malignant teratomata of the testis: a review of data on 103 tumours. *Br. J. Cancer 28:*275, 1973.

41. Khudr, G., Walsh, P. C., and Benirschke, K. Quinacrine fluorescence of testicular tumours. *Urology 2:*162, 1973.

42. Martineau, M. A similar marker chromosome in testicular tumours. *Lancet 1:*839, 1966.

43. Miles, C. P. Chromosome analysis of solid tumors. II. Twenty-six epithelial tumors. *Cancer 20:*1274, 1967.

44. Wang, N., Trend, B., Bronson, D. L., and Fraley, E. E. Nonrandom abnormalities in chromosome 1 in human testicular cancers. *Cancer Res. 40:*796, 1980.

45. Rigby, C. C. Chromosome studies in ten testicular tumours. *Br. J. Cancer 22:*480, 1968.

46. Pierce, G. B., and Kane, P. K. Nuclear sex of testicular teratomas of infants. *Nature 214:*820, 1967.

47. Linder, D., Hecht, F., Kaiser-McCaw, B., and Campbell, J. R. Origin of estragonadal teratomas and endodermal sinus tumours. *Nature 254:*597, 1975.

48. Hunter, W. F., and Lennox, B. The sex of teratomata. *Lancet 2:*633, 1954.

49. Tavares, A. S. Sex chromatin in tumors. In *The sex chromatin* Edited by L. L. Moore. Saunders, Philadelphia, 1966.

50. Kaiser-McCaw B., and Latt S. A. X-chromosome replication in parthenogenic benign ovarian teratomas. *Hum. Genet. 38:*163, 1977.

51. Lederer, B., Autengruber, M., and Mikuz, G. Statistical analysis of cytophotometric DNA measurements demonstrated on malignant testicular teratoma. *Acta Cytol. 20:*5, 1976.

52. Cavallero, G. Sulla quenza della cromatina sesuale in un caso di corionephithelioma del testicolo. *Pathologica 50:*215, 1958.

53. Tavares, A. S., Costa, J., and Costa-Maia, J. C. Correlation between ploidy and prognosis in prostatic carcinoma. *J. Urol. 109:*676, 1973.

54. Oshimura, M., and Sandberg, A. A. Isochromosome #17 in a prostatic cancer. *J. Urol. 114:*249, 1975.

55. Kaighn, M. E., Narayan, K. S., Ohnuki, Y., Lechner, J. F., and Jones, L. W. Establishment and characterization of a human prostatic carcinoma cell line (PC-3). *Invest. Urol. 17:*16, 1979.

56. Kaighn, M. C., Lechner, J. F., Babcock, M. S., Marnell, M., Ohnuki, Y., and Narayan, K. S. The Pasadena cell lines. In *Models for Prostate Cancer.* Edited by G. P. Murphy. Alan R. Liss, New York, 1980.

57. Kjaer, T. B., Thommesen, P., Frederiksen, P., and Bichel, P. DNA content in cells aspirated from carcinoma of the prostate treated with estrogenic compounds. *Urol. Res. 7:*249, 1979.

58. Mickey, D. D., Stone, K. R., Wunderli, H., Mickey, G. H. and Paulson, D. F. Characterization of a human prostate adenocarcinoma cell line (DU 145) as a monolayer culture and as a solid tumor in athymic mice. In *Models for Prostate Cancer.* Edited by G. P. Murphy. Alan R. Liss, New York, 1980.

59. Horoszewicz, J. S., Leong, S. S., Chu, T. H., Wajsman, Z. L., Freedman, M., Papsidero, L., Kim, U., Chai, L. S., Kakati, S., Arya, S. K., and Sandberg, A. A. The LNCaP cell line—a new model for studies on human prostatic carcinoma. In *Models for Prostate Cancer.* Edited by G. P. Murphy. Alan R. Liss, New York, 1980.

60. Ohnuki, Y., Marnell, M. M., Babcock, M. S., Lechner, J. F., and Kaighn, M. E. Chromosomal analysis of human prostatic adenocarcinoma cell lines. *Cancer Res. 40:*524, 1980.

61. Jellinghaus, W., Okada, K., Ragg, C., Gerhard, H., and Schröder, F. H. Chromosome studies of human prostatic tumors *in vitro. Invest. Urol. 14:*16, 1976.
62. Stone, K. R., Mickey, D. D., Wunderlei, H., Mickey, G. H., and Paulson, D. F. Isolation of a human prostate carcinoma cell line (DU 145). *Int. J. Cancer 21:*274, 1978.
63. Frederiksen, P., Thommensen, P., Kjaer, T. B., and Bichell, P. Flow cytometric DNA analysis in fine needle aspiration biopsies from patients with prostatic lesions: diagnostic value and relation to clinical stages. *Acta Pathol. Microbiol. Scand. 86:*461, 1978.
64. Leistenschneider, W., and Nagel, R. Nuclear-DNA analysis by scanning—single cell-photometry in prostatic cancer. *Aktuel Urol. 10:*353, 1979.
65. Tabata T. Karyological studies of human tumours. *Wakayama Igaku 9:*63, 1959.
66. Tabata, T. A chromosome study in some malignant human tumours. *Cytologia (Tokyo) 24:*367, 1959.

3

Oncofetoproteins and Other Markers in Genitourinary Cancer

Although the recent advances in technology including radiologic, endoscopic, and pathologic techniques, have had significant impacts on
earlier diagnosis and improved the care of cancer patients, the limits of
sensitivity of these methods still preclude the detection of cancers smaller
than 10^9 cell (1 gm). During the past several years, a number of biochemical and immunologic assays for tumor markers have made a dramatic
improvement in early detection and management of certain tumors.[1]
These markers may be measured in sera and localized in cancer cells of
cancer patients utilizing sensitive and specific radioimmunoassay and
immunocytochemical techniques. Among the important markers that
have been found in patients with urologic cancers are steroid receptors,
acid phosphatase, α-fetoprotein (AFP), human chorionic gonadotropin
(HCG), pregnancy specific β_1 glycoprotein (SP$_1$), calcitonin, and steroid
end products which are specific for certain cancers. However, a number
of other tumor markers, such as lactic dehydrogenase (LDH), carcinoembryonic antigen (CEA), placental lactogen (PL), placental alkaline
phosphatase (PLAP), γ-glutamyltranspeptidase (GGT), and other placental proteins have occasionally been helpful.

This review is a progress report on the current role of biologic markers
in urologic cancer.

CRITERIA FOR RELIABLE TUMOR MARKER

A number of criteria are essential for a marker to be useful in diagnosis
and management of cancer patients. Among these criteria are specificity
for malignant disease, lack of such markers in inflammatory disease,
detectability in body fluids and tissue extracts, a relatively short biologic

half-life, and correlation of a positive marker assay result with the presence of tumor. The assay result should reflect the tumor-bearing status and prognosis of the patients. It also is desirable to reflect the amount of tumor burden and to correlate with the effectiveness of anticancer therapeutic modalities.

False Positive and False Negative

Clinical evaluation of the efficacy of diagnostic tests often has produced misleading results, so that tests that were initially regarded as valuable were later rejected as worthless. The initial optimism and subsequent disillusionment of CEAs as a marker for different cancers serve as a classic example of such disappointment. The sensitivity and specificity of a diagnostic test may be detected by a simple algebraic formula. Sensitivity refers to the question: is this test sensitive enough to detect the minimal amount of disease, since failure to do so produces false negative results. The specificity refers to the question: if the test is negative, what is the likelihood of the patient being free of disease and, in case of failure of the test to predict this, which would produce a false positive result.

To have a low false negative initially, one should examine a large number of patients with minimal disease. To avoid false positive results also requires a large number of patients with an inflammatory disease and a number of normal controls without disease of the organ under investigation. These comparative studies should be performed in a blind fashion to avoid any bias.

Immunocytochemical Localization

Utilizing a specific antibody to a given tumor marker, one can localize the marker in cancer cells. There are several techniques of localization of tumor markers in cancer cells including indirect immunoperoxidase, peroxidase antiperoxidase, and immunofluorescence.

Radioimmunodetection of Cancer

Radioimmunodetection (RID) of cancer is based on utilization of a specific and sensitive tumor marker antiserum labeled with a γ-emitting radionuclide such as iodine-131. The deposition of radioactive antibody in tumors synthesizing a given marker such as AFP or HCG then can permit the localization of the marker-producing tumor by external scintigraphy.

TESTICULAR TUMOR MARKERS

Over the past few years, considerable progress has been made in the field of fetoplacental proteins as markers for cancer. Most studies have been on AFP, HCG, and human placental lactogen (HPL). There is also evidence that placenta secretes a chorionic thyrotropin (HCT), a chorionic follicle-stimulating hormone (HCFSH), ACTH, melanocyte-stimulating hormone, relaxin, oxytocin, vasopressin, and renin. Thus, it appears that the placenta would perform a function analogous to the hypothalamus and anterior pituitary gland, although the feedback control of this system is not clear as yet. In addition to these hormonally active peptides, the placenta also secretes a specific heat-stable alkaline phosphatase, and a number of proteins designated as pregnancy-associated proteins, including pregnancy specific β_1 glycoprotein (SP$_1$), placental alkaline phosphatase (PLAP) and γ-glutomyltranspeptidase (GGT). Testicular cancers synthesize AFP, HCG, and GGT. These tumor markers have been helpful in diagnosis and monitoring of treatment of patients with testicular cancer.

In initial studies, AFP levels were detected by the agar gel precipitation test which is simple and specific with a sensitivity of about 3000 ng/ml. With the subsequent development of specific RIA, the sensitivity was sufficient to measure 1 to 16 ng/ml of this glycopresent in normal serum.[2, 3] Utilizing this assay, 85 to 87% of embryonal carcinomas with or without teratoma have an elevated level of AFP (>20 ng/ml). None of the 160 pure seminomas had an elevated level of AFP. However, 102 of 145 patients (70%) with embryonal carcinoma, 36 of 56 (64%) embryonal carcinoma with teratoma, 3 of 4 yolk sac tumors (75%), and none of 5 choriocarcinomas had elevated levels of serum AFP in our series. The cellular localization of this glycoprotein in yolk sac tumor, embryonal carcinoma (with or without teratoma), has been reported previously. Using the RIA described by Vaitukaitis et al.,[4] the normal persons have serum values below 1 ng/ml. In our series 14 of 160 (9%) early seminomas, 87 of 145 (60%) embryonal carcinomas, 32 of 56 (57%) embryonal carcinoma with teratoma, and 5 of 5 (100%) pure testicular choriocarcinoma had elevated levels of serum HCG.

AFP and HCG in Staging and Monitoring

The most reliable technique of staging the retroperitoneum in patients with testicular cancer is a meticulous retroperitoneal lymphadenectomy.[5] However, determination of serum HCG and AFP appears to be able to stage testicular cancer more accurately than other presently available clinical tests. Utilizing these markers, we presently have decreased the staging error in stage I patients from an overall 53%, reported for embryonal carcinoma, to 9 to 14% for stage I and 5 to 10% for stage II. Interpretation of these markers requires consideration of their biologic half-lives (AFP, 3–5 days; HCG, 18–24 hours).

The important features which tumor markers add to the staging of testicular cancer are the following:

1. The clinical staging based on markers decreases the staging to appropriate diagnosis and therapy.
2. Persistently elevated serum markers after orchiectomy for testicular cancer invariably indicate stage II or III disease.
3. Persistently elevated serum markers after lymphadenectomy indicate stage III disease.
4. When lymphadenectomy is negative for tumor but postlymphadenectomy serum markers are persistently elevated, patients invariably have stage III disease. However, surgery still remains the most accurate means of assessing retroperitoneal metastasis.

5. Perhaps the most important applications of these markers are in monitoring of testicular tumor when serially measured.

The discordance between AFP and HCG is not an unusual observation during intensive chemotherapy of these tumors. This observation led to the utilization of immunocytochemical technique on the premise that the cellular origin of these two markers should be different. Utilizing an indirect immunoperoxidase technique, we were able to localize HCG in syncytiotrophoblastic giant cells of the placenta, choriocarcinomas, and AFP in embryonal and yolk sac tumor cells of the testes.

It has been shown that, by concentrating the HCG in urine specimens, HCG production can be monitored more sensitively than by measuring the serum HCG. Utilizing the kaolin-acetone precipitate from 24-hour urine specimens, the HCG was extracted, and the total volume was adjusted to 15 ml. Utilizing an H93 RIA specific to the unique carboxyl-terminal peptide of HCG-β subunit) described previously, the urinary HCG was measured in 32 specimens of 15 patients with initially HCG-producing testicular tumors. These 15 patients had simultaneous measurements of serum HCG utilizing an antisera against the HCG-β subunit (SB6) and urinary HCG concentrates utilizing H93 RIA. The initial serum HCG of these 15 patients was elevated and returned to normal levels after therapy. However, the urinary HCG was elevated in these 15 patients in spite of return of serum HCG to normal levels after therapy.

The initial five patients with elevated levels of urinary HCG but normal serum HCG were found to have recurrence. The remaining 10 patients were treated with no recurrence, confirming the sensitivity of urinary HCG. The availability of this sensitive RIA in measuring urinary HCG coupled with effective chemotherapeutic agents has made a dramatic improvement in selecting the patients in whom further therapy is warranted.

TUMOR LOCALIZATION

Localization and subsequent treatment of metastatic testicular cancer plays an important role in prolonging the survival of patients with testicular cancer. Although utilizing the conventional modalities such as computed tomography and ultrasonography have helped to detect and localize metastatic testicular cancer, these modalities are neither specific nor quantitative. In this presentation, we would like to discuss two newer modalities that have been useful in detection and localization of metastatic testicular cancer utilizing markers.

Selective Venous Catheterization

The veins draining a tissue that produce a special substance (tumor marker or hormone) should contain a significantly higher level of this substance than the veins peripheral to this tissue. The ability to measure this gradient depends on five general factors: (1) having an assay sensitive and specific enough to measure the difference (or step-up); (2) sampling close enough to the source before the substance of interest is diluted to, or close to, the concentration of the peripheral blood; (3) having a rate of blood slow enough that will not further dilute out the substance of interest; (4) the rate of production of the substance; and (5) the half-life of the substance. All of these factors are interrelated and all hinge on the sensitivity of the assay. The closer one is to the source, the slower the blood flow from the source, the greater the rate of production and the shorter the half-life; therefore, the greater will be the step-up and the higher the likelihood that the assay will be able to detect a significant increase in the draining venous blood over the peripheral blood level.

HCG and AFP Scans

Utilizing specific antisera to AFP and HCG labeled with a γ-emitting radionuclide such as ^{131}I, one may localize a solitary testicular metastasis by external scintigraphy. This noninvasive technique appears to be helpful in detection and localization of tumors that may not be clinically detectable using the conventional diagnostic modalities.

Several patients with testicular cancer received intravenous injection of between 2 and 5 mg of ^{131}I-labeled antibody to HCG or AFP, followed by total body photoscanning to visualize areas of increased radioactivity. Elevated serum AFP and HCG did not prevent tumor detection and localization by this method of radioimmunodetection. However, blood pool and nonspecific background of radioactivity were diminished by subtracting the images derived by injection of ^{99}Tc-labeled components from the ^{131}I scans to avoid false positive results. The basic mechanism of RID is utilization of a specific and sensitive radioactive antibody labeled to ^{131}I. The deposition of this labeled antibody in a tumor containing a given marker may be localized by a conventional external scintography. AFP and/or HCG are synthesized by the majority of nonseminomatous testicular cancers, and intravenous injections of between 1 and 2.5 mg of ^{131}I-labeled antibody to these markers will detect the site of extension of the tumor. We have utilized this technique in following clinical problems (1) to detect and localize tumor retroperitoneal area before the surgical ressection in patients with prior chemotherapy; (2) to detect and localize recurrent tumor after therapy. (This may accelerate or change the therapy); (3) to define the surgical resectability of the retroperitoneal and/or pulmonary metastases in patients with disseminated testicular cancer after intensive chemotherapy; and (4) to detect liver metastases in HCG-producing seminomas in order to institute chemotherapy. The role of RID in staging and possible immunoradiotherapy is under study.

Pregnancy Specific β_1 Glycoprotein in Sera and Cells of Patients with Testicular Cancer

This placental protein has recently been purified and utilized as a tumor marker by several investigators. Specific RIA and immunoperoxidase (IP) techniques have been developed to identify SP$_1$ in the sera and tumor cells of 97 men with testicular cancer. SP$_1$ was elevated at 11 to 440 ng/ml in 3 of 6 with choriocarcinomas, 5 of 17 with embryonal carcinoma

Table 3.1

Cellular origin of SP₁[a] HCG and AFP utilizing specific antisera by immunoperoxidase

Tumor	SP₁	HCG	AFP
Choriocarcinoma	+	+	−
Syncytiotrophoblastic giant cells	+	+	−
Placenta	+	+	−

[a] The abbreviations used are: SP₁, pregnancy specific β_1 glycoprotein; HCG, human chorionic gonadotropin; and AFP, α-fetoprotein.

and teratoma, and 5 of 50 with embryonal carcinoma.[6] None of 24 sera from men with seminoma and none of 5 men with orchitis had elevated SP₁. The highest value in a group of patients with nonmalignant disease was 9.1 ng/ml. The new biologic marker was identified in the syncytiotrophoblastic giant cells (STGC). STGC are seen occasionally in patients with embryonal carcinoma, teratoma, and seminomas (Table 3.1). It remains to be determined whether or not SP₁ concentrations correlate with body burden of tumor, prognosis or therapy, and whether or not other tumor cell(s) also produce this marker.

Lactic Dehydrogenase

Cancer cells have increased glycolysis leading to increased synthesis of lactate. Therefore, LDH may be utilized as a nonspecific tumor marker in several cancers including that of testicular germ cells. We have utilized LDH as a tumor marker in testicular tumor because of: (1) availability and simplicity of the assay when compared with RIA; (2) lack of frequency of other markers in seminoma; (3) bulky nonseminomatous testicular cancer with normalization of serum AFP and HCG while patients are on intensive chemotherapy when the serum LDH may monitor the therapy; and (4) monitoring the therapy of bulky seminomatous tumor. The correlation of LDH with tumor bulk and serum levels of HCG and AFP is under investigation.

TUMOR MARKERS IN SEMINOMA

HCG and AFP in Seminoma

These markers have proven helpful in diagnosis and therapy of patients with seminoma. Over the past several years we have accumulated over 160 patients with seminoma. Sixteen of these patients had elevated levels of serum HCG (Table 3.2).

One of these (case 2) proved to have an element of choriocarcinoma on further sectioning; syncytiotrophoblastic cells were found to be capping the cytotrophoblastic cells which were positive for HCG and histochemical staining. This patient underwent a retroperitoneal lymphadenectomy, and metastatic choriocarcinoma was found in the lymph nodes. Two patients with the diagnosis of pure seminoma had elevated serum levels of AFP. One of these patients (case 5) proved to have an element of embryonal carcinoma on further sections; serum AFP dropped to normal after retroperitoneal lymphadenectomy. The lymph nodes contained embryonal carcinoma. The other patient with persistently elevated serum AFP underwent debulking surgery of the retroperitoneal tumor for diagnostic and possibly therapeutic purposes. On serial sections of the multiple segments of the specimen, we were unable to find any elements of nonseminomatous testicular cancer. However, on further follow-up, he was found to have liver metastases. Biopsy examination of the liver metastases revealed pure seminoma that was negative for AFP on histochemical staining. However, the liver tissue from the vicinity of this tumor was positive for AFP by immunoperoxidase staining. These regenerative changes in the liver explain the modest but serially persistent elevated level of serum AFP (case 14). This patient refused chemotherapy and died of liver metastases. One patient underwent cytoreductive surgery of the retroperitoneal area and radiation. Fourteen of these 15 patients are alive and have been free of tumor for a mean of 3 years.

These markers are essential in establishing an accurate histologic diagnosis and, therefore, in selecting appropriate treatment in a patient with seminoma. Case 5 illustrates an accurate diagnosis made by an elevated level of serum AFP which changed the therapy from radiation to retroperitoneal lymphadenectomy. Case 14 also points to an accurate

Table 3.2
Serum and cellular HCG[a] and AFP in 16 patients with apparent seminoma: update of previous report

Patients (Case)	Serum Marker		Cellular Marker	
	AFP	HGC	AFP	HCG
1	−	4.3	−	+
2[b]	−	438.0	−	+
3	−	2.8	−	−
4	−	25.6	−	−
5[c]	152	0.4	+	−
6	−	2.3	−	+
7	−	4.9	−	+
8	−	6.4	−	+
9	−	4.8	−	+
10	−	22.0	−	+
11	−	2.7	−	+
12	−	10.0	−	+
13	−	8	−	+
14[d]	70	217	+	+
15	−	21	−	−
16		75	−	+

[a] The abbreviations used are: HCG, human chorionic gonadotropin; and AFP, α-fetoprotein.
[b] On further sectioning, an element of choriocarcinoma was found, explaining the highly elevated level of serum HCG.
[c] On further sectioning, an element of embryonal carcinoma was found, explaining the serum AFP of 152 ng/ml.
[d] Liver cells adjacent to liver metastases were positive for AFP on immunoperoxidase staining.

diagnosis of liver metastases that indicated the necessity of chemotherapy rather than conventional radiotherapy in such patients. Case 2 illustrates accurate diagnosis and treatment based on serum HCG. The finding of an elevated level of serum HCG points to the necessity for ruling out an element of choriocarcinoma. Serum markers also may be utilized to evaluate the efficacy of treatment in patients with seminoma. Case 14, which represents a patient with bulky seminoma in whom serum HCG dropped to undetectable levels after surgery and radiotherapy, reflects this finding. With tumor recurrence in this patient, the serum HCG became elevated. Although the diagnostic and prognostic implications of elevated levels of serum HCG have been reported in the literature, these cases are not acceptable as a result of the lack of serial sections and of localization of cellular HCG. Mostofi and Price[7] have reported that seminoma metastasizes as seminoma in 65% of cases. In 26% of patients, the metastases consist of embryonal carcinoma; in 4% they are teratoma. It is likely that a number of patients with seminoma and nonseminomatous metastases in these authors' series have had an element of embryonal carcinoma or teratoma in the primary tumor that could have been detected by determination of serum AFP or by histochemical staining. The high frequency of elevated levels of serum HCG in some reported series is also a matter of concern because of a lack of serial sections and histochemical staining which substantiates the absence of choriocarcinoma of the presence of STGC responsible for HCG synthesis. In the present series of 160 cases which were completely studied by serial sections and histochemical staining, 14 cases of pure seminoma with elevated serum HCG were detected. Therefore, we maintain that, although the STGC in pure seminoma may give rise to elevated serum levels of HCG, one must rule out choriocarcinoma, particularly since the conventional therapy of stage I and II choriocarcinoma with seminoma is lymphadenectomy, not radiotherapy. Although it appears that the treatment of choice for pure seminoma with elevated serum levels of HCG should be lymphadenectomy, this supposition requires confirmation in a controlled clinical trial. It has been our experience that although serum levels of HCG are highly elevated, when an element of choriocarcinoma is present in seminoma with STCG, serum HCG is only slightly or moderately elevated depending on tumor volume. Therefore, measurements of serum HCG and AFP have important roles, not only in diagnosis, but in the management and perhaps in prognostic determinations of seminoma.

Although we have not observed any elevated levels of serum AFP in patients with pure seminoma with a normal liver, we continue to obtain these markers in seminoma to rule out the presence of embryonal carcinoma with or without teratoma. Also, elevated HCG in the serum of patients with seminoma should alert physicians to rule out the presence of choriocarcinoma. For these reasons, we obtain serum levels of HCG in all patients with seminoma. Serum levels of HCG and lactic dehydrogenase also have been helpful in patients with bulky seminoma to monitor the therapy. The presence of elevated levels of serum HCG in pure seminoma may indicate a poor prognosis. The lack of a randomized study of the efficacy of radiotherapy *versus* lymphadenectomy in stage I and II seminoma makes it impossible, at present, to define the exact role of surgery, radiation, and chemotherapy in the treatment of seminoma with elevated levels of serum HCG. Although it would appear that orchiectomy and radiotherapy are adequate for the treatment of patients with stage I or II seminoma with elevated levels of serum HCG, if the level of serum HCG continued to be elevated after radiotherapy, one would have to reevaluate the patient for the possible presence of a metastatic choriocarcinoma. In addition, the poor results obtained in patients with stage III seminoma (28% to 55% rate of 2-year survival) underscore the need for intensive chemotherapy with or without surgery and/or radiotherapy.

Although the exact frequency of these markers in seminoma patients is not clear and is difficult to assess from various reported series, this should not deter the clinician from measuring these markers serially with specific and sensitive RIAs in patients with seminoma. The need for careful interpretation of these markers, considering their half-lives, the sensitivity and specificity of the assays, and other concurrent disease, has been discussed previously. Finally, utilizing a highly specific RIA system which recognizes the unique carboxyl-terminal peptide of the β subunit of HCG on a 24-hour urinary concentrate has proved to be more sensitive in patients when serum HCG is not detectable by conventional RIA.

γ-Glutamyl-Transpeptidase and Placental Alkaline Phosphatase in Seminoma

The lack of persistent tumor markers in the sera of patients with seminoma has prompted us to search for a number of tumor markers including PLAP and GGT. In a double-blind study, 89 patients were investigated. Thirty of these petients had histologic proof of seminoma and 49 patients were proven to have no detectable tumor utilizing the conventional radiologic and laboratory parameters. In the remaining 10 patients, tumors were suspected, however, due to the conventional radiation therapy after orchiectomy, pathologic staging was not feasible. PLAP, known as Regan isoenzyme, extracted from placenta has been reported[8] to be present in certain tumors including seminoma. In this study,[8] 40% (12 of 30 patients) with active seminoma had elevated serum levels of PLAP. Therefore, there is a false negative rate of 60%. Six of 49 patients without any clinically demonstrable tumor had elevated serum levels of PLAP, a false positive rate of 12%. GGT is an enzyme produced by the liver cells and an elevated serum level has been reported in liver diseases. Also, elevated serum levels of GGT have been separated to sensitive markers in hepatocarcinogenesis, thus, this marker has been considered as an oncodevelopmental marker.[9-11] GGT has been shown to be present in human seminal fluid[12] and early human placenta and in rabbit blastocyst. This oncofetal marker also has been found in human testis and in the homogenate of sacrococcygeal teratocarcinoma and in testicular seminoma. The presence of this enzyme has been reported in seminoma. In this study, 10 of 30 (33%) patients with active tumors had elevated serum levels of GGT. These 30 patients had proven to have active tumor during the period that sera were obtained for the assay. The false negative rate of 67% will preclude this marker as the only marker to be measured in the sera of these patients. The false positive happened in 2 patients out of 30 (7%). However, it should be emphasized that our patients were young and did not have clinical or laboratory evidence of liver disease. The value of serum determination in seminoma is to rule out the association of an element of choriocarcinoma. Although the elevated serum levels of HCG is uncommon (6 of 30, 20%) when it is elevated in the serum of patients with seminoma, it serves as a valuable marker in monitoring the management of seminoma.

This study indicates that when 2 or 3 of these markers are considered together the probability of finding them in the serum of a given patient with elevated levels significantly increases. When serum HCG were determined with PLAP and GGT, over 80% of patients with active tumor had elevated serum levels of one or more of these tumor markers. We were not able to serially measure these markers in all of these patients as yet or correlate GGT and PLAP in staging and monitoring of these patients. Presently, serial determination of GGT, PLAP, and HCG in patients with seminoma is under study in our laboratory and clinical program for testicular cancer.

It should be emphasized that the false positive, false negative rates of these markers, especially false positive rate for GGT in liver disease and the biologic half-lives of these markers, should be taken into consideration. A number of other markers for testicular cancer including androgen receptors[13] are under study in our laboratory at the present time.

Limitations of These Markers in Testicular Cancer

In spite of certain limitations in utilizing these markers, they appear to be the best available markers in any solid tumors. The current practices and recommendations to minimize certain problems and maximize the efficacy of RIA measurement of serum AFP and HCG from the commercial sources for testicular cancer are:

1. The physician should discuss the sensitivity and specificity of a given commercial assay with the laboratory and, perhaps, an occasional inclusion of normal serum or serum with known levels of AFP and/or HCG may serve as negative and positive controls when blindly coded.
2. These markers should not replace scrotal exploration and/or retroperitoneal lymphadenectomy for histopathologic diagnosis of the primary tumor and/ or ruling out the presence of retroperitoneal metastasis. However, the elevated levels of tumor markers are indicative of presence of tumor and necessity for further treatment. They are also helpful in monitoring the efficacy and need for changing the therapy.
3. The problem of impurity of certain antisera against the β subunit of the HCG or the possibility of high levels of luteinizing hormone (LH) in patients undergoing orchiectomy and/or chemotherapy causing a false positive result also should be kept in mind. The false positive results may be clarified by testosterone suppression test, determination of serum LH, and measurement of HCG on urinary concentrate utilizing a carboxy-terminal RIA that is currently available to all urologists through the NCI laboratories as a courtesy.

4. In monitoring the therapy or following the patients with testicular tumor, one should utilize frequent physical examination, chest x-rays, and other tests as physicians find them necessary, along with determination of serum AFP and HCG. In patients on chemotherapy, the normalization of these serum markers does not mean tumor-free status; as a matter of fact, on exploration of the retroperitoneum and chest, it is not unusual to find cystic fibrotic material with necrosis and tumor. Therefore, normalization of serum markers should not deter the surgeon from looking for tumor. Appropriate utilization of chemotherapy, surgery and radiotherapy, and tumor markers can make a dramatic improvement in prognosis and survival of these patients.

Gonadal Stromal Tumors

It also has been shown that the immunoperoxidase technique can be used to identify steroid hormones in sections of fixed embedded tissues. This advance paves the way for prospective and retrospective studies of specific sites of steroid hormone localization in a poorly understood group of gonadal neoplasms, namely, those within the sex cord-stromal category. In the past, ultrastructural and histochemical studies were inferential in assigning the function of steroid hormone synthesis to cells containing organelles thought to be associated with steroid synthesis, or in demonstrating the presence of intracytoplasmic lipid or certain enzymes, such as glucose-6-phosphate dehydrogenase and 3-β-ol-dehydrogenase, which have been shown to be present in high concentrations in cells that produce steroid hormones. The ability to localize specifically testosterone, estrogen, and progesterone has challenged many of the time-honored concepts of steroid biosynthesis by gonadal stromal tumors. In the past, specific hormone synthesis was attributed more or less to specific types of cells. Theca cells were thought to be responsible for estrogen synthesis and Leydig cells for testosterone production; granulosa and Sertoli cells were regarded as inactive generally. Utilizing highly specific antibodies for testosterone, estradiol, and progesterone, it now has been shown that all these cells are functionally active and, furthermore, that most have the capacity to synthesize both estrogens and androgens. Testosterone most frequently is localized in Leydig cells, but it also may be present in Sertoli cells and occasionally in granulosa cells. Estradiol is found not only in theca cells but also frequently in granulosa, Sertoli, and Leydig cells, whereas progesterone appears to be localized mainly in luteinized theca cells and less commonly in granulosa and Leydig cells (Table 3.3).

TUMOR MARKERS IN BLADDER CANCER

The conventional histopathologic examination of the primary or metastatic tumor rarely predicts the potentiality for recurrence or dissemination. There is some evidence that cellular differentiation in bladder cancer is reflected in the presence or absence of certain cell surface antigens. Included in the cell surface antigens are the A, B, and O(H) blood grouping antigens. These cell surface antigens can be detected easily by an immunologic technique known as specific red cell adherence

Table 3.3
Correlation of cell type and steroid localization[1]

Cell Type	Testosterone	Estradiol	Progesterone
Granulosa	+	++	+
Sertoli	+	+	−

test (SRCA). A number of investigators have demonstrated the reliability of SRCA in detecting the anaplastic potentiality of cancer of the cervix, stomach, pancreas, and lungs. Our laboratory also has applied this principle to bladder cancer and found a correlation between presence of this cell surface antigen and prognosis in stage O, A bladder cancer.[14-17] This test is not a quantitative test as are the conventional histopathologic studies, therefore, experience and judgement as well as careful attention to the detail of preparation of the sections are important. When these points are taken into consideration, it appears that there is a correlation between the absence of cell surface antigen A, B, or O(H) and invasion of bladder cancer. However, due to the weaker nature of the O(H) antigen, occasional falsely negative tests may be encountered. We recently have minimized the occasional false negative result in patients with group O blood by prolonging the incubation of tissue slide with the specific antisera and utilizing buffer solution with pH of 7.4 and fresh reagents.

Correlation of Antigens With Stage and Grade

Seventy-six bladder tumors of various stages and grades were examined for the presence of the A, B, O(H) surface antigen employing the SRCA technique. Seventy per cent of the grade I lesions studied were positive for the cell surface antigen, and none of the 26 grade III tumors retained their antigens. When correlated with clinical stage, the tumors that showed no antigens were those in stages B to D, while 12 of 18 stage A lesions were positive for the antigen. The findings of this study show that the SRCA is a valuable technique for predicting malignant potential in low grade, low stage cancer of the bladder. If supported by further investigation, this technique may offer the capability of selecting low grade, low stage bladder tumors that are destined to invade or metastasize while they are at curable stages. Several laboratories, including ours, have been interested in the cell surface antigen in urinary cytology specimens from patients with bladder cancer. The value of SRCA on cytology is not clear at the present time. Even if it proves to be valuable, it should not replace the SRCA on tissue from a bladder biopsy. In 10 consecutive patients with carcinoma *in situ* we have observed the loss of cell surface antigens. This finding confirms the natural history of bladder carcinoma in situ as has been reported by Utz and co-workers.[18]

The major role of SRCA on urinary cytology in our opinion is on carcinoma *in situ* when the cytoscopic examination of the bladder may show a normal bladder in spite of persistently positive urinary cytology. In this situation, if SRCA shows loss of surface antigens from the apparently malignant transitional cells, it not only will confirm the malignant nature of the cell, but also will predict the potential invasiveness of the flat carcinoma *in situ* of the bladder.

Chromosomal Studies

The abnormalities of cellular chromosomes in terms of number and/or structure appears to be an early marker for bladder tumor. It also appears to be of prognostic value in low grade, low stage bladder cancer to predict the rate of recurrence and invasiveness of an apparently superficial tumor, since tumors with normal chromosomes are noninvasive. In our experience, combining the SRCA and chromosomal study has been rewarding in predicting the natural history of a superficial bladder tumor.

Combined Cell Surface Antigens and Chromosomal Analysis

Malignant transformation of epithelial cell of bladder may result in quantitative and qualitative changes in the cell surface glycoprotein manifested by loss of ABO isoantigens or changes in cellular DNA manifested by chromosomal abnormalities. Utilizing these two cellular changes, we have studied 17 patients in order to correlate the grade, stage, and prognosis of these tumors to cell surface antigens and chromosomal changes in bladder cancer. These changes may not represent a specific chromosomal change similar to the Ph^1 chromosome in chronic myelocytic leukemia, nevertheless, the chromosomal changes have been proven to correlate well with grade, stage, and prognosis in the present study. Three of the four patients with grade 1 tumor had retained their antigens. These three patients also had normal chromosomes; the remaining one patient with abnormal chromosomes also had negative SRCA. Of six patients with grade II tumors, three had normal chromosomes and retained the cell surface antigens of their bladder tumors. Of six patients with grade III cancer, none had normal chromosomes and all had lost their cell surface antigens. Therefore, the grades of tumor correlates well with both chromosomal abnormalities and the loss of cell surface antigens. Although the number of patients are limited, these data indicate that SRCA and chromosomal studies may be helpful in grade I and II tumors. All patients with stage B-D had abnormal chromosomes or had lost their antigens although three of four patients with stage O or A had abnormal chromosomes and loss of cell surface antigens. These data indicate the usefulness of both SRCA and chromosomes in patients with lower stage cancer. However, as illustrated in case presentation, it appears that if SRCA and chromosomes are abnormal in an apparently low stage (O-A) the patient may be restaged. In contrast to the constancy of the diploid karyotype in normal tissue, malignant tumors may show a wide range of chromosomal abnormalities both in counts and structures. Also, ABO antigens are shown to be more predictive of the cell anaplasia and prognosis of the bladder cancer than the conventional histopathologic examination of the tumor alone. Therefore, these two modalities appear to have significant contribution in predicting the outcome of a superficial bladder cancer. The importance of these two modalities in predicting the invasion of a superficial tumor is appreciated in light of a 5-year survival of muscle-invading primary tumor treated with cystectomy and radiotherapy to be only 35–52%. However, if the potentially invading tumor is to be recognized and treatment given accordingly, the survival of the given patient should be remarkably prolonged.

From the present limited number of patients, it appears that both cell surface antigens and chromosomal abnormalities predict the potential invasiveness of a superficial bladder cancer not otherwise detectable; combining these two modalities also increases the potential predictability of invasiveness as shown in case presented in the RESULT section of this article. Presently, we are studying a larger group of patients with stage A transitional cell carcinoma of the bladder and renal pelvis to determine if these two combined modalities can be helpful in predicting which patient should have more early intensive or attenuated therapy. The prognosis of this group of patients can not be completely correlated with their survival. However, one may conclude that chromosomal abnormalities and presence or absence of the ABO antigens may be helpful in stage O and A when the conventional staging modalities, including histopathologic examination, cannot predict the anaplasia and invasiveness of a tumor.

Other Markers

A number of other markers, including CEA-like substance and β-glucuronidase have been reported in the urine and tissue of patients with bladder cancer. Recently, several investigators have reported the presence of β-glucuronidase in normal urine and bladder epithelium of rats and humans. This enzyme also has been found in urine and tumor tissue of patients with bladder cancer. However, this enzyme has not been used as a tumor marker because it is present also in urinary tract infection. Elevated levels of β-glucuronidase activity also have been reported in the urine of bilharzial and bladder cancer patients. The value of this enzyme as a tumor marker is not determined as yet.

MARKERS IN PROSTATIC CANCER

Immunoassay of Prostatic Acid Phosphatase

The human prostatic acid phosphatase is synthesized by the prostatic epithelial cells. It is a specific phosphatase isoenzyme, one of a large molecular family of phosphatases. Significant concentrations of nonprostatic acid phosphatase are normally present in red blood cells, leukocytes, platelets, osteoclasts, and the reticuloendothelial cells.

The prostatic acid phosphatase has been demonstrated to be antigenic. Therefore, specific antibody can be raised against the prostatic acid phosphatase in preparation for the specific and accurate measurement of the prostatic acid phosphatase by RIA. Such radioimmunoassay techniques have been developed by several investigators to detect the presence of prostatic acid phosphatase in the serum and bone marrow of the patients with prostatic cancer. Although there are controversial reports in reliability and specificity of such immunoassay, report from Cooper and Foti,[19] and Chu and co-workers[20] claim specificity and accuracy of their immunoassay technique.

RIA and counterimmunoelectrophoresis (CIEP) techniques have been developed through the National Prostatic Cancer Project (NPCP) of the National Cancer Institute. RIA was a conventional double antibody technique utilizing acid phosphatase from the ejaculate to raise antiserum in rabbits. The second antibody was goat antirabbit immunoglobulin G serum. The CIEP method for acid phosphatase (AP) was utilization of a specific antiprostatic AP antiserum and serum specimens from patients. Chu and associates[20] isolated AP from prostatic cancer, and the purified enzyme was used to immunize female rabbits utilizing this antisera and serum from a patient in an electric field. A positive result indicated that the serum specimen contained a detectable amount of at least 20 ng/ml of prostatic AP. An intergroup study conducted by the NPCP has claimed the relative specificity, sensitivity, and reproducibility of CIEP and recommended it to be used as the preferred method in the initial clinical staging of prostatic cancer. Comparing RIA and CIEP, the NPCP has stated that although RIA is highly sensitive, its proper performance requires highly qualified technical experts as well as sufficient funds to maintain such a costly, complex program. However, the value of CIEP and RIA as screening methods in early detection of prostatic cancer is not clear as yet. Furthermore, the superiority of RIA over enzymatic methods is questioned. Also, due to relatively frequent false positive results, RIA of PAP is not practical in early detection. The predictive value of prostatic acid phosphatase as a screening test for prostatic cancer is seriously questioned. Although the tests for prostatic acid phosphatase have played an important role in the management of prostatic cancer, its utilization in detecting the cancer as a screening test is not recommended. In comparison of 10 various diagnostic modalities, Guinan and associates[21] have concluded that rectal examination by an expert physician is the most sensitive tool to detect prostatic cancer.

Localization of Cellular Acid Phosphatase

Utilizing an antiserum to acid phosphatase as the first antibody and an appropriate second antibody conjugated with horse radish peroxidase, one may localize acid phosphatase in the epithelial lining of prostatic acini. We as well as the other investigators have localized acid phosphatase in the epithelial lining of normal, benign, and cancerous prostatic tissue utilizing immunoperoxidase. The advantage of utilization of this technique is feasibility of performing this staining on paraffin-embedded tissue that has been previously fixed in formaldehyde. Since this type of tissue preparation is the conventional method of preserving and storing prostatic cancer, one can perform any study on usually available paraffin block.

Other Markers

As far as androgen receptors are concerned, the preliminary results from Walsh *et al.*[22] suggest that the duration of hormonal response in men with symptomatic stage D prostatic cancer is related to androgen receptor content of prostatic cancer cells. If this can be confirmed in a longer follow-up, it will be helpful in selecting patients for cytotoxic agents or endocrine therapy.

Urinary hydroxyproline excretion also has been reported to be elevated in prostatic cancer with bony metastases.[23] It has been suggested that this marker should be utilized in staging and monitoring of prostatic cancer. Another nonspecific marker reported to be elevated in the serum of patients with prostatic cancer is creatinine kinase BB (CK-BB).[24] The serum levels of CK-BB have been found also in prostatic fluid and decrease with effective therapy. Whether or not multiple markers such as PAP, CK-BB, and hydroxyproline will be more accurate than a single marker remains to be determined.

RENAL CELL CARCINOMA

Some renal cell carcinomas have been reported to be associated with elevated serum renin, and these patients usually have been cured of their hypertension after nephrectomy. However, it is not clear whether the primary or recurrent tumor can actually synthesize this marker. The other marker occasionally found in patients with renal cell carcinoma is erythropoietin, assumed to be responsible for erythrocytosis.

Another group of markers found to be elevated in renal cell carcinoma and certain other urologic and nonurologic cancers are the polyamines. Putrescine, spermine, and spermidine are involved in ribonucleic acid (RNA) synthesis. The serum level may be elevated due to overproduction of these organic cations by any rapid growth of the cells such as embryonic development, regenerating tissues, and neoplasms. It has been shown that urinary polyamine excretion has increased in the urine of some cancer patients. Quantitative determination of urinary polyamines appears to be useful in the diagnosis and monitoring of patients with renal cell carcinoma, according to certain investigators. However, the exact role of these nonspecific markers remains to be clarified by more extensive investigation. A number of investigators have reported the presence of androgen receptors in renal cell carcinoma and they also stress the absence or presence of insignificant estrogen and progesterone receptors in these tumors, thus challenging the conventional use of progestational hormone. If this holds true, administration of antiandrogens will be of benefit in disseminated renal cancer rather than the conventional progesterone therapy in disseminated renal cancer. Hemstreet and associates[25] measured the binding affinities and receptor quantities in 47 pairs of normal and neoplastic kidney tissue for estrogen, progestin, and glucocorticoids utilizing a dextran-coated charcol assay. High affinity receptors were found in normal and neoplastic tissue of both sexes for all three hormones. The significance of these findings is not as yet clear.

Erythropoietin determined by new RIA may be elevated in patients with renal cell carcinoma (RCC) with normal hematocrit.[26] The value of this marker in RCC is not clear at the present time.

MARKERS IN ADRENAL TUMOR

The normal range of urinary cortisol, 17-OH corticosteroids, 17-keto-steroids, catecholamines, and 3-methoxy-4-hydroxymandelic acid (VMA) are indicated in Table 3.4. These urinary end products of adrenal hormones may be utilized as tumor markers for detection and monitoring of the therapy of adrenal tumors. Although over 50 different steroids have been isolated from the adrenal cortex, only a few are secreted into the blood stream, and the rest are intracellular intermediates. Recent studies on the biosynthetic pathway of the adrenal steroids have shown that the main steroid synthesized by the adrenal cortex are hydrocortisone, corticosterone, aldosterone, and 11-hydroxyandrostenodione and that they can be used as tumor markers.

The adrenocortical hormones are derivatives of cholesterol and are basically two structural types, those with a 2-carbon chain at the 17 position of the D ring and containing 21 carbon atoms, and those with a keto or hydroxyl group at position 17 and containing 19 carbon atoms. The 21-chain steroids are mineralocorticoid and glucocorticoid in function while the 19-carbon chains have androgenic activity. For practical purposes, the only steroids secreted in sufficient quantities to be physiologically active are aldosterone. cortisol, corticosterone, and dehydroepiandrosterone. The major excretory end products of the androgens are the 17-ketosteroids and, for practical purposes, approximately two-thirds of the ketosteroids in the male urine are derived from the adrenal or as a consequence of breakdown of cortisol in the liver, and about one-third is from the testes. About 10% of cortisol is converted in the liver to the 17-ketosteroid derivatives, but most are converted to cortisone and then tetrahydrocortisone which is soluble and rapidly excreted in the urine. Therefore, the major cortisol derivatives in the urine are 20-hydroxy derivatives of tetrahydroglucuronides (30%), tetrahydrocortisol glucuronides (25%), and tetrahydrocortisone glucuronides (15%). Orthopara-DDD blocks the secretion of all steroids.

The adrenal medulla excretes both norepinephrine and epinephrine with approximately 80% of the adrenal vein catecholamine output being epinephrine. Enzymes responsible for the formation of epinephrine from norepinephrine are present in the adrenal medulla, and the secretion of

Table 3.4
Normal range of urinary end products of adrenal hormones utilized as tumor markers[1]

Urinary Metabolites	Normal Range (Per 24 Hrs)	
	Women	Men
Cortisol	78–365 μg	108–409 μg
17-OH-Corticosteroids	2–6 mg	3–10 mg
17-Ketosteroids	6–15 mg	9–22 mg
Catecholamines	>135 μg	>135 μg
VMA[a]	0.7–6.8 mg	0.7–6.8 mg

[a] The abbreviation used is: VMA, 3-methoxy-4-hydroxymandelic acid.

the catecholamines is initiated by acetylcholine which is released from the neurons that embrace the secretory cell. The mechanism whereby acetylcholine acts to increase permeability of the cell and thereby allow calcium to induce secretion of the catecholamines is an area of active research. The catecholamines, in turn, act for only a short time in the circulation, being reduced following oxidation to 3-methoxy-4-hydromandelic acid. These substances can be detected in the urine with about 35% of the total secreted catecholamine appearing as VMA and 50% secreted as free or conjugated metanephrines, 30 μg norepinephrine, 6 μg epinephrine (700 μg of VMA).

For practical purposes, the epinephrine and norepinephrine stimulate effects that are similar to adrenergic discharge, although each has its specific actions. The effects are widespread, involving actions on the myocardium and vascular muscle, as well as multiple intermediary metabolic effects such as the mobilization of glycogen from the liver, induction of lipolysis, increase in metabolic rate, stimulation of glucagon, and inhibition of insulin.

CONCLUSIONS AND PERSPECTIVES

Although there has been encouraging progress in the area of oncofetal proteins and other markers in certain urologic cancer, this field is in its infancy. There is a great need for further investigations in this area. However, these investigations should be conducted with appropriate controls and carefully designed protocols to avoid bias or inaccurate data.

REFERENCES

1. Javadpour, N. Tumor markers in urologic cancer. *Urology 16:*127, 1980.
2. Perlin, E., Engeler, J. E., Edson, M., Karp, D., McIntire, L. R., and Waldmann, T. A. The value of serial measurement of both human chorionic gonadotropin and alphafetoprotein for monitoring germinal cell tumors. *Cancer 37:*215, 1974.
3. Waldmann, T. A., and McIntire, K. R. The use of a radioimmunoassay for alphafetoprotein in the diagnosis of malignancy. *Cancer 34:*1510, 1974.
4. Vaitukaitis, J. L., Braunstein, G. D., and Ross, G. T. A radioimmunoassay which specifically measures human chorionic gonadotropin in the presence of human luteinizing hormone. *Am. J. Obstet. Gynecol. 113:*751, 1972.
5. Javadpour, N. The role of biologic tumor markers in cancer. *Cancer 45:*1755, 1980.
6. Rosen, S. W., Javadpour, N., Calvert, I., and Kaminska, J. Pregnancy-specific B$_1$ glycoprotein (SP$_1$) is increased in certain nonseminomatous germ cell tumors. *JNCI 62:* 1439, 1979.
7. Mostofi, and Price, E. B. Tumors of the male genital system. In *Atlas of Tumor Pathology*, 2nd Series, Fasc. 8, p. 38. Armed Forces Institute of Pathology, Washington, DC., 1973.
8. Lehmann, F. G. Immunological methods for human placental alkaline phosphatase (Regan-phosphatase Regan isoenzyme) *Clin. Chim. Acta 65:*271, 1975.
9. Fishman, P. R., Krishnaswamy, Fishman, L., Millan, J. L., and McIntire, R. K. Gamma-glutamyltransferase in seminoma patients' sera carcinoembryonic proteins. In Vol. 2. Edited by F. G. Lehmann, Elsevier North-Holland, New York, 1979.
10. Laishes, B. A., Ogawa, K., Roberts, E., and Farber, E. Gamma-glutamyltranspetidase— A positive marker for cultured rat liver cells derived from positive premalignant and malignant lesions. *JNCI 60:*1009, 1978.

11. Strome, J. H., and Theodorsen, L. Gamma-glutamyltransferase: substitute inhibition kenetics mechanism and assay conditions. *Clin. Chem. 22:*417, 1976.
12. Krishnaswany, P. R., Tate, S., and Meister, A. Gamma, glutamyltranspaptidase of human seminal fluid. *Life Sci. 20:*681, 1977.
13. Shull, J. H., and Javadpour, N. Androgen receptors in testicular tumors. *Proceedings of AUA, Abstract No. 209,* 1981.
14. Bergman., S., and Javadpour, N. The cell surface antigen A, B or O(H) as an indicator of malignant potential in Stage A bladder carcinoma: preliminary report. *119:*49, 1979.
15. Emmott, R. C., Javadpour, N., Bergman, S. M., and Soares, T. Correlation of the cell surface antigens with stage and grade in cancer of the bladder. *J. Urol. 121:*37, 1979.
16. Emmott, R. C., Droller, M. J., and Javadpour, N. The A, B, O(H) cell surface antigens in carcinoma *in situ* and nonmalignant lesions of the bladder. *J. Urol. 125.*32, 1981.
17. Lange, P. H., Limas, C., and Fraley, E. E. Tissue blood-group antigens and prognosis in low-stage transitional cell carcinoma of the bladder. *J. Urol. 119:*52, 1978.
18. Utz, D. C. *et al.* Carcinoma *in situ* of the bladder. *Cancer 45:*1842, 1980.
19. Cooper, J. F., and Foti, G. A radioimmunoassay for prostatic acid phosphatase. *JNCI 49:*235, 1978.
20. Chu, T. M. *et al.* Immunochemical detection of serum prostatic acid phosphatase. Methodology and clinical evaluation. *Invest. Urol. 15:*319, 1978.
21. Guinan, et al. *N. Engl. J. Med. 303:*499, 1980.
22. Walsh, P. C., Hicks, L. L., Reiner, W. G., and Trachtenberg, J. The use of androgen receptors to predict the duration of hormonal response in prostatic cancer, abstract. 74th Annual Meeting, American Urological Association, New York, 1979.
23. Mooppan, M. M. U. *et al.* Urinary hydroxyproline excretion as a marker of osseous metastases in carcinoma of the prostate. *J. Urol. 123:*694, 1980.
24. Hindsley, J. P. *et al.* Creatine kinase BB in prostatic carcinoma. abstract 323, 75th Annual Meeting American Urological Association, San Francisco, California, 1980.
25. Hemstreet, et al. Comparison of steroid receptor levels in renal cell carcinoma and autologous normal kidney. *Proceeding of AUA, Abstract No. 254,* 1980.
26. Sherwood, J. B., and Goldwasser, E. A radioimmunoassay for erythropoietin. *Blood 54:* 885, 1979.

4

Steroid Receptors in
Urologic Cancer

The interaction between biologically active substances and cellular receptors has been known to pharmacology for many years. As long ago as 1500 Paracelsus stated that drugs should contain "spicula" (barbed hooks) with which they could become fixed to the organism and so produce an effect.[1] However, the concept that the action of steroid hormones is mediated through specific receptors dates from the late 1950s when Glascock and Hockstra[2] prepared a high specific activity, tritiated synthetic estrogen, hexestrol, and studied the tissue distribution and intracellular localization of this compound in female goats and sheep. They found specific localization of this estrogen in target organs. The accumulation of radioactivity in the reproductive tissues indicated the presence of binding components, with high affinity towards the estrogens, in the target tissues of these animals. In the decade beginning in 1960, hormone receptors and, in particular, steroid receptors received much attention. The introduction of radiolabeled steroids with high specific activity and the concurrent development of reliable techniques for both the measurement of radiolabeled compounds and the isolation and characterization of proteins provided a sound basis for the investigation of steroid receptors. This was exemplified by the work of Jensen and Jacobson[3] who demonstrated a remarkable ability for uterus and vagina, but not nontarget tissues, to retain estradiol 16 hours after the administration of tritiated estradiol to female rats. This observation, together with the finding that the retention but not the total uptake of radioactive estrogen can be saturated by the administration of increasing doses of estradiol, indicated the presence of a limited number of specific binding sites with high affinity for estradiol in target organs of the female rat.

Within a few years following these investigations, extensive research was directed towards the isolation and characterization of cellular receptors responsible for the action of different classes of steroid hormones. By the late 1960s receptor proteins with high affinity for estrogens, androgens, progestogens, and glucocorticoid were identified in their respective target organs. In the course of these investigations, a growing number of laboratories also conducted a vigorous search for steroid receptors in hormone-dependent tumors. The demonstration of the selective uptake of estradiol by hormone-dependent human breast tumor, and the isolation and characterization of estrogen receptors in this tissue, heralded a new approach in the evaluation and prediction of tumor response to the treatment.

In this chapter, an attempt has been made to review recent findings on steroid receptors in the male urological tract with particular emphasis towards the clinical significance of these receptors in malignancy. Some aspects of this work which deal with the significance of steroid receptors in relation to the diseased prostate recently have been the subject of a European[4] and an American[5] workshop, and have highlighted the necessity for a sound methodological basis for achieving a clinically meaningful tool from steroid receptor studies.

INTERACTION BETWEEN STEROID AND TARGET TISSUE

It is generally accepted that the interaction of steroid hormones with their respective target tissues involves the entry of the steroid into the cell, metabolism of the steroid in some instances, binding of the steroid or its metabolite to cytoplasmic receptor protein(s), and the subsequent translocation of the steroid receptor complex to the nuclear compartment where the complex interacts with chromatin components and results in the activation of cellular processes. This general scheme has been demonstrated in both female and male target tissues. However, the finer details of these events still require further elucidation. Indeed, considerable effort is still needed to obtain a clearer understanding of the sequence of events involved in the nuclear processes by which steroid hormones exert their biological action.[6-8]

Studies on the interaction of steroid hormones with target tissues of the male urogenital tract have lagged far behind those on female target tissues. Nevertheless, in the last decade a great deal of interest has developed towards the elucidation of the mechanism for the action of androgens in male target organs and, in particular, the prostate. The majority of our current understanding has been derived from studies carried out on the rat ventral prostate and, more recently, these studies have been extended to the human prostate and its tumors. The most significant factor in the rapid expansion of research in this field has been the high incidence of both benign and malignant tumors of the prostate. Indeed, cancer of the prostate constitutes the most common malignancy of the male urogenital tract. The hormone-dependency of the prostate and the relationship between this dependency and tumor onset in the gland has led to the development of a general scheme through which the interaction between androgens and their target tissues may be explained.

Therefore, it is most appropriate to describe the general principles by which steroid hormones interact with male target organs by reference to this scheme which has been proposed for the prostate. Thus, the discussion in this chapter will extend to the events in the cytoplasmic and nuclear fractions of the target cell and will be followed by an appraisal of our current knowledge of steroid receptors in relation to the urological tumors.

CYTOPLASMIC AND NUCLEAR EVENTS

The prostate gland is a typical example of a target organ for androgenic steroids. The growth and development of this gland is dependent on testicular androgens. This was noted as long ago as 1792,[9] when John Hunter recorded the absence of prostatic growth in the castrated male. However, it was only by the late 1960s that the cellular events associated with the action of androgenic steroids were first investigated. Early reports[10,11] suggested a selective uptake and retention of dihydrotestosterone, the main metabolite of testosterone, by the rat ventral prostate. These findings stimulated interest in the search for the cellular components responsible for the retention of steroids, as well as the relationship between these components and the metabolites of testosterone. Shortly after these initial findings, the existence of specific receptor proteins with high affinity for dihydrotestosterone in the cytoplasmic fraction of rat ventral prostate was reported by several research groups.[12-14] This protein receptor was found to have a sedimentation coefficient of either 8.5 S[14] or 3.5 S.[13] The latter group[13] found two protein components which bind dihydrotestosterone preferentially over other natural steroids. They designated these two proteins as α and β protein. The latter binds dihydrotestosterone specifically and very tightly, whereas, the former has a lower affinity but higher capacity for dihydrotestosterone and also binds estradiol. As a result of the binding of dihydrotestosterone to α and β proteins, two steroid receptor complexes designated as complex 1 and complex 11 are formed. Complex 11 formed between β protein and dihydrotestosterone corresponds to the specific steroid receptor complex reported by others and is responsible for the direct action of the hormone in the cell. The binding of the steroid to specific receptor proteins is an integral part of the cytoplasmic events. However, in the case of the prostate, this stage is preceded by the metabolism of the steroid entering the cell, *i.e.* testosterone, to its more active metabolite, dihydrotestosterone. Although this conversion has been reported as long ago as 1963 in both experimental animals and man,[15] it was only recently that a differential metabolism of testosterone has been reported in benign hypertrophied and carcinoma of the prostate.[16, 17] These studies reported that in cancer of the prostate the conversion of testosterone to dihyrotestosterone is diminished, implying a lower activity of the enzyme 5α-reductase which is responsible for this conversion. This diminished supply of dihydrotestosterone in cancer when compared to the benign and normal tissues could influence the number of steroid receptor complexes available for the subsequent nuclear events. In the rat ventral prostate, not only is testosterone rapidly converted to dihydrotestosterone but also a number of other androgens have dihydrotestosterone as their major metabolite.[18] In both experimental animal and human prostates, a further metabolism of dihydrotestosterone to androstanediols does occur. However, not only is this a reversible reaction, but also the androstanediols are not bound as tightly by the receptor proteins as dihydrotestosterone.

Thus, it can be concluded that the major events in the cytoplasm are the metabolism of testosterone to dihydrotestosterone and the binding of dihydrotestosterone to the cytoplasmic receptor proteins with the subsequent formation of the dihydrotestosterone receptor complex. The next stage is the entry of this complex into the cell nucleus. This entry, or translocation, is known to be an energy-dependent process and is hormone and tissue specific. It is possible that the steroid acts to stabilize the protein or supply an essential structural requirement so that the binding protein can transfer to its specific nuclear target site.[19] The presence of nuclear androgen receptor proteins has been demonstrated by several research groups in both animal and human prostatic tissues.[20-22] Once within the nucleus, the dihydrotestosterone receptor complex can interact with the chromatin components, but the exact manner by which this interaction occurs is not yet clear. However, there is evidence for the presence of specific receptor sites which are responsible for the retention of the steroid receptor complex.[23] It has been suggested that the acceptor can participate actively in specifying the site at which the complex binds and exerts its cellular action.[24] An alternative suggestion has been proposed that DNA is the acceptor and certain proteins act passively by restricting the receptor binding sites available on DNA.[25] Notwithstanding the mechanism of this interaction between the steroid receptor complex and the nuclear components, the ultimate result of this is the synthesis of RNA, protein, and finally cell division. It can be seen that the stages of androgen action in the prostate are interdependent, and both the metabolism of testosterone to dihydrotestosterone and the subsequent binding of dihydrotestosterone to the receptor protein in the cytoplasmic fraction of the cell are prerequisites for the final nuclear events to occur. The recognition of these events is fundamental to our understanding of not only the mechanism by which steroid hormones exert their biologic action but also the control of the growth for it's potential application in clinical practice. A simplified scheme for the interaction of steroids with their target cells is shown in Fig. 4.1.

STEROID RECEPTORS IN UROLOGIC TRACT

Prostate

In parallel to the research into the steroid receptor mechanism of the rat ventral prostate, a number of research groups directed their attention to the human prostate. Although the fundamental approach in terms of the methodological requirement for this research was common to both the animal and human tissues, the latter presented some major obstacles

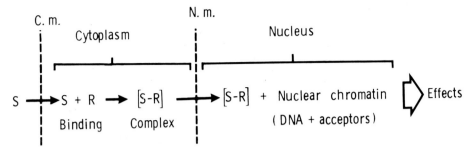

Figure 4.1. A simplified scheme for the action of steroid hormones in target cells. Steroid (S) enters through the cell membrane ($C.m$) and, in some cases, such as androgens in the prostate, undergoes metabolism. The steroid or its active metabolite binds to a specific receptor protein (R) and forms a steroid receptor complex [S-R]. The complex, then translocates to the nucleus, through nuclear membrane ($N.m.$) where it interacts with chromatin components. This interaction eventually leads to the biological effects of RNA synthesis, protein synthesis, and ultimately cell division. For more details of this scheme see the text.

to the progress of this research which were due to several inherent characteristics of the tissue under study. In general, the most commonly utilized human tissue has been benign hypertrophied human prostate. The large size of this tumor and its relative abundance were, perhaps, the major factors which stimulated the expansion of this research. The initial isolation and characterization of steroid receptors in the cytosol and nuclei of this tumor were reported by several research groups.[22, 26] The protein-binding component isolated in the cytosol was found to have a high affinity for dihydrotestosterone and was basically similar to that reported for the rat ventral prostate.[26] However, when these studies were extended to the quantitation of the receptor protein, a number of difficulties were encountered. The problems associated with the assay of androgen receptors in this tissue are mainly due to either the character of the tissue or the unstable nature of the receptor *in vitro*. Benign prostatic hypertrophied tissues contain a number of protein components; of these, sex hormone-binding globulin (SHBG) has a high concentration and a high affinity for dihydrotestosterone. This binding protein can, therefore, interfere with the assay procedure for the specific dihydrotestosterone receptor protein. Secondly, the tissue contains high levels of the two enzymes 5α-reductase and $3\alpha(\beta)$-hydroxysteroid dehydrogenase. These enzymes severely restrict the use of natural androgens in the cytoplasmic preparations of the tissue. Thirdly, the high level of endogenous androgens and, in particular, dihydrotestosterone in this tissue could interfere with the binding of radioligand to the receptor with a resultant underestimation in the true number of binding sites. Despite all these methodological considerations, several laboratories have been able to develop a number of techniques suitable for the quantitation of the dihydrotestosterone receptors in both the cytoplasmic and nuclear fractions of benign hypertrophied prostatic tissues.[27-31]

The introduction of an exchange assay using the synthetic androgen, methyltrienolone (R1881) has provided a major step forward in advancing the quantitation of androgen receptors in the prostate. This compound provides several advantages including its greater affinity for the dihydrotestosterone receptor than the natural radioligand, its lack of binding to the main interfering binding component in human prostatic tissue, namely sex hormone-binding globulin, and its stability in that it is not metabolized under the experimental conditions. Using this exchange assay at a temperature of 15°C, it has been possible to quantitate the total androgen receptor population in the cytosol fraction of the tissue.[27, 28] At a temperature of 0–4°C, this assay may be used to quantitate the free or available binding sites when a short incubation period is used.[27] The concentration of the total receptor sites in benign hypertrophied tissues has been reported to be 80–110 fmol/mg protein.[27, 32] Some laboratories have reported lower values for the receptor population in this tissue. This is possibly due to the use of a lower temperature with this technique.[29]

However, when other techniques such as agar gel electrophoresis[33] or protamine sulfate precipitation[30] have been employed, problems have been encountered with the loss of receptor and degradation, as well as incomplete labeling of the binding sites. Some of these shortcomings can lead to a gross underestimation of the total number of binding sites, and thereby give a false impression of the receptor status of the tissue. Assessment of the number of dihydrotestosterone receptors also has been performed in the nuclear fraction of the prostatic cell.[28, 29, 32] In most cases, a KCl extract of the nuclear pellet has been utilized for this measurement, although there is now evidence that a small proportion of the nuclear receptor is refractory to extraction by this technique, but may be extracted by using heparin.[34] The concentration of this receptor is reported to be (mean ± S.E.) 106 ± 14.7 fmol/mg protein.[32]

With regard to carcinoma of the prostate, there are several additional considerations which affect both the methodological approach in terms of the quantitation of steroid receptor proteins and its utilization for the clinical management of patients with this malignancy. In the first instance, the quantity of tissues available for study is much less than that of the benign tissues, and this has resulted in the necessity of developing greater sensitivity in the assay procedures. Secondly, the variability within the malignant tumors is such that the distribution of cancer within the surgical samples may vary from a few discrete foci to a diffuse spread and, additionally, the cancer cells may have from poorly to well differentiated histological characteristics. This introduces the requirement for meticulous histological study of all samples which have been utilized in the receptor assay, in order to assess both the quantity and quality of the malignancy in a given case. The aforementioned difficulties have laid a heavy burden on the attainment of reliable data which would be indicative of a correlation between the quantity of the receptor and the subsequent tumor response to hormonal manipulation. It is these factors which also make careful appraisal of the currently available data with regard to the receptor and response necessary. Despite all of these considerations, a number of research groups have been able to identify and quantitate the androgen receptor in both the cytoplasmic and nuclear fractions of the carcinomatous prostate.[32, 35, 36] Considerable variations have been reported in the quantity of androgen receptors in different cancer specimens, which makes comparison of values reported by different laboratories even more difficult. Additionally, due to the histological variation in the specimens, each receptor value needs to be considered in its own right, and prior clinical treatment, when applicable, obviously must be taken into account. The concentration of total cytoplasmic androgen receptors in untreated patients with carcinoma of the prostate has been reported to vary from 22 to 288 fmol/mg cytosol protein[32] and for the free cytoplasmic androgen receptor the value varied from 0 to 17 fmol/mg cytosol protein. In the nuclear fraction, the concentration of the total androgen receptor has been reported to range between 44 and 1123 fmol/mg protein. The concentration of the free receptor in this fraction has been reported to be negligible.[32]

An increase in the level of free androgen receptor has been reported following hormonal treatment[30, 32] but this may be attributed to the declining level of available androgens to the prostatic cells.[37] Based on the currently available data on androgen receptors in the carcinomatous prostate, and in view of the aforementioned problems in the interpretation of results, no definitive evidence has yet been produced with regard to variations in receptor concentration and the subsequent response to endocrine treatment.

As far as the role of the other steroid hormones is concerned, there is some evidence which suggests the involvement of other classes of steroid hormones and, in particular, estrogens in the development of prostatic tumors in experimental animals[38, 39] and within the human prostatic tumors.[40] In fact, the ability of prostatic tissues to take up and retain estrogens has been recognized for several years.[41] However, interest in the role of estrogens in the prostate has been overshadowed by the studies on androgens in this field. The recent evidence that estrogens play an important role in the development of canine prostatic hyperplasia[38] has added further impetus to the ongoing research as to the mechanism by which estrogens exert their biological effects and the possible interaction between estrogen receptors and those for androgens in this gland. The presence of binding protein components with high affinity for estradiol has been reported in both the rat[42] and the dog[43] prostates. Controversy still surrounds the evidence for the presence of this receptor in the normal human prostate and its tumors. Whereas some investigators have reported the presence of this receptor in human prostatic tumors,[33, 44, 45] others have failed to demonstrate specific estrogen binding in these tissues.[46, 47] The evidence so far reported both for and against the presence of estrogen receptors in prostatic tissues requires further clarification. However, based on current findings, the balance is in favor of a specific estrogen receptor in prostatic tumors.

Although it may seem premature to infer a prognostic value for the estrogen receptor, either alone or in combination with the androgen receptor, before more substantial data is obtained, it is nevertheless pertinent to note that both benign and malignant prostatic tissues contain considerable amounts of estradiol. The level of this steroid exhibits a significant negative correlation with androgen metabolites in benign hypertrophied prostate,[40] which would suggest an estrogen-androgen interrelationship in this tissue and, further, that this might encompass a receptor-mediated mechanism. Indeed, in the dog prostate, it has been demonstrated that estradiol enhances the prostatic cytoplasmic androgen binding proteins.[48]

Evidence for the presence of other classes of steroid receptors is more controversial. A number of reports have suggested the presence of progesterone-binding components, or atypical androgen receptors, with high affinity for the synthetic progesterone, R-5020.[49-52] However, other reports have not substantiated these findings.[27, 28, 53]

There is a paucity of information with regard to glucocorticoid receptors in the prostate, although in a recent study a total lack of this receptor in both the normal and benign hypertrophied prostate has been reported.[51] However, they found a glucocorticoid binding component in the metastases from several patients with carcinoma of the prostate. The significance of this finding is unclear, and further studies are required to determine the role, if any, of this steroid in the normal prostate and its tumor.

Kidney

There is good evidence to suggest that gonadal hormones influence the growth and functional activities of the kidney in both man and certain experimental animals. However, very little is known in relation to the mechanism by which these hormones exert their biological actions. Similarly, data on the effect of steroid hormones in renal tumors is both limited and inconclusive.

Both androgens and estrogens have been shown to influence this gland. Dihydrotestosterone, a reductive metabolite of testosterone, has been shown to promote prolonged enzyme induction and hypertrophy, whereas the androstanediols cause instant but transient enzyme induction, but not hypertrophy.[54] Furthermore, hypertrophy, but not enzyme induction, has been shown to be inhibited by the concomitant administration of the antiandrogen cyproterone acetate.[55] Since the androstanediols are bound exclusively in the cytoplasmic fraction and not the nucleus, these experiments have provided evidence that the nuclear events are stimulated by dihydrotestosterone, whereas cytoplasmic events are stimulated by the androstanediols. On the other hand, estrogens have been shown to reduce the weight of the kidney in experimental animals.

During the last decade, a search was conducted for different classes of steroid receptor proteins in the kidney and several laboratories have reported the existence of androgen, estrogen, and progesterone receptors in both the cytoplasmic and the nuclear fractions of the kidney from experimental animals[56-58] and man.[59, 60] Furthermore, the presence of steroid receptors has been confirmed in the natural and experimentally induced tumors of this organ.[56] In addition to the androgens, estrogens and progesterone receptors, the presence of both glucocorticoid and mineral-corticoid receptors has been reported in induced kidney tumors of experimental animals.[61] Several separation techniques, including gradient centrifugation, polyacrylamide and agar gel electrophoresis, together with Scatchard analysis, have been employed to investigate these different steroid binding components.

Although recent research has contributed somewhat toward our understanding of the mechanism of action of steroids in the kidney, data with regard to the human kidney can only be regarded as preliminary, and a great deal of additional research in this field is required before the receptor status can be fully comprehended. Indeed, controversy still exists as to the reliability criteria for the techniques which have resulted in the reports for some of the steroid-binding components of the human tissue. Therefore, in the light of our present state of knowledge of steroid receptors in human renal tumors, it would be premature to assign a predictive role for these protein-binding components in the clinical management of this urologic malignancy. It is, however, important to consider the findings in experimental animal models for the malignant tumor of the kidney. In the case of the golden hamster, the administration of synthetic estrogen induces the formation and growth of renal adenocarcinoma in which all the aforementioned species of steroid receptors have been demonstrated.[61] A significant relationship between estrogen treatment and production of the progesterone receptor component in this tumor has been observed.[58] This type of estrogen enhancement also has been observed in several other sex hormone target organs, which would suggest that, although the kidney is not generally considered to be a target organ for gonadal steroids, there are similarities in the behavior of these hormones in the experimental tumor to a number of well characterized tissues containing steroid receptor control mechanisms. This, together with a number of reports which have suggested some improvement of patients with renal tumors following hormone therapy, would emphasize the necessity for a concerted effort to clarify the involvement of steroid receptors in the pathogenesis of renal tumors.

Testis

Despite the fact that the testes are well known for being the site of production of both androgens and estrogens, less attention has been paid to the role of steroid receptors in this organ, when compared to the prostate. This may be partly explained by the low incidence of malignancy in this organ. Nevertheless, protein-binding components with high affinity for androgens, have been reported to be responsible for the retention of androgens in seminiferous tubules and the epididymis. Two types of androgen-inducing proteins have so far been described in both rat and human testes. The one corresponds to the androgen-binding protein (ABP) whose presence has been demonstrated in several androgen target organs of the rat,[62] whereas the second type corresponds to a specific intracellular receptor protein.[63] Furthermore, a receptor for androgens has been described in the nuclear fraction of the rat testicular germinal epithelial cells.[64] In addition to the androgen receptors, the presence of estrogen receptors also has been reported in the cytoplasmic and the nuclear fractions of the interstitial tissues of the rat testis, although their concentration is extremely low.[65]

In the human testis, recent reports have indicated the presence of androgen receptors in both cytoplasmic and nuclear fractions, of normal and malignant testicular tissues.[66, 67] This androgen receptor has been measured using an exchange assay with the synthetic androgen, methyltrienolone. In general, the characteristic features of this receptor protein are similar to those reported for the prostate, utilizing the same technique. The value for the concentration of the cytoplasmic androgen receptor in the normal testis has been reported to be 3 times higher than the corresponding values obtained in testicular tumors.[68] However, in the nuclei, the concentration of the receptor was noticeably greater in the tumor specimens, which had shown the lowest cytoplasmic levels. The clinical significance of these findings in both normal and malignant human testes are unclear, and the subject would require substantial experimental investigation before the role of these receptors can be determined. Information with regard to the existence of receptors for other classes of steroid hormones in this tissue is lacking.

Other Urologic Organs

With the exception of the bladder, the incidence of malignancy in other urologic tissues, such as the seminal vesicles and epididymis, is very low. In the latter two tissues, the existence of androgen receptors has been reported in experimental animals. Both of these tissues are considered androgen-dependent, and require testicular hormones for their growth and function. Androgen receptors have been isolated and characterized in both cytoplasmic and the nuclear fractions of the rat seminal vesicles[69] and the epididymis.[69, 70]

The concentration of the androgen receptors in the rat epididymis is reported to be under androgenic control during sexual development.[71] The physicochemical properties of these androgen-binding proteins are basically similar to those reported for the androgen receptors of the rat ventral prostate.[69] There is a paucity of information with regard to these receptor proteins in human tissues. The lack of information in these tissues may be due to the rarity of the tumor and consequently the limited degree to which these tissues have been investigated. However, the presence of androgen receptors in human epididymis has been reported.[72]

With regard to the bladder, little is known on the relationship between hormones and this organ which is not generally considered to be hormone-dependent and is not a target organ for steroid hormones. However, it is interesting to note that in certain species of toad, both cytoplasmic and nuclear receptors for aldosterone have been characterized in the urinary bladder epithelium.[73]

CONCLUSION

The emergence of the concept for a receptor-mediated mechanism in the action of steroid hormones heralded a new era, not only in endocrinology, but also in many related clinical disciplines of present-day medicine. This concept, which was originally pioneered for the role of estrogens in relation to female target organs, has now spread rapidly into virtually all steroid target organs, but predominantly in those in which malignancy is rife. In the course of this research, the progress has not always been equally shared by the different classes of steroid hormones. By far the greatest advancement has been achieved in the study of breast tumors, where it is now reasonably clear that a knowledge of the quantitative aspects of estradiol and progesterone receptors can contribute towards the prediction of the response of the tumor to endocrine manipulation. Thus, even in the absence of a complete knowledge of the mechanism of action of these two hormones in controlling the cellular processes, a criterion now has been established by which tumor response to treatment can be evaluated. The significance of this clinical application in relation to tumors of other steroid-dependent organs is of paramount importance. In this context, urology has a number of steroid target organs, among which the prostate has a very high record of fatal malignancy, and this has demanded a scientific approach for utilizing it as a clinical discriminant in order to provide the most satisfactory treatment of this disease. The lack of a reliable marker for assessing the response of the tumor in this field has stimulated the substantial effort which has been directed toward the elucidation of the role which steroid receptors play in prostatic tissues; however, progress has been hindered by several methodological problems, as well as the inherent difficulties which are associated with the cellular complexity of this organ. The predominant problems have been related to the extremely high enzymic activity towards androgenic steroids, the presence of other steroid-binding protein components, notably sex hormone-binding globulin, the high level of endogenous androgens, in particular dihydrotestosterone, and finally, the cellular make-up of the tissue, namely the presence of epithelial and stromal cells in a nonuniform distribution. An additional problem presented itself in this field of research through the relatively unstable character of androgen receptors when compared with those for estrogen in the breast. As outlined in the text, many of these difficulties have been overcome and reliable techniques have now been developed. As far as the present state of the published data in relation to the cytoplasmic and nuclear androgen receptor concentrations are concerned, this data is as yet, inconclusive. This is due not only to the limited number of patients in which the receptor estimation has been performed but also to the requirement for a long-term assessment of the interrelationship between the receptor content and the subsequent progress of the patients undergoing different regimes of treatment. Furthermore, the possible involvement of receptors for the other classes of steroid hormones, and in particular for estrogen, would necessitate a more comprehensive research program with a long-term view prior to the achievement of a definitive result. Although other urological tumors, in particular the kidney, but excluding the bladder, have been shown to possess receptor proteins for steroid hormones, the outlook for these tumors with regard to the development of a predictive role for receptor quantitation is less certain. The lower incidence of malignancy in these organs is the main contributory factor to the slow progress and relatively limited research effort which has been directed towards these tumors. However, it is not inconceivable to suggest that a more comprehensive understanding of the role of receptors in these tumors would contribute to their clinical management. In conclusion, it must be stressed that the value of receptor measurement for steroid hormones is now well established in breast tumors and undoubtedly has an important role to play in the management of prostatic tumors and, although much research is still required, the significance of the action of steroid receptors in the control mechanism of several other urologic malignancies must not be underestimated.

Acknowledgments—I wish to thank my staff at the Prostate Research Laboratory and in particular Mr. C. B. Smith for his utmost help and stimulating discussion in the preparation of this manuscript. Thanks are also due to Miss C. Lynch and Mrs. L. Sofras for their secretarial assistance.

REFERENCES

1. Van Rossum, J. M. Drug receptor theories. In *Recent Advances in Pharmacology*. Edited by J. M. Robson and R. S. Stacey. J. & A. Churchill Ltd., London, 1968.
2. Glascock, R. F., and Hockstra, W. G. Selective accumulation of tritium-labelled hoxoestrol by the reproductive organs of immature female goats and sheep. *Biochem. J. 72:*673, 1959.
3. Jensen, E. V., and Jacobson, H. I. Basic guides to the mechanism of estrogen action. In *Recent Progress in Hormone Research*. Edited by G. Pincus, Academic Press, London, 1962.
4. Schroder, F. H., and de Voogt, H. J. Steroid receptors, metabolism and prostatic cancer. Proceeding of the Workshop of the Society of Urologic Oncology and Endocrinology. Excerpta Medica, Amsterdam 1980.
5. Murphy, G. P., and Sandberg, A. A. Prostatic cancer and hormone receptors. *Prog. Clin. Biol. Res. Vol. 33*, 1979.
6. Gorski, J., and Gannon, F. Current models of steroid hormone action: a critique *Annu. Rev. Biochem. 38:*425, 1976.
7. O'Malley, B. W., and Schrader, W. T. Steroid hormone action: structure and function of receptor. *Prog. Clin. Biol. Res. 31:*628, 1979.
8. Liang, T., Tymoczko, J. L., Chan, K. M. B., Hung, S. C., and Liao, S. Androgen action: receptors and rapid responses: In *Androgens and Antiandrogens*. Edited by L. Martini and M. Motta. Raven Press, New York, 1977.
9. Hunter, J. Observation on certain parts of animal oeconomy. p. 44. Bibliotheca Osteriana, Ed. 2, London, 1792.
10. Anderson, K. M., and Liao, S. Selective retention of dihydrotestosterone by prostatic nuclei. *Nature 219:*277, 1968.
11. Bruchovsky, N., and Wilson, J. D. The intranuclear binding of testosterone and 5α-androstan-17β-ol-3-one by rat prostate. *J. Biol. Chem. 243:*5953, 1968.
12. Unhjem, O., Tveter, K. J., and Aakvaag, A. Preliminary characterization of an androgen macro-molecular complex from the rat ventral prostate. *Acta Endocrinol. 62:*153, 1969.
13. Fang, S., Anderson, K. M., and Liao, S. Receptor proteins for androgens: on the role of specific proteins in selective retention of 17β-hydroxy-5α-androstan-3-one by rat ventral prostate, *in vivo* and *in vitro. J. Biol. Chem. 244:*6584, 1969.
14. Mainwaring, W. I. P. A soluble androgen receptor in the cytoplasm of rat prostate. *J. Endocrinol. 45:*531, 1969.
15. Farnsworth, W. F., and Brown, J. R. Testosterone metabolism in the prostate. In *Biology of the Prostate and Related Tissues. Natl. Cancer Inst. Monogr. 12:*323, 1963.

16. Ghanadian, R., Masters, J. R. W., and Smith, C. B. Altered androgen metabolism in carcinoma of the prostate. *Eur. Urol. 7:*169, 1981.

17. Habib, F. K., Rafati, G., Robinson, M. R. G., and Stitch, S. R. Effects of tamoxifen on the binding and metabolism of testosterone by human prostatic tissues and plasma *in vitro. J. Endocrinol. 83:*369, 1979.

18. Bruchovsky, N. Comparison of the metabolites formed in rat prostate following the *in vivo* administration of seven natural androgens. *Endocrinology 89:*1212, 1971.

19. Tymoczko, J. L., Liang, T., and Liao, S. Androgen receptors interactions in target cells: biochemical evaluation. In *Receptors and Hormone action*, Vol. 2. Edited by B. W. O'Malley and L. Birnbaumer, Academic Press, New York, 1978.

20. Mainwaring, W. I. P. The binding of [1,2,^{3}H] testosterone within nuclei of the rat prostate. *J. Endocrinol. 44:*323, 1969.

21. Smith, C. B., Ghanadian, R., and Chisholm, G. D. Inhibition of the nuclear dihydro-testosterone receptor complex from rat ventral prostate by anti-androgens and stilboes-trol. *Mol. Cell Endocrinol. 10:*13, 1978.

22. Mainwaring, W. I. P., and Milroy, E. G. P. Characterization of the specific androgen receptors in the human prostate gland. *J. Endocrinol. 57:*371, 1973.

23. Liao, S., and Fang, S. Receptor proteins for androgens and the mode of action of androgens on gene transcription in ventral prostate. *Vitam. Horm. 27:*17, 1969.

24. Liao, S., Tymoczko, J. L., Liang, T., Anderson, K. M., and Fang, S. Androgen receptors: 17β-hydroxy-5α-androstan-3-one and the translocation of a cytoplasmic protein to cell nuclei in prostate. *Adv. Biosci. 7:*155, 1971.

25. Mainwaring, W. I. P., and Peterken, B. W. A reconstituted cell-free system for the specific transfer of steroid receptor complexes into nuclear chromatin from rat ventral prostate gland. *Biochem. J. 125:*285, 1971.

26. Davies, P., and Griffiths, K. Similarities between 5α-dihydrotestosterone receptor complexes from human and rat prostatic tissues: effect of RNA polymerase activity. *Mol. Cell. Endocrinol. 3:*143, 1975.

27. Ghanadian, R., Auf, G., Chaloner, P. J., and Chisholm, G. D. The use of methyltrien-olone in the measurement of free and bound cytosplasmic receptors for dihydrotestos-terone in benign hypertrophied human prostate. *J. Steroid Biochem. 9:*325, 1978.

28. Shain, S. A., and Boesel, R. W. Human prostate steroid hormone receptor quantitations: current methodology and possible utility as a clinical discriminant in carcinoma. *Invest. Urol. 16:*169, 1978.

29. Menon, M., Tananis, C. E., Hicks, L. L., Hawkins, E. F., McLaughlin, M. G., and Walsh, P. C. Characterization of the binding of a potent synthetic androgen methyltrien-olone to human tissues. *J. Clin. Invest. 61:*150, 1978.

30. Mobbs, B. G., Johnson, I. E., Connolly, J. G., and Clark, A. E. Androgen receptor assay in human benign and malignant tumors cytosol using protamine sulphate precipitation. *J. Steroid Biochem. 9:*289, 1978.

31. Castaneda, E., and Liao, S. Use of anti-steroid antibodies in the characterization of steroid receptors. *J. Biol. Chem. 250:*883, 1975.

32. Ghanadian, R., and Auf, G. Receptor proteins for androgens in benign prostatic hypertrophy and carcinoma of the prostate. In *Steroid Receptors, Metabolism and Prostatic Cancer*. Edited by F. H. Schroder and H. J. de Voogt. Excerpta Medica, Amsterdam, 1980.

33. Wagner, R. K., Schulze, J. H., and Jungblunt, P. W. Estrogen and androgen receptors in human prostate and prostatic tumor tissues. *Acta Endocr. (Suppl.) 193:*52, 1975.

34. Foekens, J. A., Bolt-de Vries, J., Romijn, J. C., and Mulder, E. The use of heparin in extracting nuclei for estimation of nuclear androgen receptors in benign prostatic hyperplastic tissue by exchange assay. In *Steroid Receptors, Metabolism and Prostatic Cancer*. Edited by F. H. Schroder and H. J. de Voogt. Excerpta Medica, Amsterdam, 1980.

35. Shain, S. A., Boesel, R. W., Radwin, H. M., and Lamm, D. L. Cytoplasmic and nuclear androgen receptors in human prostate. In *Progress in Clinical and Biological Research*, Vol. 33. Edited by G. P. Murphy and A. A. Sandberg. Alan R. Liss, New York, 1979.

36. Walsh, P. C., and Hicks, L. L. Characterization and measurement of androgen receptors in human prostatic tissues. In *Progress in Clinical and Biological Research*, Vol. 33. Edited by G. P. Murphy and A. A. Sandberg. Alan R. Liss, New York, 1979.

37. Ghanadian, R., Puah, C. M., and O'Donoghue, E. P. N. Unconjugated dihydrotestosterone and testosterone in serum of patients with carcinoma of the prostate. *Br. J. Cancer 38:*195, 1978.

38. De Klerk, D. P., Coffey, D. S., Ewing, L. L., McDermott, I. R., Reiner, W. G., Robinson, C. H., Scott, W. W., Strandberg, J. D., Talalay, J. D., Walsh, P. G., Wheaton, L. G., and Zirkin, B. R. Comparison of spontaneous and experimentally induced canine prostatic hyperplasia. *J. Clin. Invest. 64:*842, 1979.

39. Moore, R. J., Gazak, J. M., Quebbeman, J. F., and Wilson, J. D. Concentration of dihydrotestosterone and 3α-androstanediol in naturally occurring and androgen induced prostatic hyperplasia in the dog. *J. Clin. Invest. 64:*1003, 1979.

40. Ghanadian, R., and Puah, C. M. Relationship between estradiol-17β, testosterone, dihydrotestosterone and 5α-androstane-3α, 17β-diol in human benign hypertrophy and carcinoma of the prostate. *J. Endocrinol. 88:*255, 1981.

41. Ghanadian, R., and Fotherby, K. Interaction between steroids in regard to their uptake by rat ventral prostate. *Steroids Lipids Res. 3:*363, 1972.

42. Unhjem, O. Metabolization and binding of estradiol-17β by rat ventral prostate *in vivo* In *Research on Steroids.* Edited by M. Finkelstein, A. Klopper, C. Conti, and C. Cassano. Pergamon Press, Oxford, 1970.

43. Dube, J. Y., Lesage, R., and Tremblay, R. R. Estradiol and progesterone receptors in dog prostate cytosol. *J. Steroid Biochem. 10:*459, 1979.

44. Bashirelahi, N., O'Toole, J. H., and Young, J. D. A specific 17β-estradiol receptor in human benign hypertrophied prostate. *Biochem. Med. 15:*254, 1976.

45. Pertshuk, L. P., Zava, D. T., Gaetijens, R. J., Brigati, D. J., and Kim, D. S. Detection of androgen and estrogen receptors in human prostatic carcinoma and hyperplasia by fluorescence microscopy. *Res. Commun. Chem. Pathol. Pharmacol. 22:*427, 1978.

46. Ekman, P., Snochawski, M., Dahlberg, E., and Gustafsson, J. A. Steroid receptors in metastatic carcinoma of the human prostate. *Eur. J. Cancer 15:*257, 1979.

47. Hawkins, R. A., Hill, A., and Freedman, B. A simple method for the determination of estrogen receptor concentration in breast tumors and other tissues. *Clin. Chim. Acta 64:* 203, 1975.

48. Moore, R. J., Gazak, J. M., and Wilson, J. D. Regulation of cytoplasmic dihydrotestosterone binding in dog prostate by 17β-estradiol. *J. Clin. Invest. 63:*351, 1975.

49. Asselin, J., Fernand, L., Gourdeau, Y., Bonne, C., and Raynaud, J. P. Binding of methyltrienolone (R1881) in rat prostate and human benign prostatic hypertrophy (BPH). *Steroids 28:*449, 1976.

50. Cowan, R. A., Cowan, S. K., and Grant, J. K. Binding of methyltrienolone (R1881) to a progesterone receptor like component of human prostatic cytosol. *J. Endocrinol. 74:* 281, 1977.

51. Ekman, P. Clinical significance of steroid receptor assay in the human prostate. In *Steroid Receptors, Metabolism and Prostatic Cancer.* Edited by F. H. Schroder and H. J. de Voogt. Excerpta Medica, Amsterdam, 1980.

52. Gustafsson, J. A., Ekman, P., Pousette, A., Snochowski, M., and Hogberg, B. Demonstration of a progestin receptor in human benign prostatic hyperplasia and prostatic carcinoma. *Invest. Urol. 15:*361, 1978.

53. Krieg, M., Bartsch, W., Janssen, W., and Voigt, K. D. A comparative study of binding, metabolism and endogenous levels of androgens in normal, hyperplastic and carcinomatous human prostate. *J. Steroid Biochem. 11:*615, 1979.

54. Ohno, S., Dofuku, R., and Tettenborn, U. More about X-link testicular feminization of the mouse as a noninducible (i*) mutation of a regulatory locus: 5α-androstan-3α, 17β-diol as the true inducer kidney alcohol dehydrogenase and β-glucoronidase. *Clin. Genet. 2:*128, 1971.

55. Ohno, S., and Lyon, M. F. X-link testicular feminization in the mouse as a non-inducible regulatory mutation of the Jacob-Monod type. *Clin. Genet. 1:*121, 1970.

56. Li, J. J., Cuthbertson, T. L., and Li, S. A. Specific androgen binding in the kidney and estrogen dependent renal carcinoma of the Syrian hamster. *Endocrinology 101:*1006, 1977.

57. Li, J. J., Talley, D. J., Li, S. A., and Villee, C. A. An estrogen binding protein in the renal cytosol of intact castrated and estrogenized golden hamster. *Endocrinology 96:* 1106, 1974.

58. Li, S. A., Li, J. J., and Villee, C. A. Significance of progesterone receptor in estrogen-induced and dependent renal tumor of the Syrian golden hamster. *Ann. N. Y. Acad. Sci.* *286:*369, 1977.

59. Bojar, H., Maar, K., and Staib, W. The endocrine background of human renal cell carcinoma: glucocorticoid receptors as possible mediators of progestogen action. *Urol. Int. 34:*330, 1979.

60. Concolino, G., Di Silverio, F., Marocchi, A., and Bracci, U. Renal cancer steroid receptors: biochemical basis for endocrine therapy. *Eur. Urol. 5:*319, 1979.

61. Li, J. J., Li, S. A., and Cuthbertson, T. L. Nuclear retention of all steroid hormone receptor classes in the hamster renal carcinoma. *Cancer Res. 39:*2647, 1979.

62. Hansson, V., Djoseland, O., Reusch, E., Attramadal, A., and Torgersen, O. An androgen binding protein in the testis cytosol fraction of adult rats; comparison with the androgen binding protein in the epididymis. *Steroids 21:*457, 1973.

63. Hansson, V., McLean, W. S., Smith, D. J., Tindall, S. C., Weddington, S. C., Nayfeh, S. N., French, F. S., and Ritzen, E. M. Androgen receptors in rat testis. *Steroids 23:*823, 1974.

64. Sanborn, B. M., Elkington, J. S. H., Steinberger, E., and Meistrich, M. L. Androphilic proteins in the testis. In: *Regulatory Mechanism of Male Reproductive Physiology.* Edited by C. H. Spilman, T. J. Lobl, and K. T. Kirton. Excerpta Medica, Amsterdam, 1976.

65. De Borc, W., Mulder, E., Van Beurden, W. M. O., Peters, M. J., and Van der Molen, H. J. Steroid hormone receptors in rat testicular tissue. *J. Endocrinol. 64:*21P, 1975.

66. Hoisaeter, P. A., Hekim, N., Dahl, O., and Stoa, K. F. Androgen binding in normal and malignant testis tissues. *Scand. J. Urol. Nephrol. (Suppl.) Vol. 48,* 1978.

67. Hsu, A. F., and Troen, P. An androgen binding protein in the testicular cytosol of human testis: comparison with human plasma testosterone-estrogen binding globulin. *J. Clin. Invest. 61:*1611, 1978.

68. Stoa, K. F., Hekim, N., Dahl, O., and Hoisaeter, P. A. Binding of androgens and progestins in the human testis. *J. Steroid Biochem. 11:*261, 1979.

69. Hansson, V., Tveter, K. J., Unhjem, O., Djoseland, O., Attramadal, A., Reusch, E., and Torgersen, O. Androgen binding in male sex organs with special reference to the human prostate. In *Normal and Abnormal Growth of the Prostate.* Edited by Goland, M., Charles C Thomas Publisher, Springfield, Ill., 1975.

70. Blaquier, J. A., and Calandra, R. S. Intranuclear receptor for androgens in rat epididymis. *Endocrinology 93:*51, 1973.

71. Calandra, R. S., Podesta, E. J., Rivarola, M. A., and Blaquier, J. A. Tissue androgens and androphilic proteins in rat epididymis during sexual development. *Steroids 24:*507, 1974.

72. Attramadal, A., Weddington, S. C., Naess, O., Djoseland, O., and Hansson, V. Androgen receptors in male sex tissues of rats and humans. In: *Prostatic Disease.* Edited by H. Marberger, H. Haschek, H. K. A. Schirmer, J. A. C. Colston, and E. Witken. Alan R. Liss, New York, 1976.

73. Kusch, M., Farman, N., and Edelman, I. S. Binding of aldosterone to cytoplasmic and nuclear receptors of the urinary bladder epithelium of bufo marinus. *Am. J. Physiol. 253:*82, 1978.

5

Immunology of Genitourinary Cancer

The study of tumor immunology was based on the observation that tumors have antigens which stimulate a host immune response. Since the early observation in the methylcholanthrene-induced sarcoma, tumor-associated antigens have been extensively studied and have been identified in every adequately studied animal tumor. Detection of human tumor-associated antigens has been more difficult, since antigenicity is weak and variable compared to other surface antigens such as transplantation antigens. Identification of those antigens which are specific for the tumor cells is further complicated by the expression of a variety of antigens by the tumor cell, some of which may be unique to the tumor, but some of which may be common to other tumors and to normal tissue. Recent evidence suggests that at least some tumor-associated antigens may be found in more than one histologic tumor type.[1] A variety of tumor-related antigens have thus far been identified.

Oncofetal antigens may reappear in the process of genetic transformation into malignancy. While these antigens have no specific therapeutic significance, they have been invaluable diagnostic and prognostic indicators. The carcinoembryonic antigen (CEA) is expressed in patients with carcinoma of the gastrointestinal tract, pancreas, and lung. α-Fetoprotein is a fetal liver glycoprotein. It is elevated in the adult with hepatocellular carcinoma and in the presence of germ cell tumors. The human blood group antigens seem to be lost in the process of malignant transformation. This has been well documented in transitional carcinoma of the bladder, and is becoming an important prognostic indicator in early stage tumors (see below).

Tumors also possess antigens which they share in common with the organ of origin. Alternatively, tumors of similar origin may lack antigens of the normal tissues from which the tumor arose, yet share antigens with normal tissue in another organ system. What was originally perceived to be tumor-specific antigen was often later identified as a histocompatibility antigen (HLA). Virus-related antigens pose a particular problem in sorting out antigens population in human tumors. Most humans are exposed to many viruses, some of which may belong to classes of tumor-related viruses. Antigens to various components may incite specific antibody responses in the human host.

In addition to these multiple tumor-related antigens, the existence of tumor-specific antigens still seems plausible to most investigators. Tumors such as renal carcinoma appear to have both these nonspecific shared antigens, as well as unique antigens which are related to malignant transformation (see below). The specific identification of these peculiar antigens may be markedly advanced by the new technology of monoclonal antibody production. Tumor-associated antigens have been commonly defined by repeated absorption of cytotoxic antisera with normal tissue constituents. Kohler and Milstein[2] described a technique of hybridizing splenocytes from immunized animals with myeloma cells. The resultant hybridomas produced antibodies specific to tumor antigens. The hybridoma could then be cloned and antibody could be produced in large amounts, without the need for absorption against normal tissue. This technique provides a tool for identification of varied and specific tumor antigens. More attractive to the clinician, however, are the diagnostic and therapeutic implications. Specific antibody to a tumor antigen or to a marker hormone elaborated by a tumor may be radiolabeled for detection of subclinical tumor deposits, or complexed with cytotoxic or radioactive compounds which are then directly carried to the tumor target.

Convincing evidence of tumor-specific antigens has not been reported for most human tumors, however, even in the existing state of knowledge, the hosts responses to "nonself" tumor-related proteins has provided an impetus for further studies in human immunobiology. The character and magnitude of the response to these tumor antigens has been examined in many aspects and by a multitude of assays. Although the host immune response is an integrated series of events, separation into a cellular and humoral response is appropriate for discussion and analysis.

The macrophage is probably the initiating and pivotal cell in the host immune response. The macrophage facilitates the processing of antigen and promotes the T cell response. Macrophage, therefore, may process antigen or may evolve into a sensitized effector cell. Processed antigen then stimulates thymus-derived lymphocytes (T cells) to become killer or effector cells. The cells specifically attack and lyse the tumor or produce lymphokines which attract other lymphocytes and macrophages to the tumor site by preventing dispersal of macrophages through production of migration inhibition factor.[3] Some of the activated lymphocytes react with thymus-independent lymphocytes (B cells) which are thereby transformed either into effector cells or into antibody-producing plasma cells. Multiple factors, many of which as yet unidentified, clearly effect this process in a regulatory fashion.

Suppressor cells and helper cells, respectively, inhibit and potentiate the transformation of B cells into plasma cells. Suppressor cells are probably a distinct subset of T cells. These immunoregulatory cells may be specific or nonspecific, and seem to have a role in modulating response to antigens and preventing autoimmune disease. This subject has been succinctly reviewed by Broder and Waldman.[4]

Natural killer cells (NK cells) also have been identified. These lymphoid cells display cytotoxicity *in vitro* to many cell types, both malignant and normal. They represent part of a complex interaction of cellular and soluble factors, including type I interferon, which may represent the mechanism of natural immunity to cancer. The precise role of the NK cells and associated mechanisms *in vivo*, however, has not been determined.[5] The origin of the cells is unclear, and many have Fc receptors. Although these may represent altered T cells, natural killer activity can be independent of T cell immune function and appears to be different from the antibody dependent cellular cytotoxicity (ADCC) effector cells. In addition to suppressor and NK cells, circulating factors such as antigen· antibody complexes, specific and nonspecific antibodies, and free tumor-associated circulating antigen, modify the immune response in largely unknown ways.

GENERAL IMMUNOLOGY

Humoral Immunity

Numerous sophisticated techniques have been employed for the identification of tumor-related antibodies and antibodies to tumor cell fractions. Antibodies to melanoma, sarcoma, and renal carcinoma (see below) have been reported. Specificity remains a problem in all of these assays, and will only be solved by the identification of tumor-specific antigen targets. Also, it is possible other immunoglobulins or immune complexes have been attached to tumor cells by Fc receptors and do not represent binding to tumor-specific antigens. Finally, response to tumor-specific antigens in contrast to tumor-associated antigens is difficult to determine and remains a major problem in the study of antibodies.[6] The identification of tumor-specific antigens, possibly with the aid of monoclonal antibody techniques, will greatly aid the study of circulating factors in tumor patients. Even in the present state of knowledge about circulating immune factors, antibodies seem to have promise as diagnostic and therapeutic agents. Passive infusion of antibody effectively suppresses *in vivo* growth of only a small number of tumor cells, a fact which limits, but does not preclude, this form of cancer therapy in the future. The treatment of experimental tumors with antiserum combined with cytotoxic drugs suggests an additive effect of the two modalities.[7, 8] Conjugation of drugs to antibodies allows targeting of the drug to the tumor and more effective, less toxic chemotherapy. Clinical application of macroglobulin as drug carriers will depend on solution of a number of problems, but is a plausible expectation. Radioimaging with isotopes conjugated to specific antibodies which target the isotope to subclinical tumor deposits has been attempted, with some success, in animal systems and human tumors. The current status of antibodies in tumor immunity has been admirably reviewed by Economous.[9]

Cellular Immunity

Following the demonstration of altered response to skin test antigens in cancer patients,[10] cellular immunity was thoroughly investigated both *in vivo* and *in vitro*. Numerous assays have been devised to study the circulating peripheral blood lymphocytes and macrophages *in vitro* and to correlate their functions with disease progression or regression. The results of such tests have not been consistent in reflecting the true disease status of the patient although these assays have provided evidence for the presence of tumor-associated antigens in human tumors. The principals and interpretations of these assays have been thoroughly reviewed.[11] Three main types of assays have been employed: blastogenic response to antigen, lymphokine production, and assays of *in vitro* cytotoxicity. The last, which proportedly measures the degree of destruction of the tumor cell *in vitro* by peripheral blood leukocytes, has been the most widely applied. Interpretation of the results of these assays is complicated by nonspecific reactivity and multiple logistic factors such as the multitude of cells, types in tumor specimens minimal reactivity of cells in culture to cytolysis necessitating use of long-term tumor cell lines, and lack of availability of tumor specimens. Specificity of the reaction is difficult to establish. It is often difficult to establish tumors and normal tissue controls in cell culture, and allogeneic tumor cell lines have been employed with the obvious expression of nontumor-specific reactions. Even when autochthonous tumors are used as the target cell, the test leukocyte often shows reactivity against other tumors or nontumor target cells, Secondly, assessment of the degree of target cell destruction is often subjectively determined when individual colonies or cells are counted. In assays employing the incorporation or release of radioactively labeled markers, the labeled marker may itself influence cell adherence to the test plates or introduce variability in the assay by virtue of varying degrees of radioactivity in varying batches of the marker substances. Thirdly, errors may be introduced by virtue of differences in the peripheral blood leukocytes. Methods of separating and freezing leukocytes vary and may alter cell surface reactions. Specific populations of leukocytes which either effect or inhibit cytotoxicity have been identified. The degree of cytotoxicity observed in the studies mentioned above was an expression of the heterogeneous peripheral leukocytes rather than specific effector cells. Finally, in serially determined assays, many events not related to the tumor influence the degree of activity of the peripheral blood leukocytes. These multiple factors have seriously limited the contribution of the various cytotoxicity assays to the study of renal carcinoma. Reservations regarding the specificity of these reactions have been summarized by Bean *et al.*[12] and the relationship of peripheral blood leukocyte cytotoxicity to the disease status or prognosis awaits further sequential studies. The variety of classes of peripheral blood leukocytes also may complicate interpretation of these cytotoxicity assays. Assays of suppressor cell function and NK activity are not commonly included in assessment of immune status of cancer patients, since the clinical implications of these functions are still unclear.

Clinical Evidence for Host Immunity

An equally compelling, though poorly understood, clinical body of evidence attests to the significance of host immunity to cancer. First, the incidence of cancer is increased in patients with congenital immune deficiency states. Children with hypogammaglobulinemia have a marked increased incidence of lymphoreticular neoplasms.[13] Patients with Wiskott-Aldrich syndrome have a much higher incidence of malignancy than the general population as well as an increased incidence of recurrent infections. Second, patients with artificially induced immunosuppression, such as renal transplantation patients, have a higher probability of developing malignancy.[14] Such patients receive immunosuppressive agents, mainly azathioprine steroids, or antilymphocyte serum. The tumor types are mainly lymphoreticular neoplasms which seem to be approximately 100 times greater than in the general population. Third, spontaneous regression of cancer has been documented many times.[15] This suggests, but does not prove, the presence of some form of intrinsic tumor control mechanism which is presumed to be immunologic, but may be related to other regulatory mechanisms. Fourth, evidence exists to support the theory that humans frequently encounter tumor-associated antigens of many types but only rarely develop clinical manifestations of tumor.[16] Infiltration of tumors by effector cells such as macrophages and lymphocytes suggest an attempt by the host to police his own environment. The detection of antibodies to proportedly tumor-specific antigens in normal controls has been noted repeatedly. If indeed this represents a specific response to tumor antigen, it provides further evidence that these subjects at some time came in contact with the antigen. The observation of Klein.[17] that the capacity of the immune system does deal with viral-induced neoplastic transformation and is greatly superior to its ability to deter chemically induced neoplastic transformation also suggests the presence of immunologic surveillance. Spontaneous regression, mentioned above, may also be a product of the host immune surveillance mechanisms.

The concept of immunologic surveillance has not been embraced by all investigators.[18] The possibility exists that genetic influences may be a more important determinant and the variability of tumor response and tumor antigenicity make the adoption of a single unified surveillance theory somewhat difficult to support. However, the theory is useful in postulating why humans, endowed with formidable defense mechanisms, develop malignant diseases.

A number of escape mechanisms have been postulated. First, cells of greater antigenicity might be immunoselected, thereby allowing proliferation of less antigenetic cells. Second, modulating factors such as blocking antibodies, circulating antigen·antibody complexes, and suppressors T cells might modulate the effect of circulating antibody and effector cells. Thirdly, the tumor may modify to avoid detection by the host mechanisms.[19] Fourth, immunocompetence might be impaired. This is reflected in the decline of immune reactivity in the aged. Fifth, various forms of therapy such as chemotherapy and radiation therapy suppress certain aspects of host immunity. Finally, although some tumors may ellicit an immune response, this does not necessarily equate with tumor rejection. In experimental systems, a transplanted portion of a tumor may regress or fail to grow while the primary tumor continues to proliferate.[20] Similarly, variable growth and regression of metastases has been observed in renal carcinoma—while some tumor foci grow, others may simultaneously regress.

RENAL MALIGNANT TUMORS

Renal cell carcinoma often behaves contrary to the expected course of malignancy. Tumors may remain dormant for years before rapidly progressing, and metastases (especially pulmonary lesions) may partially or completely regress. Although these clinical peculiarities do not necessarily indicate host immunological control of the tumor, this remains a plausible explanation, stimulating clinical and laboratory research of immune response in renal carcinoma patients.

Cutaneous response to skin test antigens in patients with renal cell carcinoma has produced varying results. Morales and Eidinger[21] reported a correlation between the degree of cutaneous reactivity to dinitrochlorobenzene (DNCB) and the stage of renal carcinoma. Catalona et al.[22] reported a similar association. Patients with early stage tumors retained reactivity to DNCB which was lost in patients with advanced disease. We have studied 37 renal carcinoma patients by means of serial testing with DNCB and common skin tests antigens. After initial sensitization with DNCB, patients were challenged at 1 or 2 monthly intervals. The response was quantitated by an arbitrary method and assigned an index number. Initial response to DNCB was surprisingly poor, even in patients with limited metastases. We could, therefore, find no correlation between DNCB response and tumor stage or prognosis. The findings were in general agreement with those of Schellhammer et al.[23] and DeCenzo et al.[24] Serially measured absolute lymphocyte counts similarly showed no consistent correlation with stage of disease or prognosis. In vitro assays of cell-mediated immunity (CMI) to renal cell carcinoma have been mainly measurements of lymphocyte cytotoxicity. Specific cytotoxicity of peripheral leucocytes from renal carcinoma patients to autochthonous or allogeneic cell cultures of renal tumor using the colony inhibition assay or its variations has been reported.[25, 26] Cole et al.,[27] demonstrated a significant level of cytotoxicity against autochthonous cells in patients with limited metastatic disease which was lost when the disease became far advanced. Patients who were apparently cured by surgery also lost lymphocyte cytotoxicity as well as detectable levels of blocking factor. Elhilali and Nayak,[28] similarly found a correlation between limited renal tumor volume and the capacity for in vitro lysis of renal tumor cells. Montie et al.[29] could not determine a correlation between microcytotoxicity and tumor stage. The reaction also was not specific for renal carcinoma, since lymphocytes from normal subjects also caused target cell lysis. This is not surprising in view of the probable incompatibility of the lymphocytes and allogeneic renal tumor cells.

We studied 31 patients with renal carcinoma in various stages by means of serially determined lymphocyte cytotoxicity as measured by the ^{125}I-IDU method. Patients were arbitrarily categorized into three groups: patients recently rendered tumor-free, patients with limited metastatic disease and patients with advanced metastases. Cytotoxicity levels varied in each group, but the mean cytotoxicity of patients who were tumor free and those with minimal tumor burden were significantly higher than in patients with advanced disease. An increase in cytotoxicity following the development of metastases was associated with improved survival. However, the CMI measured by the assay was not specific. Since allogeneic renal tumor cell lines served as target cells, the cytotoxicity observed was not solely on the basis of CMI to renal carcinoma antigens.

Regardless of the inherent shortcomings, discussed above, these assays provide evidence of an altered cell-mediated response in patients with renal cell carcinoma. Perhaps the quantitative leukocyte cytotoxicity assay as suggested by Hakala[30] by means of the lymphocyte titration method may prove to be a more objective and quantitative method of measuring cell-mediated immunity.

Other in vitro methods of measuring CMI in renal carcinoma patients have been reported. Stjernsward et al.[31] presented evidence of a cell-mediated tumor-distinctive response in renal carcinoma patients by means of the mixed lymphocyte-target cell interaction test. Peripheral blood lymphocytes from patients with renal cell carcinoma which were exposed to autochthonous renal carcinoma cells in vitro were stimulated to proliferate and divide. Such stimulation, as measured by incorporation of tritiated thymidine, was not detected when the lymphocytes were incubated with antigen from autologous kidney cells. Daly et al.,[32] reported lysis of both autochthonous and allogeneic renal cell carcinoma cells in vitro by lymphocytes from patients with renal cell carcinoma. This cross-reactivity among the cell lines provided suggestive evidence that tumors of the same histologic type share some tumor-associated antigens (see below).

Other than the leukocyte cytotoxicity assays, the assay of leukocyte migration inhibition (LMI) has been the most widely applied to the study of renal carcinoma. Kjaer and Christensen[33] obviated a major problem with the standard cytotoxicity assays by use of soluble tumor extracts rather than whole tumor cells as the source of target antigen and demonstrated cell-mediated immunity in renal carcinoma patients by use of this LMI assay. Subsequently, Wright et al.[34] employed 3M KCl extracts of renal cell carcinoma in the LMI assay of 30 patients with renal carcinoma. Sixty-three percent of these patients had a positive LMI test in contrast to 7% of normal donors, 30% of patients with other tumors, and 36% of patients with benign kidney disease. Only 33% of renal carcinoma patients reacted to a KCl extract of normal kidney. These data suggest that CMI to a renal carcinoma-associated antigen was indeed measured by the assay. These authors[34] further correlated the LMI response with stage of the disease. Seventy-one percent of patients who were clinically free of recurrence 1 year or more after nephrectomy lost the LMI response. However, untreated patients with metastases developed or retained the reaction to renal carcinoma antigen in the LMI assay, suggesting that the cell-mediated immunity determined by the LMI correlates with the presence of renal tumor. We observed a similar relationship of tumor presence to levels of complement-fixing antibodies (see below). Hemstreet and Richardson[35] showed a decreased peripheral blood monocyte chemotactic response to lymphocyte-dependent chemotactic factor in renal carcinoma patients, which was restored to normal by removal of the primary tumor. An inhibitor of monocyte chemotaxis was identified in the serum.

In summary, altered CMI seems to exist in patients with renal cell carcinoma. Although specificity of the *in vitro* reactions is still questioned, the weight of evidence suggests that the reactions observed are stimulated by renal carcinoma-associated antigens.

The relationship of levels of cell-mediated immunity to clinical stage of prognosis has been suggested in some studies, but not others. Thus far, no assay of cell-mediated immunity has been proven to be of clinical value.

Humoral immune functions of renal carcinoma patients have not been extensively studied, although the demonstration of circulating antitumor antibodies in the sera of patients with cancer suggests that humoral immunity may be an important component of the host response to malignancy. The degree to which circulating factors influence the growth and dissemination of renal carcinoma is unknown, but antirenal carcinoma antibodies have been detected using various methods. It is important to qualify the term "antibodies" in this discussion, since the target preparations in most of these assays were not isolated, specific, tumor-associated antigens.

Evidence for circulating antibodies against renal carcinoma was provided by Hakala *et al.*,[36] who reported autochthonous tumor-specific cytotoxicity in the sera of renal carcinoma patients. Five out of 11 patients with the tumor had serum factors which were cytotoxic to autochthonous renal carcinoma, but not to autologous normal kidney. This cytotoxicity could be abrogated by absorption of the serum with tumor, but not with normal tissue.

We analyzed the sera of 75 patients with various stages of renal cell carcinoma in an attempt to detect the presence of antirenal carcinoma antibodies. The microcomplement fixation assay was employed.

Initially, the target antigen was a cell wall extract of autochthonous tumor produced by hypotonic cell lysis. Attempts to initiate long-term culture of autochthonous tumor were insufficiently successful to permit long-term serial assays. We therefore used the renal carcinoma cell-line, A948, as a constant target antigen.

Ninety-four percent of patients with recently resected, localized, or metastatic renal cell carcinoma had detectable antibody levels (greater than 1:4). The reaction was not specific in that 40% of patients' sera also reacted with allogeneic normal kidney cells. Also, the sera from five renal carcinoma patients reacted positively against cultures of melanoma, sarcoma, breast, colon, and lung carcinoma. However, results of absorption studies strongly suggest that the assay indeed measured a reaction to tumor-associated antigens. The level of antibody also varied with clinical status.[37]

A major limitation in the interpretation of assays of antibodies to renal carcinoma or other tumors is the difficulty in identifying and purifying tumor-associated antigens. Although the data from studies of cell-mediated immunity and circulating factors suggest the presence of tumor-associated antigens, few attempts to isolate renal tumor-associated antigens have been reported. Ueda et al.[38] identified autologous antibody to cell surface antigens of cultured renal carcinoma cells by means of mixed hemadsorption and anti-C3 mixed hemadsorption assay. Using absorption studies as an autologous typing system, the authors defined three types of renal tumor surface antigens: individually specific, shared surface renal tumor antigens, and nonspecific. Belitsky et al.[39] in an immunofluorescence assay, reported reactivity of antirenal carcinoma antibodies from immunized goats with renal cell carcinoma from 20 patients. Normal adult tissue showed no immunofluorescence. These authors subsequently coupled the goat antibody to ^{131}I and demonstrated preferential binding of the isotope to the renal carcinoma. LeBlanc et al.[40] employed the staphylococcal protein A assay to detect reactivity of renal carcinoma patient sera with two renal carcinoma cell lines. As in other studies, specificity was not proven, since sera from nonrenal carcinoma patients also reacted in some instances.

In summary, considerable evidence supports the presence of tumor-associated surface antigens of human renal cell carcinoma. Individually specific as well as shared antigens seemed to be present. Further purification of these tumor-associated antigens will greatly improve the sensitivity and specificity of the immunologic assays discussed above, and perhaps increase the role of these assays in the diagnosis and treatment of renal carcinoma patients.

BLADDER CARCINOMA

In contrast to the studies in renal carcinoma, skin test reactivity to DNCB has been extensively studied, and early reports suggest that it correlates with prognosis in patients with transitional carcinoma of the bladder. Catalona et al.[41] demonstrated a close correlation between DNCB response and prognosis in 38 patients with potentially curable transitional cell carcinoma of the bladder. Thirteen of 19 patients with impaired reactivity developed tumor recurrence, 11 of whom died within 1 year. Of 19 patients who initially responded to DNCB, only 5 have had a recurrence and none have died during the same interval. Fahey, et al.,[42] in a larger study of 130 patients with bladder cancer, confirmed the prognostic value of DNCB skin test response. Seventy-two percent of their patients with metastatic disease who were unresponsive to DNCB died within 1 year, while all five of those who reacted to the reagent were alive at 20 months. The degree of reaction to DNCB was related to tumor burden, and increased following surgical resection. Response was impaired by radiation therapy, even after small doses. Skin test reactivity to another antigen, keyhole limpet hemocyanin (KLH), has been studied by Olsson and associates,[43] who reported decreased reactivity in bladder cancer patients.

The prognostic significance of all skin test responses to topically applied antigens recently has been challenged and currently remains in question. Schellhammer et al.[23] showed depression of skin test response in patients with invasive bladder cancer, but could not correlate initial response with prognosis. DeCenzo and Leadbetter[44] were unable, however, to identify a correlation between initial skin tests in patients with bladder cancer and their ultimate prognosis, and contended that tumor aggressiveness was more important then host immune defenses.

In vitro studies of host immunity to bladder cancer have been numerous. O'Toole et al.[45] identified significant cytotoxicity to a bladder tumor cell line in patients with bladder cancer. The presence and level of cytotoxicity changed as disease status changed, and the presence of cytotoxicity seemed to correlate with presence of a growing tumor. Loss of cytotoxicity was secondary to either advanced tumor burden or total absence of disease. Bean et al.,[46] using a different cytotoxicity assay, demonstrated specific cytotoxicity in 56% of the patients with superficial bladder tumors and only 18% significant cytotoxicity in patients with advanced bladder cancer.

Hakala and associates[30] modified the conventional cell-mediated lymphocytotoxicity assay to quantitate the number of effector cells necessary to destroy specific percentages of the tumor target cells. In contrast to other studies that suggested that cytotoxicity was found when tumor burden was low and disappeared after removal of the tumor, these authors indicated that elevated cytotoxic levels were found after the removal of the tumor and decreased levels were found associated with tumor recurrence.

Clearly, lymphocyte cytotoxicity against bladder cancer cell lines is greater than normal in patients with early stage bladder tumor. However, there is a marked variability in the degree of cytotoxicity. Furthermore, as indicated above, specificity of these reactions is difficult to ascertain. It is increasingly obvious that many types of effector and suppressor cells are present in the circulation of cancer patients and in those with no apparent malignancy; and that these cells direct their activity against a broad range of antigens.

Evidence from other types of in vitro assays also supports the importance of the cellular immune response in patients with bladder cancer. Depression of lymphocyte responsiveness to in vitro stimulation in lymphocytes of patients with bladder cancer has been reported.[47] Alteration in the percentage of circulating T cells also has been noted in patients with invasive bladder cancer.[48] Monocyte chemotaxis, an in vitro test of macrophage antitumor function, has been shown to be significantly depressed in patients with all stages of bladder cancer.[49] Furthermore, removal of tumor was correlated with the return to normal levels in patients with invasive carcinoma. Bean et al.[50] reported a decreased mixed leucocyte culture (MLC) response and decreased response to concanavalin A (Con A) and photohemagglutinin (PHA) of leucocytes from the peripheral blood of bladder cancer patients. Responsiveness to Con A decreased with disease progression. Stimulatory function of the leucocytes in the one-way MLC was restored in some patients by tumor removal. Leucocyte migration inhibition in bladder cancer patients has also been reported.[51]

Perhaps the most comprehensive study of immune function and bladder cancer patients was reported by Fahey and Zighelboim.[48] Multiple assays for immune functions, including numbers of circulating T cells, proliferative response to PHA, and assays for nonstimulated cellular toxicity were serially measured in a large number of patients with various stages of bladder carcinoma. Although the results usually varied from the normal controls, no significant correlation with prognosis or tumor burden could be made.

Recently, histology of the regional lymph nodes of patients undergoing cystectomy for invasive bladder cancer was correlated with ultimate prognosis.[52] In this important work, Herr and associates reported significantly greater survival in patients whose regional lymph nodes showed evidence of stimulation (prominent germinal center and expansion of the central cortex), as compared with patients whose regional nodes were not stimulated. This correlation was based not only on the stage but also the grade of the tumor. Herr[53] later reported inhibition of normal and autologous peripheral blood leucocytes by cells from the regional nodes of some patients with locally invasive bladder cancer. They invoke the presence of lymph node suppressor cells as an explantation. Extracts from the regional lymph nodes of patients with bladder cancer have been shown to suppress toxic immune mechanism (antibody-dependent cytotoxicity) in three of four patients tested.[54] The implications of this finding with respect to the role of regional lymphadenectomy for bladder cancer are purely speculative at this time.

The clinical importance of suppressor cell function in human malignancy is unclear (see above), but it may be assumed that changes in suppressor cell function are associated with tumor progression. Weingurtner et al.[55] demonstrated decreased suppressor cells in the peripheral blood of patients with bladder and renal carcinomas. Tumor dissemination was associated with increased suppressor activity. Spina et al.[56] detected depressed cell-mediated immunity in bladder cancer patients, and attributed this in part to a circulating suppressive macrophage-like cell.

The evidence for humoral immune factors in patients with bladder cancer is less convincing. Pesce et al.[57] were unable to identify specific antibodies to bladder carcinoma in the sera of 31 patients by immunofluorescence techniques. However, Hakala et al.[58] identified a complement-dependent antibody in the sera of patients with transitional cell carcinoma that produced specific lymphocyte toxicity. They also showed cross-reactivity among patients' sera, thereby supporting the evidence that tumors of similar histologic types share some common tumor-associated antigens. *In vitro* cytotoxicity mediated by serum factors has been described, but identification of specifically tumor antigen-directed antibodies awaits isolation of tumor-specific bladder tumor antigens.

Immunodiagnosis

The sensitivity and potential specificity of immunologic methods suggest their role in diagnosis and staging of tumors, and in measuring the biologic potential of individual tumor. The presence of shed tumor antigens in the urine of bladder cancer patients has been demonstrated, but distinguishing these from other antigens has been difficult. O'Brien *et al.*[59] identified a unique, low molecular weight, component in the urine of bladder cancer patients which was not present in normal subjects or those with inflammatory bladder conditions. DeFazio *et al.*[60] produced rabbit antisera to a tumor-associated antigen found only in the urine of bladder cancer patients. The implication of these and other studies of urinary tissue-associated antigens are clear, but their place in the diagnostic armamentarium has not been established.

Davidsohn,[61] postulating an altered expression of blood group antigens in tissues which had undergone malignant degeneration, reported loss of the ABO antigens from certain human tumors. In recent years, numerous authors have shown a correlation between presence or absence of surface blood group antigens on bladder carcinoma and survival. Limas *et al.*[62] studied 60 patients with noninvasive bladder tumors. Only 19% of those whose tumors retained blood group antigens developed invasive tumors within 5 years, whereas 62% of patients whose tumors were ABO antigen depleted developed invasive tumors. Recurrence rate was 3 times as high in those whose first tumor was ABO antigen negative. Similar results have been reported by Johnson and Lamm.[63] The technical complexity of the test, especially with respect to "H" antigen detection, has thus far discouraged its routine clinical application.

CARCINOMA OF PROSTATE

The investigation of *in vivo* abnormalities of cellular immunity in patients with prostatic carcinoma provide rather convincing evidence of depressed cell-mediated immunity. Brosman *et al.*[64] found impaired ability of patients with prostate cancer to respond to DNCB and to mount an inflammatory response to the irritant croton oil. Furthermore, this delayed cutaneous hypersensitivity response correlated with the clinical stage of the disease. No correlation between disease status and skin test response to DNCB was found by Schellhammer *et al.*,[23] and all patients with prostatic cancer, regardless of stage, showed a depressed response.[23]

As has already been noted, most evidence for cellular and humoral immune responses in patients has been dependent upon *in vitro* lymphocyte cytotoxicity assays. Such assays require reliable tumor target cell lines that can be maintained in tissue culture for many generations. Establishment and maintenance of prostatic carcinoma cell lines has been difficult, probably due to complex hormonal interrelationships. Characterization of malignant cell lines from normal or hyperplastic cells is difficult due to the lack of prostate-specific markers, but properties peculiar to prostate cancer may become useful research tools.[65, 66] For example, Okabe et al.[67] demonstrated decreased cell-mediated cytotoxicity in patients with advanced prostate cancer using the EB 33 cell line as a target cell. Defective cellular immunity in patients with prostatic cancer also has been demonstrated by the use of other in vitro assays such as monocyte chemotaxis.[64] McLaughlin and Brooks[68] incubated lymphocytes from prostate cancer patients in autologous sera, and noted decreased lymphocytes response to PHA. This impaired immunologic reactivity was thought to be secondary to an α_2-globulin.[68] Thomas et al.[69] also suggested that a serum factor may depress cellular immunity in prostate cancer patients. A recent study identified depressed spontaneous cytotoxicity and depressed antibody-dependent cell-mediated cytotoxicity (K cell functions) in prostate cancer patients.[70]

Little data is available regarding humoral immunity and B cell function in prostate cancer patients. Conflicting results have been reported regarding the levels of immunoglobulins in prostate cancer patients.[71, 72] Antigen ·antibody complexes have been identified in the sera of prostate cancer patients but their relationship to other immunologic function is unknown. Starling et al.[73] prepared monoclonal antibodies against a human prostate carcinoma cell line (DU145). One hybridoma preferentially, but not specifically, bound to the DU145 cell line.

Humoral immunity to prostatic cancer has been suggested to explain the regression of metastatic foci following cryosurgery in prostatic cancer. Ablin[71] identified circulating antibodies (by fluorescent microscopy) to autologous prostate tissue in a patient with metastatic carcinoma of the prostate, and noted the disappearance of distant metastases following cryosurgery in six patients. Soanes et al.[74] also reported regression of distant metastases in three patients after cryosurgery and demonstrated an antibody that specifically precipitated prostatic fluid in patients after cryosurgery. The subject of the immunologic phenomena associated with carcinoma of the prostate and reactions to freezing of prostate tissue has been thoroughly reviewed.[75]

Immunodiagnosis

Immunodiagnosis is becoming an important part of evaluation of the prostate cancer patient. Prostatic acid phosphatase is secreted by malignant prostate cells and is immunologically distinct from acid phosphatases released from other tissues. Radioimmunoassay (RIA) and counterimmunoelectrophoresis (CIEP) methods have been developed, and are much more sensitive and specific than the standard enzymatic assay.

In a national trial comparing RIA and CIEP, CIEP was found to be more easily reproducible in multiple centers, and perhaps more sensitive.[76]

The CIEP method detects elevated serum acid phosphatase in a large percentage of patients with localized prostate cancer but has not been proven sufficiently sensitive to use as a routine screening technique. Also, a small, but important number of normal patients have elevated levels of CIEP. While sensitivity of these assays increase, their utility as staging tests for detection of skeletal metastases decreases, since elevation does not necessarily indicate the presence of disseminated tumor.

Using immunoelectrophoresis and radial immunodiffusion, Grayhack et al.[77] measured levels of various immunoproteins in the expressed prostatic fluid of prostate cancer patients and controls. Levels of C3, C4, and transferrin were significantly elevated in prostate cancer patients, providing a potential for identification of early prostate cancer in high risk patients.

CONCLUSION

Study of the immunology of urologic tumors now parallels that in other human tumors. The complexity of the host immune response is increasingly appreciated, and identification of new functions of lymphoid cells (i.e. suppressor cells, and NK activity) has opened new areas of rewarding research. The identification and isolation of tumor-specific antigens may now be practical for many urologic tumors by monoclonal antibody techniques. In turn, the application of monospecific antibodies in diagnosis and therapy may become a reality. Most importantly, the basic tenets of human tumor immunology host response to tumor-specific antigen, and resultant influence on tumor growth and dissemination, can finally be adequately tested.

REFERENCES

1. Erie, R., Erie, K., and Morton, D. L. A membrane antigen common to human cancer and fetal brain tissues. *Cancer Res. 36:*5310, 1976.
2. Kohler, G., and Milstein. C. Continuous cultures of fused cells secreting antibody of pre-defined specificity. *Nature 256:*495, 1975.
3. David, J. R. Lymphocyte mediators and cellular hypersensitivity. *N. Engl. J. Med. 288:* 143, 1973.
4. Broder, S., and Waldmann, T. A. The suppressor-cell network in cancer. *N. Engl. J. Med. 299:*1281, 1978.
5. Peter, H. H., and Heidenreich, W. Spontaneous cell-mediated cytotoxicity. *Cancer Immunol. Immunother. 8:*79, 1980.
6. Green, I., Cohen, S., and McClusky, R. T. *Mechanisms of Tumor Immunity.* John Wiley & Sons, New York, 1977.
7. Economou, J. S. Therapy of a murine lymphoma with tumor-specific anti serum in combination with adriamycin cyclophosomide or L-aspharginase. *Surgery 87:*190, 1980.
8. Kröger, H., Stutz, E., and Rother, M. The effect of anti serum on the metastases of ascites cells as a function of time. *Eur. J. Cancer 3:*165, 1977.
9. Economou, J. S. The role of antibody in tumor immunity. *Surg. Gynecol. Obstet.* In press, 1980.
10. Eilber, F. R., and Morton, D. L. Impaired immunologic reactivity and recurrence following cancer surgery. *Cancer 25:*362, 1970.
11. Golub, S. Host immune response to human tumor antigen. In *Cancer—A Comprehensive Treatise*, Vol. 4. Edited by F. Becker. Plenum Publishers, New York, 1975.

12. Bean, M. A., Blum, B. R., Herberman, R. B., *et al.* Cell-mediated cytotoxicity for bladder carcinoma evaluation of a work shop. *Cancer Res. 35:*292, 1975.
13. Good, R. A. The lymphoid system, immuno deficiency, and malignancy. *Adv. Biosci. 12:*123, 1974.
14. Penn, I., and Starzl, T. Malignant tumors arising de novo in immune-suppressed organ transplant recipients. *Transplantation 14:*407, 1972.
15. Everson, T. C., and Cole, W. H. *Spontaneous Regression of Cancer.* W. B. Saunders, Philadelphia, 1966.
16. Burnet F. M. The concept of immunological surveillance. *Prog. Exp. Tumor Res. 13:*1, 1970.
17. Klein, G. Immunological Surveillance Against Neoplasia. *Harvey Lect. 69:*71, 1975.
18. Möller, G., and Möller, E. Immunological surveillance against neoplasia. *Immunological Aspects of Cancer,* Edited by J. E. Castro, University Park Press, Baltimore, 1978.
19. Biano, G. Clinical aspects of cancer immunotherapy. In *Immunity and Cancer In Man,* Edited by A. E. Reif. Marcel Dekker, New York, 1975.
20. Prehn, R. T. Do tumors grow because of the immune response of the host? *Transplant. Rev. 18:*34, 1976.
21. Morales, A., and Eidinger, D. Immune activity in renal cancer: a sequential study. *J. Urol. 115:*510, 1976.
22. Catalona, W. J., Chretien, P., and Trahan, E. Abnormalities of cell-mediated immuno-competence in genitourinary cancer. *J. Urol. 111:*229, 1974.
23. Schellhammer, P. F., Bracken, R., Bean, M. A., *et al.* Immune evaluation with skin testing. *Cancer 38:*149, 1976.
24. DeCenzo, J. M., Allison, R., and Leadbetter, G. W., Jr. Skin testing in genitourinary carcinoma: two year follow up. *J. Urol. 114:*271, 1975.
25. Cummings, K. B., Peter, J. B., Kaufman, J. J. Cell-mediated immunity to human antigens in patients with renal cell carcinoma. *J. Urol. 110:*31, 1973.
26. Hellström, I., Hellström, K., and Sjörgren, H., *et al.* Demonstration of cell-mediated immunity to human neoplasms of various histological types. *Int. J. Cancer 7:*1, 1971.
27. Cole, A. T., Avis, I., Fried, F., *et al.* Cell-mediated immunity in renal cell carcinoma-preliminary report. *J. Urol. 115:*234, 1976.
28. Elhilali, M. M., and Nayak, S. K. *In vitro* cytotoxicity studies in bladder and renal cell cancer. *Urology 7:*488, 1976.
29. Montie, J., Straffon, R., Deodhar, S., *et al. In vitro* accessed with cell-mediated immunity in patients with renal cell carcinoma. *J. Urol. 115:*239 1976.
30. Hakala, T. R. Transitional cell and renal cell carcinoma; cell-mediated immunity as determined by the lymphocyte titration technique. *Natl. Cancer Inst. Monogr. 49:*151, 1978.
31. Stjernsward, J., Almgrad, L. E., Frawzen, S., *et al.* Tumor-distinctive cellular immunity to renal carcinoma. *Clin. Exp. Immunol. 6:*963, 1970.
32. Daly, J. J., Prout, G. R., Jr., Ahl, C. A., and Lyn, J. C.: Specificity of cellular immunity to renal cell carcinoma. *J. Urol. 111:*448, 1974.
33. Kjaer, M., and Christensen, N. Ability of renal carcinoma tissue extract to induce leukocyte migration inhibition in patients with nonmetastatic renal carcinoma: correlation with clincial histopathological findings. *Cancer Immunol. Immunother. 2:*41, 1977.
34. Wright, G. L., Jr., Schellhammer, P. R., Rosato, R. E., *et al.* Cell-mediated immunity in patients with renal cell carcinoma as measured by leukocyte migration inhibition test. *Urology 12:*525, 1978.
35. Hemstreet, G. P., and Richardson, G. Inhibitors of monocyte chemotaxis from kidney cancer compared to autologous normal kidney. *Fed. Proc. 39:*898, 1980.
36. Hakala, T. R., Castro, A. E., Elliott, A. Y., *et al.* Humoral cytotoxicity in human renal cell carcinoma. *Invest. Urol. 11:*405, 1974.
37. deKernion, J. B., Ramming, K. P., and Gupta, R. K. The detection and clinical significance of antibodies to tumor-associated antigens in patients with renal cell carcinoma. *J. Urol. 122:*300, 1979.
38. Ueda, R., Shiku, J. Whitmore, W. F., *et al.* Seriological analysis of cell surface antigens of human renal cancer. *Proc. Am. Assoc. Cancer Res. 19:*198, 1978.
39. Belitsky, T., Ghose, T., Aquino, J., *et al.* Radionuclide imaging of primary renal cell carcinoma by ^{131}I-labeled anti-tumor antibody. *J. Nucl. Med. 19:*427, 1978.

40. LeBlanc, P. A., Taffet, S. M., Fried, F. A., and Avis. F. T. Staphylococcal protein A assay for detection of antibody directed at renal cancer cells. *J. Urol. 121:*724, 1979.

41. Catalona, W. J., Smolev, J. K., and Harty, J. I. Prognostic value of host immunocompetence in urologic cancer patients. *J. Urol. 114:*922, 1975.

42. Fahey, J. L., Brosman, S. and Dorey, F. Immunological responsiveness in patients with bladder cancer. *Cancer Res. 37:*2875, 1977.

43. Olsson, C. A., Rao, C. N., Menzioan, J. O., and Byrd, W. E. Immunologic unreactivity of bladder cancer patients. *J. Urol. 107:*607, 1972.

44. DeCenzo, J. M., and Leadbetter, G. W., Jr. The interaction of host immunocompetence and tumor aggressiveness in superficial bladder carcinoma. *J. Urol. 115:*262, 1976.

45. O'Toole, C., Unsgaard, B., and Almgrad, L. E., and Johansson, B. The cellular immune response to carcinoma of the urinary bladder. Correlation to clinical stage and therapy. Br. J. Cancer (Suppl. 1) *28:*266, 1973.

46. Bean, M. A., Pees, H., Vogh, J. E., Grabstald, H., and Oetgen, H. F. Cytotoxicity of lymphocytes from patients with cancer of the urinary bladder: detection by a H^3-prolene microcytoxicity tests. *Int. J. Cancer 14:*186, 1974.

47. McLaughlin, A. P., III, Kessler, W. O., Triman, K., and Gittes, R. F. Immunologic competence in patients with urolgoic cancer. *J. Urol. 111:*233, 1974.

48. Fahey, J. L., and Zighelboim, J. Tumor immunology. In *Clinical Immunology*, Edited by C. W. Parker, W. B. Saunders, Philadelphia, 1980.

49. Hausman, M. S., and Brosman, S. A.: Abnormal monocyte function in bladder cancer patients. *J. Urol. 115:*537, 1976.

50. Bean, M. A., Schellhammer, P. S. Garr, H. W., Pinsky, C. M., and Whitmore, W. F., Jr. Immunocompetence of patients with transitional cell carcinoma as measured by dinitrochlorobenzene skin tests and *in vitro* lymphocyte function. *Natl. Cancer Inst. Monogr. 49:*111, 1978.

51. Schellhammer, P. F., Wright, G. L., Jr., Rosato, F. E., and Faulconer, R. J. Leukocytic migration inhibition assay in patients with bladder cancer. J. Urol. *122:*746, 1979.

52. Herr, H. W., Bean, M. A., and Whitmore, W. F., Jr. Prognostic significance of regional lymph node histology in cancer of the bladder. *J. Urol. 115:*264, 1976.

53. Herr, H. W. Suppressor cells in pelvic lymph node regional to bladder cancer. *J. Surg. Oncol. 11:*289, 1979.

54. Catalona, W. J., Feldman, A. T., Ratliff, T. L., and McCool, R. E. Suppressive effects of regional lymph node cells and extracts on antibody-dependent cellular cytotoxicity. *J. Urol. 119:*396, 1978.

55. Weingurtner, F., Hammer, C., Chaussy, C., Schuller, J., and Wieland, W. Suppressor cell activity in the peripheral blood of patients with carcinoma of the bladder and the kidney. *Immunobiology 156:*275, 1979.

56. Spina, C. A., Dorey, F., Vescera, C., Brosman, S., Fahey, J. L. Depress cell-mediated cytotoxicity in patients with bladder carcinoma: presence of macrophage-like suppressor cells. *Proc. Am. Assoc. Cancer Res. 21:*250, 1980.

57. Pesce, A. J., Evans, A., Ooi, B. S., Ooi, Y. M. Specific antibodies to bladder carcinoma tumor antigen. Proceedings of 18th National Bladder Cancer Conference, Miami, December, 1976.

58. Hakala, T. R., Castro, A. E., Elliott, A. Y., and Fraley, E. E. Humoral cytotoxicity in human transitional cell carcinoma. *J. Urol. 111:*382, 1974.

59. O'Brien, P., Gozzo, J. J., Monaco, A. P. Detection of a less than 50,000 dalton tumor associated antigen in urine from patients with bladder cancer. *Fed. Proc. 39:*351, 1980.

60. DeFazio, S. R., Gozzo, J. J., and Monaco, A. P. Fractionation of tumor-associated antigens from urine of bladder cancer patients by hydroxyapatite chromatography. *Fed. Proc. 39:*1143, 1980.

61. Davidsohn, I. Early Immunologic Diagnosis and Prognosis of Carcinoma. Am. *J. Clin. Pathol. 57:*715, 1972.

62. Limas, C., Lange, T., Fraley, E. E., Vessela, R. N. A,B,H, antigens in transitional cell tumor of the urinary bladder: correlation with the clinical course. *Cancer 44:*2099, 1979.

63. Johnson, J. D., and Lamm, D. L. Prediction of bladder tumor invasion with the mixed cell agglutination tests. *J. Urol. 123:*24, 1980.

64. Brosman, S., Hausman, M., Slacks, S. Immunologic alteration in patients with prostatic carcinoma. *J. Urol. 113:*841, 1975.

65. Kaighn, M. E. Human prostatic epithelial cell culture models. *Invest. Urol. 17:*382, 1980.
66. Lubaroff, D. M. H T C—36: epithelial tissue cultural line derived from human prostate adenocarcinoma. *Natl. Cancer Inst. Monogr. 49:*35 1978.
67. Okabe, T., Ackerman, R., Wirth, M., and Frohmuller, J. G. Cell-mediated cytotoxicity in patients with cancer of the prostate. *J. Urol. 122:*628, 1979.
68. McLaughlin, A. P., III, and Brooks, J. D. A Plasma factor inhibiting lymphocyte reactivity in urologic patient. *J. Urol. 112:*366, 1974.
69. Thomas, J. W., Jerkins, G., Cox, C., and Lieberman, P. Defective cell-mediated immunity in carcinoma of the prostate. *Invest. Urol. 14:*72, 1976.
70. Catalona, W. J., Ratliff, T. L., McCool, R. E. Discordance among cell-mediated cytolytic mechanisms in cancer patients: importance of the assay system. *J. Immunol. 122:*1009, 1979.
71. Ablin, R. J. Serum antibody in patients with prostatic cancer. *Br. J. Urol.* 48:355, 1976.
72. Schmidt. J. D., Feldbush, T. L., Weinstein, S. H. and Bonney, W. Serum immunoglobulins in genitourinary malignancies. *J. Urol. 115:*293, 1976.
73. Starling, J. J., Sieg, S. M., and Wright, G. L. Monoclonal antibodies against human prostate adenocarcinoma cells. *Proc. Am. Assoc. Cancer Res. 21:*234. 1980.
74. Soanes, W. A., Ablin, R. J., and Condor, M. J. Remission of metastatic lesions following cryosurgery in prostatic cancer. *J. Urol. 104:*154, 1970.
75. Prout, G. R., Jr., and Ornelles, E. P. Immunology of the prostate. *Urol. Clin. North Am. 2:*93, 1975.
76. Wajsman, Z., Chu, T. M. Saroff, J., Slack, M., and Murphy, G. P. Two new direct, and specific methods of acid phosphatase determination. National field trial. *Urology 13:*8, 1979.
77. Grayhack, J. T., Wendel, E. F., Oliver, L., and Lee, C. Analysis of specific proteins in prostatic fluid for detecting prostatic malignancy. *J. Urol. 121:*295, 1979.

6

Use of Electron Microscope in Diagnosis of Genitourinary Neoplasms

Scanning electron microscopy (SEM) and transmission electron microscopy (TEM) studies of genitourinary neoplasms have been randomly reviewed and reported.[1-3] The majority of these neoplasms are usually of specific interest to certain groups depending either on the medical or surgical problems encountered in terms of diagnosis and/or therapy. We are, therefore, going to attempt to provide an overall broad survey of the genitourinary tract with a combined SEM and TEM overview.

RENAL TUMORS

Neoplasms of the kidney are usually surveyed by TEM and less frequently by SEM. Recent literature has revealed that primary renal parenchymal tumors arise from the tubular epithelium of the kidney and, therefore, should be termed "renal cell carcinomas."[4,5] This evidence has been supported by numerous studies which show that the renal cell carcinomas in many ways mimic normal tubular structure and/or exhibit transitions from normal tubules to those that are arranged in a papillary or cordlike fashion. Further proof for this concept of tumor cell origin has been substantiated by electron microscopy. TEM studies demonstrate that there are many striking similarities between renal cell carcinomas and normal epithelium of the proximal convoluted tubules.[6-12] In man, the normal appearance of the different parts of the tubules does not differ markedly in any important diagnostic way from those found in animals.[5, 13-15] The main distinguishing features of proximal convoluted tubules of the kidney are: (1) The presence of a brush border containing numerous tightly packed microvilli, (2) invaginations of the apical plasma membrane provided with membrane coatings, (3) the occurrence of vesicles or vacuoles with characteristic structure in the apical cytoplasm, (4) an abundance of mitochondria, and (5) deep invaginations of the basilar plasma membrane which create slender cytoplasmic compartments. The cells of the distal tubules do not demonstrate any of these specializations in the apical plasma membrane. However, they do contain abundant mitochondria and may show deep basilar plasma membrane invaginations. The cells in other parts of the tubular system are less well specialized and show a simpler structure of the plasma membrane as well as of the cytoplasm.

CLEAR CELL CARCINOMAS OF KIDNEY

When examined by electron microscopy, clear cell carcinomatous cells are found to grow in cords or tubules that are surrounded by a basement membrane. They have abundant cytoplasm with sparse numbers of mitochondria, endoplasmic reticulum, and Golgi apparatus. In the cytoplasm of many of these cells are dense particles measuring from 200 to 400 Å units and they are believed to be particulate glycogen (Fig. 6.1). Many of the clear cell carcinomas characteristically contain large numbers of clear vacuoles in the cytoplasm. However, many of these cells are attached to each other by various types of intercellular junctions. In their studies of these tumor cells, several schools of pathology[16] have noted that in some foci there are special local surface structural alterations which have the appearance of brush border-like structures or microvilli. There are also numerous vesicles associated with the plasma membrane. Some authors[16] have also noted that the numbers of microvilli and the area of the plasma membrane alteration showing these specializations vary greatly from one part of the tumor to the other. More detailed ultrastructural descriptions by TEM have been delineated elsewhere.[1]

Some of the main aspects of these tumors are very quickly characterized on the freshly cut surfaces and can be fixed immediately in normal TEM fixatives. These can then be scanned and they reveal a very distinctive surface alteration. The complexity and variability of the microvilli can be described not only by TEM, but also by SEM. For the clear cell carcinomas, TEM demonstrates the variability in spacing of these microvilli. On the other hand, there is compactness of the microvilli in granular cell carcinomas of the kidney. SEM of these tumors demonstrates much more quickly, readily, and with greater ease, the variability in cell patterns as it relates to the microvilli. Great multiplicity of pattern and configuration is generally the rule for kidney carcinoma. If metastatic tumor from the kidney to the bone or lung is diagnosed and an aspiration biopsy is obtained which reveals a sarcomatous appearance, then TEM and SEM can distinguish whether the tumors are of epithelial renal cell origin rather than some bizarre sarcomatous pattern of unknown origin.

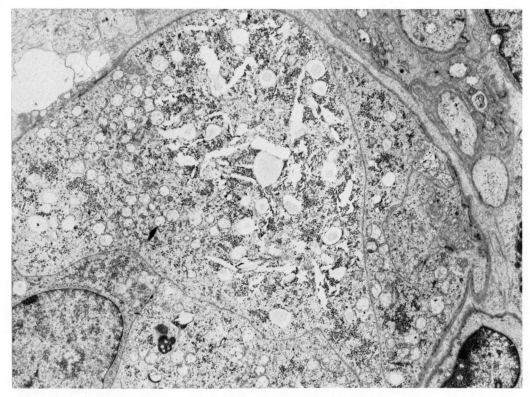

Figure 6.1. Clear cell carcinoma of the kidney. Tumor cells contain predominantly fat globules and glycogen, with very few mitochondria. There are numerous cell junctions and few microvilli (transmission electronmicroscopy ×3,625).

GRANULAR CELL CARCINOMAS OF KIDNEY

Light microscopy (LM) of these tumors reveals a granular cell type where the cytoplasm is either deeply basophilic or eosinophilic. The cells are arranged in a cord or papillary configuration with, not infrequently, cells of the clear cell type interposed between them. However, when these cells are examined by TEM, their cytoplasm is excessively rich in mitochondria and devoid of numerous fat vacuoles. When compared to the clear cell carcinomas of the kidney, these cells possess a more basilar plasma membrane infolding (Fig. 6.2). The precise mechanism by which these laminations of the basement membrane are formed among these tumor cells is not understood. It is possible that the neoplastic cells in certain areas have lost their polarity and have produced this basement membrane-like material in an excessively haphazard fashion.

URINARY BLADDER

The classification and histopathology of the urinary bladder carcinomas have been well documented by numerous authors. By light histology,

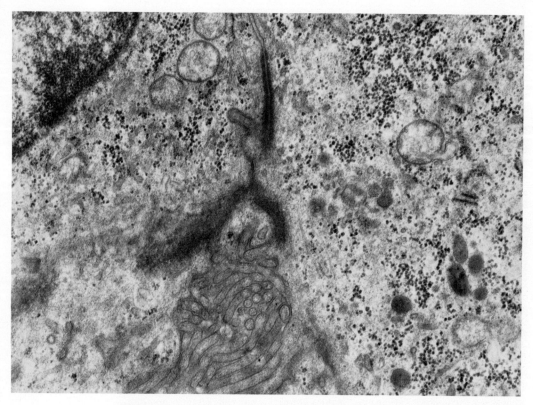

Figure 6.2. Granular cell carcinoma of the kidney. Transmission electronmicroscopy shows numerous short, blunted, closely packed, microvilli on cell surfaces (×18,125).

Mostofi[17] has classified histologically the numerous patterns demonstrated by urothelial cancers. Despite this, there is much about the urinary tract neoplasm that remains an enigma to many devotees of the problem, namely the urologic surgeon, the surgical pathologist, the chemotherapist, the radiologist and now, especially, the environmentalist. However, it is possible with the aid of TEM and SEM to clarify the areas of diagnostic confusion.

In retrospect, there are very few ultrastructural descriptions or studies of normal human and neoplastic urothelia. When such studies are reevaluated or future ones contemplated, the manner in which the urothelium is obtained is consequently of great importance. In any research or histological descriptive paper, it should be explicitly stated how the tissue specimen is obtained for morphological analysis by LM, SEM, and TEM. The urologist is certainly aware of the fact that biopsies of the bladder mucosa are exposed to cytoscopy fluids with very low osmotic pressure. The surgical pathologist and researchers who do ultrastructural analysis of bladder mucosa are not aware of how long the bladder urothelium is exposed to these cystoscopy fluids of low osmotic pressure before the biopsy is obtained and put into the proper fixatives.

NORMAL UROTHELIUM

In many specimens, notably those obtained from surgical specimens of the ureter and renal pelvis, as well as of the human bladder, the urothelium comprises a very tight arrangement of a compact layer of cells. When these cells have disruptive interdigitations, then some attention must be paid to the manner in which the specimen is collected. These features are not noted to occur with any frequency in animal bladders or ureters which are isolated and fixed very rapidly.

The normal urothelium is composed, for the most part, of three different layers of cells which can be ultrastructurally described as a layer of superficial cells, one or more layers of intermediary cells and, finally, a layer of basal cells (Fig. 6.3). These latter cells are attached to the basement membranes by means of numerous hemidesmosomes.

Superficial Cells

The luminal surface of the bladder or other portions of the genitourinary system are lined by superficial cells. From a morphological point of view, these cells are very characteristic of the urothelial system. The superficial cells may measure from 20 to 30 μm in width and half that in height. The cytoplasm of the cells contains numerous mitochondria as well as numerous profiles of thick-walled, round, or fusiform vesicles which vary greatly in size and number.[18-20] In man, these vesicles are not as prominent in number as they are in the rodent. In this instance, it is extremely important to consider what is meant by normal urothelium. Bladder mucosa which is not inflamed nor involved in a neoplastic process, or which is obtained during a suprapubic prostatectomy, is the type of bladder biopsy that should be obtained. In the latter instance, the urothelium is almost similar to that which is described in the rodent.[21] However, care must be taken to ensure that these specimens are from nontraumatized or noninflamed areas. This can be easily doublechecked by doing a histological analysis by LM after the specimen is first examined by SEM. In favorable sections of these superficial cells, a tripartite junctional complex may be seen. As revealed by SEM the superficial cells are covered by asymmetrical membranes or microridges (Fig. 6.4). TEM of these superficial cells will reveal tripartite junctional complexes. The function and interrelationship of these junctional complexes with the vesicles and the surface of the normal urothelium with its asymmetrical membranes is not clearly understood at the present time. The exact role of the vesicles and the asymmetrical membranes may be associated with fluid transport and consequently, systemic hydration of the individual. It has been speculated that the vesicles may represent structures for storage or transport of the plasmalemma or transitional epithelial cells. It also has been suggested that these vesicles in the normal surface cell may function as part of the excretory system for the excessive fluid that might enter through the cells. In the normal human material, these vesicles can also be seen in the intermediary layers of cells.

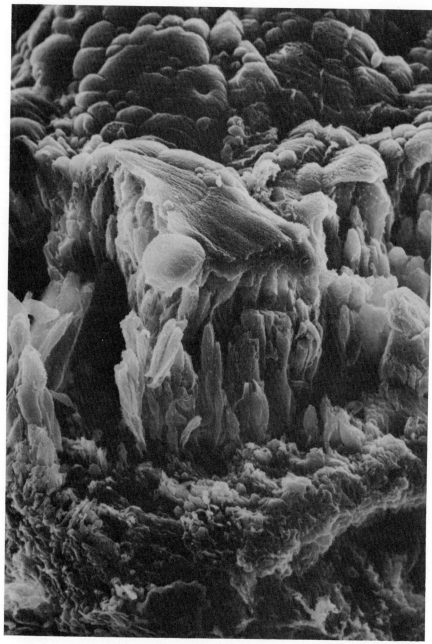

Figure 6.3. Normal bladder mucosa from left lateral wall. The *upper one-third* of the picture demonstrates normal surface cells with microridges. The *middle one-third* reveals a few intermediary cells, and the *lower one-third* consists of basal cells with a basement membrane (scanning electronmicroscopy ×600).

Intermediary and Basal Cells

These layers of cells show much of the same ultrastructural morphology as the surface cells, but to a lesser degree as one progresses from the intermediary to the basal cell layer.

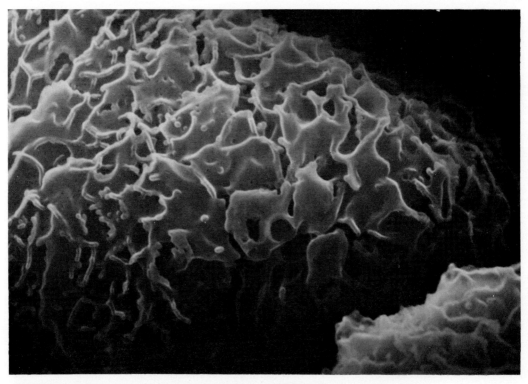

Figure 6.4. Surface cell of normal urothelium. Surface shows prominent microridges and very rare microvilli. (scanning electronmicroscopy ×11,760).

PAPILLARY TUMORS

SEM of the surface of papillary exophytic tumors which are in contact with urine usually reveals microvilli rather than a microridge pattern, as is seen on the surface of normal noninflamed urothelial cells. Depending on the grade of tumor that is mixed with the normal cells, the majority of the surface cells are covered with microvilli (Fig. 6.5). The higher the grade of the tumor, the greater will be the number of surface cells that have numerous pleomorphic microvilli on their luminal side. These surface cells then usually cover in a very loose fashion the intermediary and basal cells which for the most part also have microvilli that may not be of the pleomorphic type. When there is tumor, there is a great tendency for the spatial relationship of differentiation of these three different layers to disappear with respect to the basement membrane. This also occurs with its morphological relationship to the fibrovascular core in the center of these papillary tumors. The blood vessel is devoid of smooth muscle in the fibrovascular core. If LM reveals any tendency toward squamous cell change or metaplasia, then numerous tonofilaments are usually found in the cytoplasm of many of the cells comprising these tumors. If the tumor is biologically breaking out of tissue architecture, careful examination may show that many of these tumors at their base will exhibit, at one time or another, a tendency to ultrastructurally halt the formation of

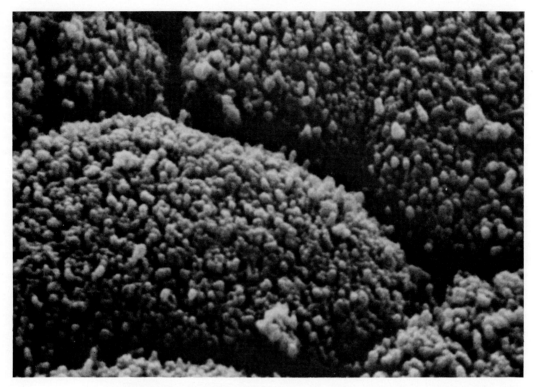

Figure 6.5. Scanning electronmicroscopy of surface of tumor. Surface covered by pleomorphic microvilli (×14,000).

basement membranes. When this occurs, either with an invading papillary tumor or carcinoma *in situ*, ultrastructurally, an electron-dense floccular material can be seen interposed between the underlying stroma and the invading transitional cell tumor. This deposit is very similar to that observed in the basement membranes of various immune glomerular nephropathies. Quite often the urologists do not take their biopsies cold *i.e.*, without an electrical cutting current. As a consequence, many pathologists will see extremely cauterized cells that are of inflammatory cell origin, and which can be readily misdiagnosed as tumor cells that are invading the lamina propria. Frequently the cells are so distorted that it is impossible to differentiate them as being tumor as opposed to a tissue macrophage or histiocyte. Many of the squamous cell and urothelial tumors of the bladder not only exfoliate tumor cells into the urine but also exfoliate histiocytes with cytologically malignant nuclei. On numerous occasions, we have noted a crush or cautery artifact in our extensive surgical pathology material. Thus, a false diagnosis easily can be obtained for the presence or absence of tumor in the biopsy unless one is continually on guard against this mishap.

Not only can the invading urothelial cells be destroyed beyond recognition, but also the multinucleated cells can be distorted to such an extent that they can be misdiagnosed as tumor cells. These multinucleated cells are ubiquitous and seem to increase in number in the lamina propria and muscularis of the urinary bladder when there has been (1) previous biopsies of the urinary bladder, (2) prior radiotherapy to the bladder, (3) chemotherapeutic instillation into the bladder, and (4) invading tumor. TEM of these cells shows that they are very distinctive and different from those that compose the invading bladder tumor. The syncytium of histiocytes or macrophages has several nuclei and a markedly vacuolated cytoplasm. The numerous vesicles are lined by either a single or double layer of membranes. The cytoplasm may contain mitochondria, dense bodies and phagolysosomes, but the Golgi apparatus is hard to find in these cells. The giant cells are almost always adjacent to collagen and tumor cells but they do not appear to fuse to them. The nuclei have prominent chromocenters, sometimes several, with margination of some of the chromatin at the nuclear membrane. There are also fine granular dense bodies in their nuclei. When prominent sinus histiocytosis is present, these histiocytes or macrophages are morphologically identical to those found in lymph nodes. What then is the function of these macrophages or nonattached cells? Are they then processing tumor antigen or are they a form of cell-mediated immunity?[2]

CYTOLOGIC MONITORING OF NEOPLASTIC UROTHELIUM

The human urinary bladder offers the scientific investigator interested in carcinogenesis a unique opportunity for monitoring the induction, conversion, and progression of the urothelium to a cancer that eventually invades and kills. All of these observations can be accurately viewed by means of urinary cytology and electron microscopy as employed by the surgical pathologist.

Table 6.1 provides a correlation between urinary cytology and cystoscopic findings of biopsies taken from patients at high risk or with a previous history of bladder tumors. The cytological findings can alert the urologist to visualize the bladder cystoscopically and, if there is an exophytic urothelial lesion, it can be treated by surgery or other forms of therapy. There are numerous occasions where there is positive urinary cytology and no positive cystoscopic findings i.e., no papillary exophytic tumor. However, with the use of electron microscopy, the urologist can be speedily alerted if the urothelium is at high risk for cancer by means of the specific surface morphological markers as previously described.

Thus, the human bladder cancer problem may be better comprehended with the potential aid of TEM and SEM as applied to urinary bladder biopsies obtained under maximal cystoscopic conditions along with urinary cytology. It can be carefully monitored both before and after its inflection point in the cancer growth curve. This multidisciplined approach can only improve our understanding of the problem, its causes and its effective treatment.

Table 6.1
Correlation of urinary cytology, cystoscopy and bladder biopsies[a]

Cytology	Cystoscopy	Bladder Biopsy Interpretation
Negative	Visible papillary lesion	Papillary lesion of low grade. No significant epithelial atypia.
Marked atypia (suspicious)	Visible papillary lesion	Papillary lesion of moderate grade, or peripheral epithelial atypia, or both.
Positive (cancer cells present)	Visible papillary lesion	Papillary lesion of low grade with peripheral carcinoma *in situ.*
		Papillary lesion of high grade with or without carcinoma *in situ.*
	Visible nonpapillary lesion	Invasive carcinoma with or without carcinoma *in situ.*
	No visible lesions	Carcinoma *in situ* (common)
		Metastatic carcinoma (rare)
		Carcinoma in diverticulum (very rare)

[a] Modified from L. G. Koss, *Diagnostic Cytology and Its Histopathologic Bases.* J.B. Lippincott, Philadelphia, 1979.

ULTRASTRUCTURAL PATHOLOGY OF MALE ACCESSORY ORGANS

As most urologists know, cancer of the prostate is one of the foremost causes of death in men over the age of 70; however, prostate carcinoma deaths in males past 50 are only exceeded by lung cancer.[22]

The histological criteria for diagnosis of prostatic adenocarcinoma have been well documented, and relatively effective methods of treatment have been developed yielding a 5-year survival rate of greater than 75%.[23, 24] Even though LM of the more common types of tumor is well illustrated, few studies have been specifically directed toward the ultrastructural study of these tumors by combined TEM and SEM. There have been a few scattered reports on the study of surface topography of these variegated patterns of prostatic carcinoma using SEM.[25-30]

When carcinoma of the prostate is suspected after a rectal examination, or when there is an elevation of serum prostatic acid phosphatase, the urologist frequently obtains a needle biopsy, either through the rectum or the perineum. Many times when obtaining prostatic tissue, the needle will encounter a portion of seminal vesicle which the pathologist then has to pathologically evaluate.[24]

The seminal vesicles are evaginations of the vasa deferentia, which are also of a similar histological nature. The seminal vesicle is known to have the ability to secrete a fluid which is then added to the sperm from the testes. This fluid manifests itself as a yellowish, thick, viscous substance in surgical and autopsy specimens. By LM, the cytoplasmic findings of a yellow-brown pigment or lipofuscin is of immense help in differentiating seminal vesicle epithelium from carcinomatous prostatic epithelium.

SEM of these structures reveals that the seminal vesicle epithelium is arranged in a papillary form. The epithelium covers an outer tube of musculature. The papillary configuration may be in the form of ridges where the surfaces are covered by many cells (Fig. 6.6). The epithelium covering is next to the secretion. There are many cells that have an apocrine-type snout or marked bleb secretions that project from the cell surface. These are pinched off to form the secretions of this structure. Some of these surface cells may be studded with, or devoid of, long pleomorphic microvilli. SEM reveals considerable variation in the epithelium of the seminal vesicle or vasa deferentia. This variability also depends upon the age of the patient and the functional state of the epithelium.

The human prostate consists of a tubular, aveolar, branching of glands which opens into the urethra through a series of periurethral prostatic excretory ducts. The glandular elements of these glands are surrounded by varying amounts of stroma, which are composed primarily of smooth

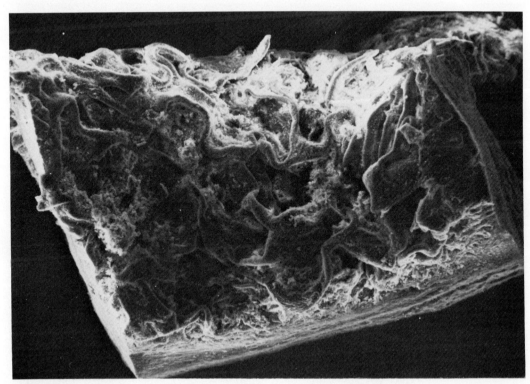

Figure 6.6. Seminal vesicle. Note wall and numerous papillary folds of epithelium (scanning electronmicroscopy ×38).

muscle and fibroblasts. SEM of tissue obtained from suprapubic or retropubic prostatectomy specimens presents varying results depending upon the age of the patient.

Benign prostatic hyperplasia (BPH) is a smooth muscle fibroblastic proliferation which begins in the late 20s. The epithelium examined from this age group can demonstrate a pattern quite different from that seen in the late 40s. SEM of tissue from this age group reveals numerous branching and tubular aveolar glands adjacent to blood vessels (Fig. 6.7). Numerous types of inflammatory cells, small or large in size, are scattered throughout the fibromuscular tissue. They are also adherent to the walls of the different blood vessels that course through the fibromuscular tissue. When examined histologically, the various kinds of prostatic epithelia that are seen in the ducts or acini are usually lined by either low cuboidal or columnar cells (Fig. 6.8). These cells then cover a basal or reserve cell.

Adjacent to the ducts are acini which are filled with numerous surface cells. LM shows that these acinar cells also cover basal or reserve cells but are fewer in number than in the ducts. Fibromuscular tissue surrounds all of this glandular or tubular epithelium. As part of the normal aging process, numerous corpora amylacea are lodged in the center of some of these ducts. Ductal epithelium surrounds the corpora amylacea which then blocks the ducts and prevents the egress of secretions produced by

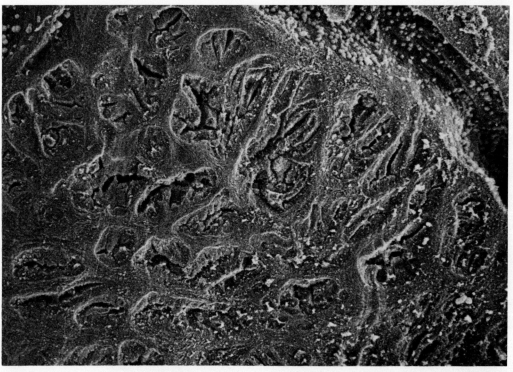

Figure 6.7. Benign prostatic hyperplasia (BPH). Scanning electronmicroscopy shows hypertrophic glands and surrounds fibromuscular tissue and blood vessels (×70).

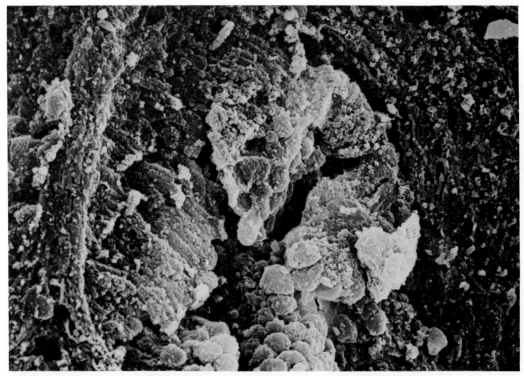

Figure 6.8. Acinus of prostatic gland. Fibromuscular tissue surrounds the acinus consisting of surface and basal cells (scanning electronmicroscopy ×799).

these surface cells. The secretions which accumulate behind the corpora amylacea tend to cause dilatation of these ducts. At times, rupture of the ducts may occur and the secretions escape into the surrounding connective tissue, eliciting a granulomatous reaction. Granulomatous prostatitis may clinically simulate carcinoma of the prostate. When the biopsy procedure is not taken with great care, it can be easily distorted and may be misread as carcinoma of the prostate. Fortunately, the type of carcinoma which has a similar cell type is extremely rare. Therefore, distortion of these cells histologically should not cause much trouble.

Examination of the surface of corpora amylacea shows that it is covered by a large number of granular secretory debris which, on higher magnification, is nodular and coarse in appearance. There is a great similarity between this material and the granularity of the surface of the individual prostatic surface cells (Fig. 6.9). TEM demonstrates the fibrillar, proteinaceous matrix of the corpora amylacea. The surface is covered with coarse granular secretions which are partially embedded in the proteinaceous matrix. SEM reveals that many acini are surrounded by fibromuscular stroma and the acini, at higher magnification, reveal many papillary projections covered by small nodular excrescences or prostatic secretions in the lumen of the gland. SEM of these excrescences reveals a marked compact nest of nodularity on the surface of many of the prostatic surface cells (Fig. 6.10). TEM of similar nodular material reveals that several of

ELECTRON MICROSCOPE IN DIAGNOSIS   113

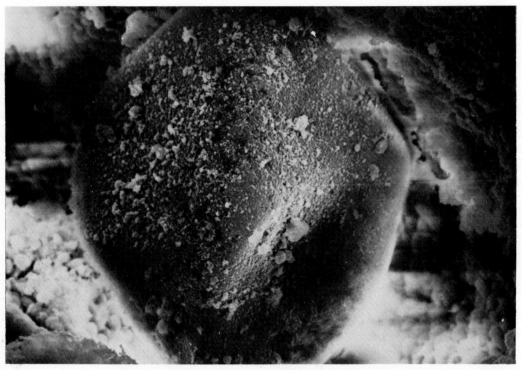

Figure 6.9. Corpora amylacea lodged in a duct. The walls are on the *left* and *right* of the corpora amylacea. The surface of this is covered by secretory debris (scanning electronmicroscopy ×689).

these cells are associated with secretory vesicles partially filled with small secretory granules. The prostatic surface cell has a tripartite junctional complex similar to that described in the bladder, allowing these surface cells to adhere closely to each other.

Many of the surgical specimens examined from the younger age group (under 30) are composed of surface acinar cells covered by coarse excrescences with very few microvilli interposed between the nodular excrescences. In the older age group, there is a great tendency for many of the surface cells to have less compactness of the coarse nodular excrescences, and many portions of the prostatic surface are now associated with loose arrays of microvilli.

Ultrastructural characteristics of prostatic carcinoma are quite dependent on the variation in patterns associated with most prostatic carcinomas. One should attempt to relate these structural changes to the various grades of the Gleason or Mostofi[17] classifications, which has not been done at the present time. It is well documented that carcinomas of the prostate may vary from one high power microscopic field to another in the same specimen. When comparing the normal to the malignant prostatic cancer cell, the major theme is that of a significant loss in ultrastructural organization of the cytoplasmic organelles within the prostatic cancer cell. Such structural changes become more accentuated as the tumor progresses

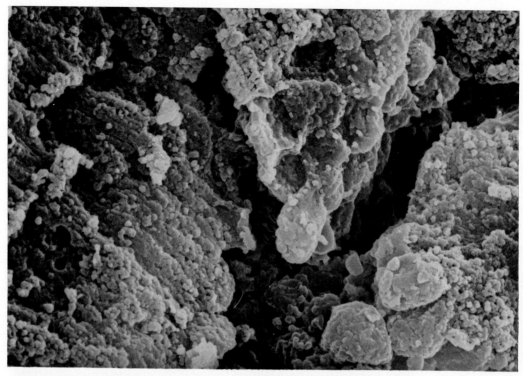

Figure 6.10. Portion of the acinus. Small papillary projections into the lumen of the gland with individual cells showing secretory granules. (scanning electronmicroscopy ×2,100).

to a higher grade. This is characteristically reflected in an alteration in its polarity of secretion. The cancer cell tends to secrete toward the direction of the basement membrane instead of toward the lumen. Many of the proliferating prostatic tumor cells also fail to form adequate junctional complexes. There is a defective communication between the lumen of the malignant acini and the larger normal prostatic ducts. The malignant acinar secretions may not empty into the normal prostatic ducts. Morphologically, this is very characteristic of infiltrating or metastatic tumors of the prostate gland. Acid phosphatase or other secretory products can no longer be channeled into the excretory ducts and, as a consequence, many of these secretions accumulate inside the cell or, as often happens, leak out into the surrounding interstitial connective tissue. Diffusion may be the mechanism by which this occurs but, ultrastructurally, these cells often demonstrate actual breakdown of degenerative cells that have outgrown their blood supply. This probably is the most frequent mechanism whereby intracellular products eventually reach the interstitium and then into the vascular channels, thereby causing an elevation of acid phosphatase in the blood stream.

SEM of the prostatic tissue has not been extensively correlated with TEM. TEM, however, has been correlated with the grade of tumor. Characteristic of most carcinomas of the prostate is the disturbance of tissue architecture, whereby small glands are back to back. Like the light microscope, SEM can readily reveal such a focus of carcinoma of the prostate. Many of these glands are well differentiated. SEM of such a cluster of cells in one of these glands will reveal that the surface is very irregular and pitted with numerous excavations and sparse microvilli. Occasionally an operculum-like structure will cover the surface of the tumor cells. There is extreme variation even when the glands of the well differentiated carcinomas of the prostate are examined. Characteristically, the secretory excrescences seen by the electron microscope have almost gone and some cells are almost always covered by microvilli.

Another variation around the central theme is that one prostatic carcinoma cell may have one or two secretory excrescences on its surface whereas the adjacent cells are covered by numerous microvilli. The junctional complexes are not present and, as a consequence, these prostatic carcinoma cells are well separated from each other. Many well differentiated prostatic tumor cells still have the capacity to secrete acid phosphatase and this can be readily demonstrated by histochemical techniques. Correlative TEM of well differentiated carcinomatous glands may show marked variability in each carcinomatous cell; some of the cells lining the lumen have numerous microvilli whereas others do not. Many well differentiated prostatic carcinomas have the capacity to cleave the smooth muscle cells apart. It is not uncommon to find instances where some portions of the gland have a basement membrane and other parts of the gland do not. The surface cells are lighter in density and have well formed Golgi apparatus and mitochondria. However, there is a reversal of polarity of cell secretion, being now toward the basement membrane instead of toward the luminal portion of the cell. TEM of poorly differentiated carcinomatous patterns demonstrates marked deviation away from what is normal in terms of alteration of cytoplasmic components. Here, there are increased numbers of mitochondria with or without extreme variability in the mitochondrial size and shape. Tumor cells also are known to be in close proximity to blood vessels, and the surrounding extracellular space is very edematous and filled with a large amount of cytoplasmic debris. This is a finding which correlates well with the elevations of acid phosphatase in the blood stream. Characteristically, this is found in many of the invading tumors, but not in the well differentiated carcinomas.

TESTICULAR TUMORS

The majority of testicular tumors are readily characterized by LM. However, a small percentage of tumors can be histologically confused with each other and combined SEM and TEM can help with the differential diagnosis. If these tumors are not placed in the proper pathobiologic category, the surgical procedures or the medical management of these patients will be altered and the prognosis for the patient will be drastically affected. This confusion can sometimes occur among the undifferentiated embryonal carcinomas, anaplastic seminomas, and reticulum cell sarcomas. The latter frequently occurs as a testicular tumor after the age of 55.

Seminomas

Seminomas are not always composed of cell patterns that are easily separated from either embryonal carcinoma or reticulum cell sarcoma. The seminoma cells are not always found in association with inflammatory cells revealing the typical light histology appearance of seminoma or the spermatocytic type of seminoma. In several cases of anaplastic seminoma and regular seminoma, a consistent pattern begins to unfold when they are examined by SEM. Under low magnification, all the testicular tumors appear alike. At high magnification, the surface topography of the anaplastic seminomas, as well as the regular seminomas, all reveal numerous long tubular tortuous structures attached to the cell bodies. These are similar in size to the midtail piece and tail of the sperm and are seen to connect one cell to the other. Also covering these cells are focal tufts of microvilli which may be found in concentrated clusters on the surface of some of these cells.

TEM of the seminoma cells does not always easily demonstrate these structures as observed by SEM.[31] It is very difficult to visualize the tufted, stellate collection of microvilli as well as the tubular connections between or over the surface of these tumor cells. As seen by TEM, seminoma cells do demonstrate a rare cellular connection.[32] Ultrastructurally, the cells have scattered lysosome-like material, Golgi apparatus, and focal accumulations of glycogen and/or polyribosomes. They may be surrounded by inflammatory cells and/or macrophages. They do not demonstrate ultrastructurally the tripartite junctional complexes that are commonly seen between the differentiated and the undifferentiated cells of the embryonal carcinoma type of germ cell tumor.

Embryonal Carcinoma

Embryonal carcinoma may be a pure epithelial lesion or may be associated with teratocarcinomatous change. The latter has a fibromyxomatous stroma and is associated with the teratocarcinomatous portion of the germ cell tumor. The embryonal carcinomas may or may not have papillary embryonal patterns or embryoid bodies. However, when the papillary portions and/or the embryoid bodies of the undifferentiated portions of the embryonal carcinoma are examined by SEM or TEM, other ultrastructural characteristics begin to unfold which are quite distinctive and different from the anaplastic or the undifferentiated seminomas. SEM of these tumors will usually reveal smooth surface of the embryonal carcinomatous portion with few if any microvilli or tubular structures seen in the seminomatous cells. These cells are usually tightly adherent to each other. TEM of these tumors is very characteristic in that they have numerous cell attachments and/or tripartite junctional complexes and they tend to form small lumens with microvilli (Fig. 6.11). They will also form many more tight junctions and attenuated desmosomes than can be found in the majority of seminomas. Internal cytoplasmic components are not that radically different from those found in seminomas.

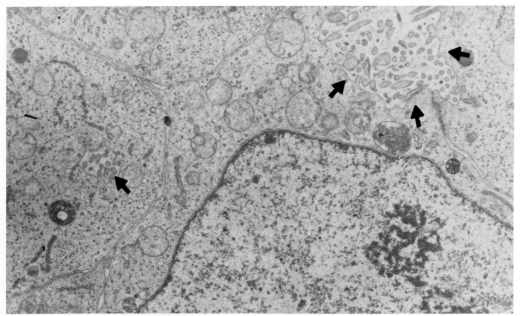

Figure 6.11. Transmission electronmicroscopy of embryonal carcinoma of the testis. *Arrows* point to lumina that are not seen by light microscopy. They contain microvilli and tripartite junctional complexes which the seminomas do not have (×11,050).

In summary, the characteristic findings of the embryonal carcinoma are tripartite junctional complexes and an attempt at the formation of extracellular or intracellular cytoplasmic lumina. There is also the absence of tubular structures and microvilli commonly seen in seminoma.

Reticulum Cell Sarcomas of Testis

SEM of these tumors under low power are quite similar to that seen in seminoma. There is a scant amount of stroma which is not absolutely characteristic for this type of tumor. When the cell surfaces are examined under high magnification, they are seen to have a very irregular ruffled surface. The surface morphology shows that they are not similar to the anaplastic seminomas or the undifferentiated embryonal carcinomas. TEM of these tumors reveals irregular clusters of cells surrounded by a very small, or else a large, amount of collagen and reticulum fibers that may surround not only clusters of these cells, but also individual cells (Fig. 6.12). It is very difficult to discern whether there are any cell connections similar to those seen in the seminoma or embryonal carcinoma. TEM of these tumor cells shows light and dark cell types with varying amounts of lysosomal material in their cytoplasm.

Briefly, the testicular tumors that are undifferentiated may be categorized by means of the combined use of SEM and TEM when they are not able to be distinguished from each other by LM. The pathology of these testicular tumors, therefore, can be clarified in a significant number of cases where LM cannot put them into the proper categories.

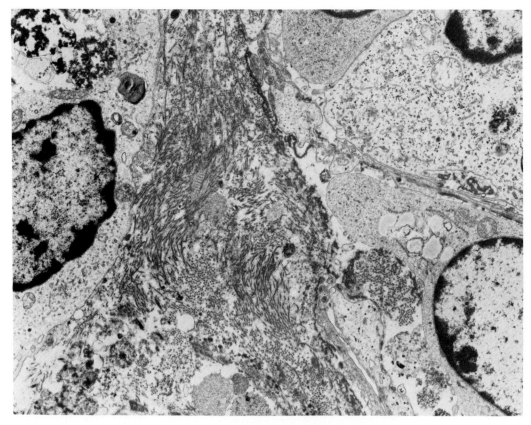

Figure 6.12. Transmission electronmicroscopy of reticulum cell sarcoma of the testis. Elastic fibers are interposed between malignant cells on the *left* and *right* of electron micrograph. There are no microvilli, tripartite junctional complexes, or cell processes. (×6,375).

CONCLUSION

We have attempted to provide a brief ultrastructural survey of the genitourinary system in terms of what is currently being investigated in several different laboratories throughout Europe and various other parts of the world. These basic ultrastructural studies will, in due time, serve as a baseline for more definitive treatment, whether it be chemotherapy, radiation, or perhaps effective hormonal therapy for various forms of urogenital disease.

In addition to clinical impressions, we can specifically observe what might be happening to normal as well as cancer cells with this type of methodology. Thus, with new instrumentation, which is now commercially available, we can have more finite quantitation as it relates to definitive therapies and, hopefully, eradicate some aspects of the various types of urogenital neoplasms.

REFERENCES

1. Tannenbaum, M. Renal tumors. In *Electron Microscopy in Human Medicine, Vol. 9: Urogenital System and Breast*, p. 166. Edited by J. V. Johannessen. McGraw-Hill, New York 1979.

2. Tannenbaum, M. Lower urinary tract. In *Electron Microscopy in Human Medicine, Vol 9: Urogenital System and Breast*, p. 193. Edited by J. V. Johannessen. McGraw-Hill, New York, 1979.

3. Tannenbaum, M. Male accessory organs: seminal vesicle, prostate, and testis. In *Electron Microscopy in Human Medicine, Vol 9: Urogenital System and Breast*, p. 227. Edited by J. V. Johannessen. McGraw-Hill, New York, 1979.

4. Evans, R. W. *Histologic Appearances of Tumors*, p. 663. Livingston Book Co., London, 1956.

5. Hanssen, O. E., and Herman, L. The presence of an axial structure in the microvillus of the mouse convoluted proximal tubular cell. *Lab. Invest. 11:*610, 1962.

6. Bennington, J. L., and Beckwith, J. B. Tumors of the kidney, renal pelvis and ureter. In *Atlas of Tumor Pathology, Series 2, Vol. 12.* Armed Forces Institute of Pathology, Washington, 1975.

7. Ericsson, J., Seljelid, R., and Orrenius, S. Comparative light and electron microscopic observations of the cytoplasmic matrix in renal carcinomas. *Virchows Arch. Pathol. Anat. 341:*204, 1966.

8. Oberling, C., Riviere, M., and Haguenau, F. Ultrastructure of the clear cells in renal carcinomas and its importance for the demonstration of their renal origin. *Nature 186:* 402, 1960.

9. Okada, K., Yokoyama, M., Tokue, A., and Takayasu, H. Ultrastructure of renal cell carcinoma. *Urol. Int. 36:*1, 1969.

10. Seljelid, R., and Ericsson, J. An electron microscopic study of mitochondria in renal clear cell carcinoma. *J. Micros. 4:*759, 1965.

11. Seljelid, R., and Ericsson, J. Electron microscopic observations on specializations of the cell surface in renal clear cell carcinoma. *Lab. Invest. 14:*435, 1965.

12. Lucké, B., and Schlumberger, H. G. Tumors of the kidney, renal pelvis and ureter. In *Atlas of Tumor Pathology*, Sec. VIII. Armed Forces Institute of Pathology, Washington, 1957.

13. Ericsson, J. Absorption and decomposition of homologous hemoglobin in renal proximal tubular cells. An experimental light and electron microscopic study. *Acta Pathol. Microbiol. Scand. 168:*Suppl. 1, 1964.

14. Miller, F. Hemoglobin absorption by the cells of proximal convoluted tubule in mouse kidney. *J. Biophys. Biochem. Cytol. 8:*689, 1960.

15. Rhodin, J. Electron microscopy of the kidney. In *Renal Disease*, p. 117. Blackwell Scientific Publications, Oxford, 1962.

16. Tannenbaum, M. Ultrastructural pathology of human renal cell tumors. In *Kidney Pathology Decennial 1966–1975,* p. 647. Edited by S. C. Sommers. Appleton-Century-Crofts, New York, 1975.

17. Mostofi, F. K. Pathology of malignant tumours of urinary bladder. In *The Biology and Clinical Management of Bladder Cancer*, p. 87. Edited by E. H. Cooper and R. E. Williams. Blackwell Scientific Publications, Oxford, 1975.

18. Firth, J. and Hicks, R. M. Interspecies variation in the fine structure. *J. Anat. 116:*31, 1973.

19. Koss, L. G. The asymmetric unit membranes of the epithelium of the urinary bladder of the rat. An electron microscopic study of a mechanism of epithelial maturation and function. *Lab. Invest. 21:*154, 1969.

20. Staehelin, L. A., Chlapowski, F. J., and Bonneville, M. A. Luminal plasma membrane of the urinary bladder. I. Three-dimensional reconstruction from freeze-etch images. *J. Cell Biol. 53:*73, 1972.

21. Walker, B. E. Electron microscopic observations on transitional epithelium of the mouse urinary bladder. *J. Ultrastruct. Res. 3:*345, 1960.

22. Franks, L. M. Etiology and epidemiology of human prostatic disorders. In *Urologic Pathology: The Prostate*, p. 23. Edited by M. Tannenbaum. Lea & Febiger, Philadelphia, 1977.

23. Murphy, G. P. Current status of therapy in prostatic cancer. In *Urologic Pathology: The Prostate*, p. 225. Edited by M. Tannenbaum. Lea & Febiger, Philadelphia, 1977.

24. Tannenbaum, M. Histopathology of the prostate gland. In *Urologic Pathology: The Prostate*, p. 303. Edited by M. Tannenbaum. Lea & Febiger, Philadelphia, 1977.

25. Brandes, D. Fine structure and cytochemistry of male sex accessory organs. In *Male Accessory Sex Organs: Structure and Function in Mammals*, p. 18. Edited by D. Brandes. Academic Press, New York, 1974.

26. Fisher, E. R., and Sieracki, J. C. Ultrastructure of human normal and neoplastic prostate. In *Pathology Annual 1970*, p. 1. Edited by S. Sommers. Appleton-Century-Crofts, New York, 1970.

27. Mao, P., Nakao, K., and Angrist, A. Human prostatic carcinoma: an electron microscope study. *Cancer Res. 26:*955 1966.

28. Gaeta, J. F., Bergen, J. E., and Gamarra, M. C. Scanning electron microscopic study of prostatic cancer. *Cancer Treat. Rept. 61:*227, 1977.

29. Heidger, P. M., Jr., Feuchter, F. A., and Hawtrey, C. E. Scanning and transmission electron microscopy of human prostatic adenocarcinoma. In *Male Reproductive System*, p. 185. Edited by R. D. Yates, and M. Gordon. Masson Publishing, New York, 1977.

30. Takayasu, H., and Yamaguchi, Y. An electron microscopic study of the prostatic cancer cell. *J. Urol. 87:*935, 1962.

31. Pierce, G. B., Jr.: Ultrastructure of human testicular tumors. *Cancer 19:*1963, 1966.

32. Rosai, J., Khodadoust, K., and Silber, I. Spermatocytic seminoma. II. Ultrastructural study. *Cancer 24:*103, 1969.

7

Experimental Cancer Models in Urology

Numerous experimental models for urological malignances have been described and characterized over the years. Several have provided fundamental new knowledge relevant to the biology and/or clinical management of their human counterpart. This chapter will review the animal models that have been well characterized. We will not include information on human tumor cell lines or heterotransplants. The organ sites will include kidney, bladder, prostate, and testis.

KIDNEY TUMOR MODELS

Renal adenomas are frequently discovered in large animals (horse, cow) but spontaneously occurring renal malignant tumors are rare in laboratory animals.[1, 2] Renal cell carcinomas have been described in a variety of animals including rat, mouse, hamster, frog, and fowl.[3, 4] A variety of chemical agents can induce renal neoplasms in rodents. β-Anthraquinoline, 4-fluoro-4-aminodiphenyl (4-F-4-BAA) and formic acid 2-[4-(5-nitro-2-furyl)-2-thiazolyl]hydrazine (FNT) have all produced carcinoma in rats.[2, 5–9] In addition, 30 to 40% of Sprague-Dawley rats receiving greater than 450 rads will develop renal cell or transitional cell carcinoma. A diet containing 0.1% lead acetate produces malignant renal tumors in more than 30% of rats.[7, 8] Transplantable, nonmetastasizing tumors occur after 46 weeks of a diet containing FNT in Sprague-Dawley rats. Three transplantable kidney tumors were produced in 4-F-4-BAA-fed Buffalo strain rats by Morris et al.[10] The better characterized models are listed in Table 7.1. Murphy and Hrushesky[11, 12] have characterized a spontaneous, transplantable, metastasizing renal cell carcinoma in BALB C/Cr mice. This well differentiated adenocarcinoma can be transplanted subcutaneously, intravenously, intramuscularly, and intraperitoneally. Intrarenal transplantation produces accelerated tumor growth and early

Table 7.1
Renal tumor models

Species	Induced	Sponta-neous	Trans-plantable	Comments
BALB C/Cr	No	Yes	Yes	Murphy and Hrushesky[11,12]; well differentiated adeno-carcinoma, hormone de-pendent, growth enhanced by testosterone; metas-tases: lung, liver
Wistar rats	DMN[a]	NO	Yes	Hard and Butler[26]; anaplas-tic, mesenchymal tumor 100% incidence after single dose; metastases: perito-neal cavity, lung, liver
Syrian golden hamster	Estrogen		Yes	Bloom et al.[19,22]; well differ-entiated transplanted tu-mors, not dependent on ex-ogeneous estrogens, hor-mone responsive; metas-tases rare
Leopard frog	Herpes virus			Lucke[15]; viral induced, wide range of histology, trans-missable; metastases: lung, liver, peritoneal cavity
Fürth-Wistar rat	No	Yes	Yes	Tomashefsky et al.[32]; neph-roblastoma, well character-ized, elevated erythropietin levels; metastasizes

[a] The abbreviation used is DMN, dimethylnitrosamine.

metastases. A tumor nodule is palpable within 21 days of transplantation and metastases to lung and liver are detectable by day 28. The animals survive for approximately 50 days. These intervals permit chemothera-peutic agent screening. Tumor growth is enhanced by testosterone and estrogens but not by progesterone.[13] Vinblastine and 1-(2-chlorethyl)-3-cyclohexyl-1 (CCNU) delay tumor growth and prolong survival. Clinical trials have been reported in humans with these agents.[11,13,14]

Lucke Adenocarcinoma

Baldwin Lucke at the University of Pennsylvania originally described a kidney tumor in the leopard frog (*Rana pipiens*) in 1934.[15] These tumors occur in almost all of the wild *Rana pipiens* population in north central and northeastern United States and are generally multicentric, bilateral and metastasize to lung, liver and other viscera.[16] Ultrastructure analysis suggests a proximal tubular cell origin and herpes virus has been impli-cated etiologically.[17] Frogs captured during the cold winter months con-tain Cowdry type A nuclear inclusions but these cannot be detected in tumors from animals gathered during the summer months. Interestingly, housing the latter frogs at 4°C will result in the appearance of these inclusions. Virus replication appears to be temperature dependent. Inoculation of cytoplasmic fractions from inclusion-bearing cells produce tumors in immature frogs.[18] Lucke herpes virus has been cultured *in vitro* and found to be oncogenic for frog embryos resulting in renal tumors in early adulthood. The Lucke tumor provides an opportunity to study the natural history of a prevalent, naturally occurring, virally induced neoplasm.

Syrian Golden Hamster Renal Cell Carcinoma

An estrogen-induced renal cell carcinoma in male Syrian golden hamsters was first described by Matthews et al. (in Bloom et al.[19]) at Stanford University in 1947. Subcutaneous implantation of a 20-mg estrogen pellet in hamsters 6 to 8 weeks of age induces a palpable renal tumor within 12 months in 80% of animals. The incidence can be increased to 100% if the pellet is renewed at 4 months. Neoplasms are often multiple and appear to rise from the proximal convoluted tubule. Distant metastases are extremely rare. Subcutaneous innoculation of tumor cells in syngeneic hamsters produces a 100% take and tumor growth does not require exogenous estrogen. Testosterone will inhibit tumor transplantation but has no effect on an established primary or a transplanted and growing renal tumor. Bilateral orchiectomy inhibits tumor growth. Provera was found to have an inhibitor affect on tumor transplants and cortisone produced marked growth inhibition directly proportional to dosage.[20] Combining cortisone and Provera results in almost complete suppression of growth.[20] Bloom[20] and Bloom et al.[21, 22] reported the response of this tumor to various hormonal agents and endocrine ablation. Bloom has extended his investigations to clinical trials. Administration of high doses of progesterone to patients with widespread renal adenocarcinoma claimed to produce a 55% subjective, but only 16% objective, response rate.[20] Men responded more frequently than women (40% *versus* 80%) and patients showing an objective response survived longer. Fluorouracil (5-FU), adriamycin, and actinomycin D have been tested and produce inhibition of tumor growth in tumor-bearing hamsters.[23-25]

Dimethylnitrosamine-Induced Renal Cell Carcinoma

Dimethylnitrosamine (DMN) is a nitro compound capable of producing mesenchymal tumors in rats. A single high dose of DMN produces renal lesions in virtually 100% of surviving rats.[26, 27] Histologically, the tumors resemble nephroblastoma, adenosarcoma, and hemangioendothelioma. This provides an ideal model to study chemical carcinogenesis in the kidney and the relevant biology of human neoplasia.

Wilms' Tumor Model

Nephroblastoma or Wilms' tumor constitutes 1% of tumors in laboratory animals.[28-30] The first transplantable Wilms' tumor was reported by Olcott in Sherman-Mendel rats.[31] Other transplantable tumors have been described since and the Fürth-Wistar model is the best characterized.[32-34] Originally described by Tomashefsky et al. in 1972,[30] it has been characterized by Murphy and associates.[35–38] Growth characteristics, metastatic spread, animal survival times, and response to various chemotherapeutic agents have been documented and this model expresses many of the characteristics found in the human counterpart.[39–42] Histologically identical to human Wilms' tumor, it metastasizes to the lung and contralateral kidney. Erythropoietin also has been detected as in the human counterpart.

BLADDER TUMOR MODELS

A number of potent carcinogens can produce bladder neoplasms in laboratory animals.[43–58] The more widely used agents at present include FANFT, BBN, BF, and MNU listed in Table 7.2. Few spontaneous bladder tumor cancer models are available.

Brown Norway Rat

The brown Norway rat has a high indicence of spontaneous urothelial tumors with 20% of males developing bladder and 6% ureteric neoplasms.[59] The proportion is reversed in females. Bladder tumors are multiple, papilliary, and exhibit a wide rate of grade and stage. These tumors are transplantable.

Table 7.2
Bladder Tumor Models

Carcinogen	Species	Histology	Transplantability	Metasases	Comments
FANFT[a]	Rat, Mouse, Hamster, Dog	Transitional cell	Rat, mouse; MBT-2 cell line	Yes None Demonstrated in dog	Greater than 90% incidence; very specific for bladder; multiple chemotherapeutic trails using induced and transplanted tumours (Soloway[64, 65])
DBN BBN	Rat, mouse, hamster, rabbit, guinea pig	Poorly differentiated transitional cell with squamous cell elements	Rat, mouse: FCB line: anaplastic, rapid growth, transplants readily NBT II: *in vitro* cell line, transplants to syngeneic rats	Rats, mice	DBN also produces high proportion of liver tumours (50% of animals) BBN very specific for bladder, 90% of animals, more potent by weight than FANFT
MNU	Rat	Poorly differentiated	Not attempted; transitional cell and squamous cell	No	Intravesical administration; rapid induction—20 weeks; tumors develop in 100% of animals
BF	Cow	Transitional and squamous cell	Not well documented	Squamous cell only	Bracken Fern (BF): popular foodstuff in some countries; carcinogen not known, milk from BF-fed cows carcinogenic for rats; rapid induction—12 weeks, 80% of animals

[a] The abbreviations used are: FANFT, *N*-[4-(5-nitro-2-furyl)-2-thiazolyl]formamide; DBN, dibutylnitrosamine; BBN, butyl-(4-hydroxybutyl)nitrosamine; MNU, *N*-methyl-*N*-nitrosourea; and BF, bracken fern.

FANFT

Rats, mice, hamsters, and dogs are susceptible to the highly specific carcinogenic action of FANFT on the urothelium.[60, 61] For example, 100% of Sprague-Dawley rats surviving more than 9 weeks develop bladder tumors when fed 0.188% by weight FANFT. The exact nature of the carcinogen produced after injection is not known but Croft and Bryan[57] suggest that the 5-nitro group on the furan ring of FANFT and related compounds plays a major role.

Bladder tumors induced by FANFT resemble their human counterpart grossly and histologically. FANFT-fed rats initially develop hyperplasia of the bladder mucosa with progression to sessile or papillary carcinoma. Hyperplasia produced by FANFT feeding for up to 6 weeks is reversible but after 8 weeks the changes are irreversible and result in carcinoma in all animals by 84 weeks. Urothelial changes are not restricted to the bladder and some animals develop carcinoma in the renal pelvis. The bladder tumors progress to muscle invasion and widespread metastases.[62]

A FANFT-induced, serially transplanted, poorly differentiated transitional cell tumor in C3H/He mice, has been characterized and designated MBT-2.[63] Subcutaneous transplantation of tumor cells produces a measureable tumor mass that can be used to evaluate response to chemotherapeutic agents. Cyclophosphamide produces inhibition of tumor growth in 100% of the animals if administered prior to the tumor becoming palpable. Hydroxyurea, CCNU and 5-FU alone are ineffective in slowing tumor growth rate.[64] Cyclophosphamide, dactinomycin, cis-platinum, and Adriamycin (doxorubicin) alone or in combination were all effective in reducing the mean bladder weight in animals who had received 10 months of FANFT. Implantation of transplantable cells directly on the bladder surface has provided evaluation of intravesical antineoplastic agents thio-TEPA and Epodyl.[65] This model has provided a foundation for several clinically used chemotherapeutic protocols.

BBN, DBM

The N-nitrosamines comprise a major class of chemical carcinogens. First characterized by Magee and Barnes,[66] Druckrey et al.[66a] reported the activity of 65 N-nitro compounds in the BD strain of rat.[66–68] Two compounds, dibutylnitrosamine (DBN) and its hydroxylated derivative, butyl-(4-hydroxybutyl)nitrosamine(BBN) were found to be highly potent and specific bladder carcinogens. DBN, when added to the drinking water of C57BL6 mice produces tumor of the liver, stomach and esophagus, as well as of the bladder.[69] Subcutaneous injection of DBN to IF × C57 mice produced only liver and bladder tumors; this difference probably relates to the route of administration. DBN is metabolized in the liver, possibly to BBN, and eventually excreted into the urine.[70, 71] BBN is a potent carcinogen and has been found to produce only bladder carcinoma in rats, mice, hamsters, guinea pigs, and rabbits.[70, 72] BBN-induced tumors are multifocal, poorly differentiated, transitional cell carcinomas, with areas of squamous metaplasia, that readily metastasize to peritoneal lymph nodes.[70] Rats fed BBN develop hyperplastic bladder mucosal changes at 8 weeks which progress to papillomas by 16 weeks. Frank carcinomas are generally not evident until 20 weeks, with 100% of animals developing tumors after this time.[72] The latent period of bladder tumor induction is shorter in male than females. This sex difference can be abolished by castrating males or by treating females with testosterone.[70] BBN tumors in Wistar rats can be cultured *in vitro*. A cell line, designated NBT II, can be grown *in vitro* and then transplanted into syngeneic rats with stable histology. Flaks and Flaks[73] have characterized a transplantable DBN-induced anaplastic transitional cell carcinoma in IF × C57 F1 hybrid mice, designated FCB I. This was originally a well differentiated transitional cell carcinoma, but with passage now appears anaplastic but stable. IF or C57 black mice develop rapid subcutaneous tumor growth after transplantation and are dead at 3 weeks. The microscopic development of DBN rabbit bladder tumors has been documented by Cohen *et al.*[74] endoscopically. This animal model conveniently allows for direct bladder visualization.

MNU

The *N*-nitrosamide, *N*-methyl-*N*-nitrosurea (MNU) produces tumors in a wide variety of organs, except bladder, if given orally or intravenously.[75] Hicks and Wakefield[75] induced transitional bladder carcinoma in Wistar rats by intravesical installation. Administration of 6 mg in divided doses over 6 weeks produce malignant tumors in all animals surviving for more than 20 weeks. They are histologically similar to the BBN-induced tumors. Both squamous cell and transitional cell carcinomas are found. Metastases have not been observed and the tumor has not been transplanted. This system provides a simple and rapid method of inducing bladder cancer and does not appear to depend on host activation for its carcinogenic effect.

Braken Fern

Braken fern (*Pteris aquilina*) is a human food delicacy and salad green consumed in Japan, New Zealand, and North America. It is known to produce a high incidence of bladder tumors in cows, and milk from these cows is carcinogenic to rats resulting in intestinal and bladder neoplasms.[76-81] A majority (80%) of albino rats fed braken fern will develop intestinal and bladder neoplasms.[73] Both transitional cell and adenocarcinomas are observed, but metastases have occurred only in rats with squamous cell carcinomas. Pamukca[82] *et al.* examined tumor morphology and found that epithelial hyperplasia was present in all test animals after 3 weeks, with tumor present as early as 12 weeks. Transitional cell carcinomas were found to originate from the hyperplastic epithelium and squamous cell carcinomas from metaplastic squamous epithelium. The majority of tumors were papillary and infiltrating, and carcinoma *in situ* was not observed before the appearance of infiltrating tumors.

PROSTATE TUMORS

The ideal properties of an animal model for prostate cancer include: (1) spontaneous appearance in an aged animal, (2) presence and secretion of acid phosphatase, (3) metastasis to the lymph nodes and bone, and (4) hormonal sensitivity to androgens for maximal growth, and to estrogens or castration for inhibition, with a subsequent relapse to a hormonal-insensitive state. Any model should represent the wide range and variability encountered in human prostate tumors.[83-90]

Spontaneous prostatic carcinoma is rare in laboratory animals. In 1940, Engle and Stout[91] noted the appearance of a spontaneous prostatic adenocarcinoma without metastases in an old Rhesus monkey. This was the first primary prostatic malignancy reported in primates. A number of spontaneous neoplasms in a variety of laboratory animal species have been described since, but few are suitable as models for human disease (Tables 7.3 and 7.4). In 1963, Dunning[92a] described a spontaneous prostatic adenocarcinoma, R3327, in a Copenhagen rat that was transplantable and produced acid phosphatase. Pollard reported the cell lines PA I, PA II and PA III in an aged germ free Wistar rat.[106]

Dunning Prostate Model

First described by Dr. W. F. Dunning[92a] of the University of Florida in 1963 the original tumor arose spontaneously in the prostate of a male

Table 7.3
Prostatic Tumors in Animals

Species	Investigators	Tumor	References
SPONTANEOUS			
Rat	W. F. Dunning, 1963	Adeno, Copenhagen rat designation R3327 (H, HI, AT)	93–104, 107
	M. Pollard 1973	Adeno, aged Germ Free Wistar rat, designation PA, II, III	109–112, 115, 116
	S. A. Shain, B. McCullough, A. Seagaloff, 1975	Adeno, aged AXC rat	89
Hamster	J. G. Fortner, J. W. Faunkhauser, M. R. Cullen, 1963	Adeno, Syrian golden hamster	4
Mastomys	K. C. Snell, H. L. Stewart, 1965; J. Holland, 1970	Adeno, aged female African rodents	86, 90
Monkey	E. T. Engle, A. P. Stout, 1940	Aged *Macaca mulatta*	91
Dog	I. Leav, G. V. Ling, 1969	Aged mongrels	87
INDUCED			
Rat	R. Noble, 1977	Nb rats, tetosterone, and estrone induced.	113, 114
	B. Fingerhut, R. O. Veenema, 1977	Fischer/Fürth rats (also mice and hamsters); castrated animal administered DMBA[a]	85
	W. F. Dunning, M. R. Curtis, A. Seagaloff, 1963	Fischer rats, intraprostatic, MCA induced	92

[a] The abbreviations used are: DMBA, 7,12-dimethylbenz(a)anthracene; and MCA, methylcholanthrene

Table 7.4
Prostatic Tumor Models

Model	Species	Origin Designation	Metastases	Other Characteristics
Dunning	Copenhagen	Spontaneous, rat	Lung, liver, R3327, other viscera, no bone, 30% metastases	Multiple sublines, variety of histology, androgen-dependent, autonomous lines; slow growing (doubling time 20 days); Transplantable, responds to hormonal manipulation and various chemotherapeutic agents; produces acid phophatase; has hormonal receptors.
Pollard (Wistar)	Lobund	Spontaneous, cell lines PA I, PA II, PA III	Lymph nodes, lung, other viscera, no bone, very predictable, 100% metastases	Homogeneous population, three separate lines, hormone dependent, fast growing, transplantable, good model to examine mechanisms of metastases
Noble rat	Nb (Noble)	Hormone induced	Lymph nodes, lung, liver, other, no bone, 15–60% metastases	Variety of tumor types; hormone dependent, transplants to nude mice; various chemotherapeutic agents tested; fast growing

Copenhagen rat. This tumor, designated R3327, has been preserved by serial subcutaneous transplantation to syngeneic animals or Copenhagen-Fisher F1 hybrids.[93] Histologically, this neoplasm is a well differentiated adenocarcinoma almost identical to its human counterpart. Subsequent investigators have found this tumor to be hormonally responsive and it metabolizes testosterone *via* the 5-α reductase system.[94, 95] Subcutaneous or intraprostatic transplantation produces good tumor growth in normal males but poor growth in females or castrated males.[96, 97] Intraprostatic lesions exhibit a pattern of growth similar to that observed in humans. Initially intracapsular, the tumor spreads outside the capsule, to lymph nodes and metastasizes to lung, liver, and peritoneal cavity. The only site where metastases have not been demonstrated is bone, unlike the human tumor.[98] Numerous sublines have been cloned, exhibiting a wide range of hormonal sensitivity and growth rate.[97, 99] It is important that investigators monitor the histologic pattern and hormonal sensitivity of the Dunning tumors to ensure the degree of homogeneity within each subline.[100] It is this apparent heterogeneity that has attracted criticism regarding the usefulness of this system as a predictive tumor model, although, human tumors may be similar.

The first subline R3327A is an androgen-insensitive squamous cell carcinoma described by Voigt *et al.*[94, 95] Growing equally well in male and female rats, this subline has an accelerated growth rate when compared to the parent tumor and exhibits almost no 5-α reduction of testosterone. Issacs *et al.*[96] has characterized 3 sublines: R3327H, a well differentiated hormone-sensitive tumor; R3327I, a similar, slow growing hormone insensitive line; and, R3327AT, an anaplastic hormone-insensitive line similar to R3327A. All tumors have been well characterized with respect to morphology, histochemistry, growth properties, and therapeutic response.[88, 93, 99, 101]

Scott et al.[88] have examined in detail the growth characteristics and hormonal requirements of the Dunning tumors. To parallel a clinical situation encountered in advanced human prostatic cancer, R3327H was grown in intact male rats for 20 days before castration or diethylstilbestrol (DES) therapy. Seventy-two percent of the animals responded with an average 37% decrease in tumor volume. After the initial response, the tumor relapsed and was found to have a growth rate similar to the original transplant. It is unknown whether this was due to the presence of hormone-insensitive cells in the original cell population or a new clone of tumor cells.

Markland et al.[93] have demonstrated both androgen and estrogen receptors in the Dunning tumors. Correlating well with the hormonal responsiveness of the particular subline, high levels of receptors are present in R3327H cells and virtually none in the R3327AT subline. Serum acid phosphatase levels are elevated in rats bearing long-term subcutaneous R3327HI implants. Consistently elevated acid phosphatase has not been demonstrated after intraprostatic transplantation nor in rats bearing R3327A tumors. Subcutaneous transplants produce metastases to retroperitoneal lymph nodes, lung, and peritoneal cavity in 5 to 10% of animals.[101] This low incidence can be increased by intraprostatic transplantation.[97] Block et al.[104] have evaluated various chemotherapeutic regimes in the Dunning tumor model and the various immunologic aspects of prostatic cancer, particularly in the field of cryosurgery, have been well documented by Lubaroff et al.,[97] Lande et al.[103] and Block et al.[104]

Pollard Tumors

A spontaneous, transplantable, metastasizing, prostatic adenocarcinoma in germ free (GF) Wistar rats was first described by Pollard in 1973.[106] Spontaneous prostatic carcinoma in Wistar rats were thought to be relatively rare prior to this time, with only one previous report in the literature.[92a] Rats examined in earlier series were relatively young at the time of autopsy, usually less than 24 months of age. Pollard's rats were older, ranging from 32 to 40 months of age which may account for the higher incidence of carcinoma.[106] Further characterization of the Pollard tumors have yielded three cell lines (PA I, PA II, PA III). Each of these tumors originated from different GF rats and have been transplanted, without change, through several generations of Lobund-Wistar rats.

Prostatic tumors PA I and PA III are both scirrhous adenocarcinoma. Within 10 days of subcutaneous implantation from either line in the hind footpad, metastatic lesions appear in the ipsilateral nodes, followed by discreet lung secondaries within 3 weeks. Bone, heart, and kidney lesions have been found in animals surviving more than 60 days. Both tumors can be propagated in vitro and successfully transplanted.[108] PA II differs histologically, although still an adenocarcinoma, growing to a greater size at the site of implantation than PA I and PA III, which more commonly ulcerate through the skin. Metastatic spread of PA II tumors is through ipsilateral nodes with eventual involvement of lung, heart, and kidneys. Hematogenous spread has been documented with detectable tumor cells in the rat blood growing PA II for a period greater than 14 days.[109] PA II cells are activated by estrogens while PA I and PA III cells are not modified by DES administration. The pattern of mestastases is predictable on all tumors and, to some extent, does not depend on the site of initial transplantation. These tumors provide a methodology to examine the therapeutic effects of hormonal and chemotherapeutic agents and the various factors which regulate the occurrence of metastases.[110] Pollard has reported the effect of several agents on the metastatic spread of the PA models.[111, 112]

Noble Prostate Model

The Noble rat prostatic adenocarcinoma provides a well characterized, hormonally induced, family of tumors. First described by Robert L. Noble[113, 114] at the University of British Columbia, this model has been further characterized by Drago and associates.[115-118] The Nb rat is an inbred strain with a low incidence of spontaneous prostatic adenocarcinoma (0.45%). Suitable hormonal treatment increases this to 20%. After subcutaneous testosterone implants, tumors appear in 59 to 64 weeks. These neoplasms transplant to syngeneic rats and athymic mice (nude). Androgen-dependent, estrogen-dependent, and autonomous cell lines have been described. Growing equally well in male or female rats, the autonomous tumor is composed of large, solid sheets of malignant cells with few glandular structures. Lung and liver metastases can be demonstrated in 50 to 60% of rats bearing this tumor. Well defined trabeculae of malignant cells with glandular formation characterize the hormonally dependent tumors. Metastases occur in 15 to 20% of tumor-bearing rats. Unlike the Dunning tumors, Noble tumors are homogeneous and none of their sublines have been cloned. Acid phosphatase is produced by all tumors, although serum levels are generally not elevated. Bone metastases have not been demonstrated.

Drago and associates have further characterized the androgen-dependent and autonomous tumors in athymic (nude) mice.[119, 120] Heterotransplants maintain their hormonal dependence or autonomy. Chemotherapeutic agents employed with some success in human prostate cancer produce similar response in both Nb rats and nude mice.[115] A combination of these two systems provides an excellent opportunity to evaluate tumor response in both normal and immunosuppressed animals.

Several induced tumors have been described in castrated rats, mice, and hamsters with the intravenous administration of 7,12-dimethylbenz(a)anthracene (DMBA) by Fingerhut and Veenema.[85] Dunning et al.[92] implanted methylcholanthrene (MCA) crystals in the prostate of Fischer rats and induced squamous cell carcinomas that metastasized to bone.

GERMINAL TESTICULAR TUMOR MODELS

Nonmurine Models

Spontaneous, clinically benign seminomas occur frequently in dogs and have been reported in monkeys, birds, fish, and jungle cats.[121] Seminomas have been induced in albino rats by the injection of zinc salts, but this model has not been reproduced.[122] Spontaneous nonseminomatous tumors are extremely rare but they have been induced in fowl and Syrian hamsters by intratesticular injection of metal salts.[121-123] None of these models have been extensively studied to date.

Murine Models

In 1954, Stevens and Little[124] found a spontaneous testicular teratoma in strain 129 mice that has spawned the most useful model system for testicular tumors. The tumor incidence is subject to genetic and environmental influences.[125] With the introduction of a mutant gene, a subline with a spontaneous incidence of 30% has been developed. These congenital tumors arise within the seminiferous tubule and rupture into the interstitium of the testis with progressive growth. Histologically, the initial tumor cells are embryonal carcinoma (EC), however, complete differentiation to somatic tissues almost always occurs with spontaneous cessation of growth. Very rarely, EC cells persist and transplantable lines have been developed which can be converted in the ascitic fluid to yolk sac carcinoma and embryoid bodies. Manipulation by transplantation of fetal genital ridges into adult testes produces teratocarcinoma in 80% of the male grafts. Interestingly, the transplantation site is important for successful growth. Genital ridges from a subline with few germ cells results in a much lower incidence of tumor, supporting the concept that the germ cell is the cell of origin.

A second technique to induce tumor is embryo transplantation.[126] Most embryos harvested prior to implantation can be implanted into extrauterine sites with growth as teratocarcinoma. Such embryo-derived tumors continue to grow only if they contain EC cells which are similar to the genital ridge grafts and the spontaneously occurring murine tumors in strain 129 mice. These observations are notable as, clinically, the presence of mature teratoma results in cessation of tumor growth unless there are one or more persistent clones of EC cells. Furthermore, one of the original theories of the origin of teratomas proposed by Askanzy (in Jewett[127]) was that a misplaced embryo had escaped control and grew as a tumor. The growth patterns of the embryo transplants appear to be dependent on escaped embryo development rather than genetics, although environmental factors may be important.

The rare spontaneous tumor and the induced tumors (by genital ridge grafting or embryo transplantation) have provided clonable cell lines that have contained undifferentiated EC cells. Although the principal application has been as a model system for normal differentiation, interesting data have been collected that may be pertinent to human germinal testicular tumors. EC cells have been characterized in several ways.

MORPHOLOGY AND DIFFERENTIATION

As in human tumors, the murine EC cells are small, undifferentiated, epithelioid cells which grow in monolayers in tissue culture. The undifferentiated EC cell appears to be the stem cell of the differentiated somatic tissues in teratocarcinomas.[128] Transplantation of single murine EC cells intraperitoneally produce tumors with a variety of somatic cell types. The presence of EC cells is necessary to continue tumor growth. Pierce and Wallace[129] suggested, therefore, that the optimum therapy would be induction of differentiation, and attempts have been made with a number of substances including retinoids and substituted dioxins.[130, 131] It is well documented that retinoids strongly influence the pattern of epithelial cell differentiation. Vitamin A (retinoic acid) and related compounds greatly increase the probability of differentiation of EC cells *in vitro*.[132] The effect is irreversible and dependent on exposure time. Retinoic acid increases the survival time of mice following a challenge by a threshold number of tumorigenic F9 cells. The differentiation of F9 cells was suggested by an analysis of SSEA-1 and H2 antigen expression.

Independent clones of cultured lines and transplantable tumors vary with respect to ability for differentiation. Multipotential lines have established with both 129/SV and C3H mice. The nullipotential cell line F9 may be induced to differentiation to parietal endoderm. The genetic and environmental influence is important in EC cell differentiation and is poorly understood.

CHROMOSOMES

Most murine EC cells are diploid or near diploid although the incidence of chromosome abnormality may increase with the loss of ability to differentiate. Spontaneous tumors and those induced by gential ridge grafting are male by karyotype, suggesting that they arise premiosis. Embryo transplant tumors are both male and female suggesting that embryonic cells produced by fertilization are still capable of producing a tumor.

BIOCHEMISTRY

The tumor marker α-fetoprotein (AFP) was first detected in mice with teratocarcinoma.[133] Undifferentiated murine EC cells do not produce AFP but *in vitro* differentiation along endodermal lines results in AFP synthesis.[134] Specific antiAFP has been used for active and passive immunization with the suggestion that tumor growth may be inhibited after passive administration.[135] Immunologically, human AFP is slightly different from the murine counterpart. There are several well characterized enzyme activities which change upon transition of EC cells to a differentiation pathway. EC cells have high levels of alkaline phosphatase and characteristic isoenzyme patterns of lactate dehydrogenase, and creatine kinase. EC cells do not produce plasminogen activator or AFP and do not secrete fibronectin.[136]

ANTIGENIC MARKERS

The production of monoclonal antibodies to cell surface and organelle antigenic markers by hybridomas is an exciting new field.[137] A well characterized panel of such monoclonal antibodies may be used to define the molecular state of marker expression: a series of points in a particular differentiation pathway. EC cells share determinants with early embryonal cells which are not expressed with somatic differentiation. The major histocompatibility complex cell surface antigens are absent on EC cells. An antigen SSEA-1 detected by monoclonal antibody is a glycolipid and it is present in several multipotent EC cell lines as well as preimplantation embryo.[138]

INTERACTION OF EC CELLS WITH VIRUS

EC cells differ from somatic cells by their ability to support the growth and replication of murine virus.[139] They may have different patterns of RNA synthesis than normally differentiated cells. RNA markers may be characterized to better understand the mechanism by which normal cells control integrated viral genes and their own genetic material during differentiation.

ENVIRONMENTAL INFLUENCE OF BLASTOCYST ON DEVELOPMENT OF EC CELLS

In 1974, Brinster[140] reported the formation of chimeric mice from blastocysts that were injected with one EC cell. The EC cell may participate in normal development when directed by the field of the blastocyst. To date, four independent *in vitro* EC cell lines and three *in vivo* transplantable tumors may participate in normal development with a low frequency of chimerism.[141] Histologic examination of tumors from chimeric mice show that EC cells are not always present, so that the blastocyst may not always control EC cell growth. It is not clear whether these tumors develop from injected cells which remain quiescent or develop *de novo* from their differentiation progeny. However, the growth of EC cells in blastocysts provides a dramatic demonstration of the control of a malignant phenotype.

REFERENCES

1. Murphy, G. P., Johnston, G. S., Melby, E. C. Comparative aspects of experimentally induced and spontaneously observed renal tumors. *J. Urol.* 97:965, 1967.
2. Grabstald, H. Experimental aspects of renal tumors. *J. Surg. Oncol.* 29:509, 1973.
3. Epstein, S. M., Bartus, B., Farber, E. Renal epithelial neoplasms induced in male Wistar rats by oral aflatoxin B. *Cancer Res.* 29:1045, 1969.
4. Fortner, J. G., Funkhauser, J. W., Cullen, M. R. Spontaneous adenocarcinoma in the Syrian hamster. *Natl. Cancer Inst. Monogr.* 12:371, 1963.
5. Reuber, M. D. A model for carcinoma of the kidney in buffalo strain rats ingesting *N*-4-(4′-fluorobiphenyl) acetamide, *Gan* 65:389, 1974.
6. Heatfield, B. M., Hintor, D. E., Trump, B. F. Adenocarcinoma of the kidney. II. Enzyme histochemistry of renal adenocarcinoma induced in rats by *N*-(4-fluoro-4-biphenylyl) acitamide. *JNCI.* 57:795, 1976.

7. Van Esch, G. J., Van Genderen, H., Vink, H. H. The induction of renal tumors by feeding of basic lead acetate to rats. *Br. J. Cancer 17:*289, 1963.

8. Boyland, E., Dukes, C. E., Grover, P. L., Mitchley, B. C. V. The induction of renal tumors by feeding lead acetate to rats. *Br. J. Cancer 16:*283, 1962.

9. Dees, J. H., Reuber, M. D., Trump, B. F. Adenocarcinoma of the kidney. I. Ultrastructure of renal adenocarcinomas induced in rats by *N*-(4-fluoro-4-biphenyl) acetamide. *JNCI. 57:*779, 1976.

10. Morris, H. P., Wagner, B. D., Meranze, D. R. Transplantable adenocarcinomas of the rat kidney possessing different growth rates. *Cancer Res. 30:*1362, 1970.

11. Murphy, G. P., Hrushesky, W. J. A murine renal cell carcinoma. *JNCI. 56:*1019, 1973.

12. Hrushesky, W. J., Murphy, G. P. Investigation of a new renal tumor model. *J. Surg. Res. 15:*327, 1973.

13. Hrushesky, W. J., Murphy, G. P. Evaluation of chemotherapeutic agents in a new murine renal carcinoma model. *JNCI. 52:*122, 1974.

14. Murphy, G. P., Williams, P. D. Testing of chemotherapeutic agents in murine renal cell adenocarcinoma. *Res. Commun. Chem. Pathol. Pharmacol. 9:*265, 1974.

15. Lucke, B. A neoplastic disease of the kidney of the frog *Rana pipiens. Am. J. Cancer 20:*352, 1934.

16. Rafferty, K. A. Kidney tumors of the leopard frog: a review. *Cancer Res. 24:*169, 1964.

17. Bloom, H. J. G., Hendry, W. F. Influence of cytotoxic drugs and hormones. In *Scientific Foundations of Urology*, Vol. II, p. 272, edited by D. I. Williams and G. D. Chisholm, Year Book Publishers, Chicago, 1976.

18. Morek, D. M. An organ culture study of frog renal tumor and its effects on normal frog kidney *in vitro. Oncology 28:*536, 1973.

19. Bloom, H. J. G., Dukes, C. E., Mitchley, B. C. V. Hormone dependent tumors of the kidney I. *Br. J. Cancer 17:*611, 1963.

20. Bloom, H. J. G. Medrox progesterone in treatment of metastatic renal cancer. *Br. J. Cancer 25:*250, 1965.

21. Bloom, H. J. G., Roe, F. J. C., Mitchley, B. C. R. Sex hormones and renal neoplasia. *Cancer 29:*2118, 1967.

22. Bloom, H. J. G., Baker, W. H., Dukes, C. E., Mitchley, B. C. V. Hormone dependent tumors of the kidney II. *Br. J. Cancer 17:*646, 1963.

23. Dekernion, J. B., Resnick, M. L., Persky, L. The response of the stilbesterol-induced renal tumor to chemotherapeutic agents. *J. Surg. Oncol. 5:*53, 1973.

24. Soloway, M. S., Myers, G. H. The effect of hormonal therapy on a transplantable renal cortical adenocarcinoma in syngeneic mice. *J. Urol. 109:*356, 1973.

25. Williams, P. D., Burdick, J., Murphy, G. P. Evaluation of hexamethylmelamine in a murine renal cell carcinoma model. *Res. Commun. Chem. Pathol. Pharmacol. 8:*399, 1978.

26. Hard, G. C., Butler, W. H. Ultrastructure study of the development of interstitial lesions leading to mesenchymal neoplasia induced in the rat renal cortex by DMN. *Cancer Res. 31:*337, 1971.

27. Murphy, G. P., Mirand, E. A., Johnston, G. S., Schmidt, J. D., Scott, W. W. DMN-induced renal cell carcinoma. *Invest. Urol. 4:*39, 1966.

28. Saroff, J., Chu, T. M., Gaeta, J. F., Williams, P., Murphy, G. P. Characterization of a Wilms' tumor model. *Invest. Urol. 12:*320, 1975.

29. (Deleted in proof)

30. Tomashefsky, P., Lattimer, J. K., Priestly, J., Fürth, J., Vakili, B. F., Tannenbaum, M. An experimental Wilms' tumor suitable for therapeutic and biologic studies: II The inhibition of renal compensatory hypertrophy by a transplantable tumor. *Invest. Urol. 11:*141, 1973.

31. Olcott, C. T. A transplantable nephroblastoma (Wilms' tumor) and other spontaneous tumors in a colony of rats. *Cancer Res. 10:*625, 1950.

32. Tomashefsky, P., Fürth, J., Lattimer, J. K., Tannenbaum, M., Priestly, J. The Fürth-Columbia rat Wilms' tumor. *J. Urol. 107:*348, 1972.

33. Babcock, U. L., Southam, C. M. Transplantable renal tumors of the rat. *Cancer Res. 21:*130, 1961.

34. Jasmin, G., Reopelle, J. C. Nephroblastomas induced in ovarectomized rats by dimethylbenzanthracene. *Cancer Res. 30:*321, 1970.

35. Murphy, G. P., Williams, P. D., Mirand, E. A. Erythropoietin levels in Wistar-Fürth Wilms' tumor rats. *J. Surg. Oncology 8:*131, 1976.
36. Murphy, G. P., Williams, P. D. Beneficial effects of adriamycin on Wistar-Fürth Wilms' tumor. *Urology 5:*741, 1975.
37. Murphy, G. P., Williams, P. D. The effects of chemotherapy on the Wistar-Fürth Wilms' tumor. *J. Med. 6:*401, 1975.
38. Murphy, G. P., Williams, P. D., Klein, R. The growth characteristics of the metastatic Wistar-Fürth Wilms' tumor model. *Res. Commun. Chem. Pathol. Pharmacol. 12:*397, 1975.
39. Mount, B. M., Themo, W. L., Husk, M. A re-examination of the renal blastema graft model for Wilms' tumor production. *J. Urol. 111:*738, 1974.
40. Murphy, G. P., Mirand, E. A., Staubetz, W. J. The value of erythropoietin assay in the follow-up of Wilms' tumor patients. *Oncology 33:*154, 1976.
41. Wajsman, Z., Williams, P. D., Murphy, G. P. The value of levamisol in a Wilms' tumor animal model. *Oncology 35:*212, 1978.
42. West, C. R., Wajsman, Z., Williams, P., Murphy, G. P. A study of the effect of environmental CO_2 on experimental Wilms' tumor. *J. Med. 9:*91, 1978.
43. Foulds, L. The induction of tumors in mice of the R3 strain by 2-acetylamenofluorene.
44. Koss, L. G., Lavin, P. Studies of experimental bladder carcinoma in Fischer 344 rats. I. Induction of tumors with a diet low in vitamin B6 containing *N*-2-fluoramglacetamide. *JNCI. 46:*585, 1971.
45. Lavin, P., Koss, L. G. Studies of experimental bladder carcinoma in Fischer 344 female rats. II Characteristics of three cells lines derived from induced urinary bladder carcinoma. *JNCI. 46:*497, 1971.
46. Melicow, M. M., Uson, A. C., Price, D. T. Bladder tumor induction in rats fed 2-acetamedofluorene (2-AAF) and a pyridoxine-deficient diet. *J. Urol. 91:*520, 1969.
47. Allen, M. J., Boyland, E., Dukes, C. E., Horning, E., Watson, J. G. Cancer of the urinary bladder induced in mice with metabolites of aromatic amines and tryptophan. *Br. J. Cancer 11:*212, 1957.
48. Bryan, G. T., Brown, R. R., Price, J. M. Mouse bladder carcinogenicity of certain tryptophan metabolites and other aromatic nitrogen compounds suspended in cholesterol. *Cancer Res. 24:*596, 1964.
49. Cohen, M. S., Price, J. M., Bryan, G. T. Pathogenesis, histology and transplantability of urinary bladder carcinoma induced in albino rats by oral administration of *N*[4-(5-nitro-2-furyl)-2-thiazole]formamide. *Cancer Res. 29:*2219, 1969.
50. Clayson, D. B., Bonser, G. M. The induction of tumors of the mouse bladder epithelium by 4-ethimylsulphonynapathalene l-sulphonamide. *Br. J. Cancer 10:*531, 1956.
51. Stula, E. F., Barnes, J. R., Sherman, H., Reinhardt, C. F., Zapp, J. A. Urinary bladder tumors in dogs from 4,4-methylene-BCS (2-choranilene) MOCA. *J. Environ. Pathol. Toxicol. 1:*31, 1977.
52. Taranger, L. A., Chapman, W. H., Hellstrom, I., Hellstrom, K. E. Immunologic studies on urinary bladder tumors of rats and mice. *Science 176:*1337, 1976.
53. Tiltman, A. J., Friedell, G. H. The histogenesis of experimental bladder cancer. *Invest. Urol. 9:*218, 1971.
54. Walpole, A. L., Williams, M. H. C., Roberts, D. C. Tumors of the urinary bladder in dogs after ingestion of 4-adminodephenyl. *Br. J. Ind. Med. 11:*105, 1954.
55. Wahlstrom, T., Chapman, W. H., Hellstrom, K. E. Long term transplantability and morphological stability of three experimentally induced urinary bladder carcinomas in rats. *Cancer Res. 36:*4652, 1976.
56. Williams, P. D., Murphy, G. P. Experimental bladder tumor induction, propagation and therapy. *Urology 8:*36, 1976.
57. Croft, W. A., Bryan, G. T. Production of urinary bladder carcinomas in male hamsters by *N*-[4-(5-nitro-2-furyl)-2-thiazolyl]formamide, *N*-[4-(5-nitro-2-furyl)-2-thiazolyl] acetamide or formic acid 2-[4-(5-nitro-2-furyl)-2-thiazolyl]hydrazide. *JNCI. 51:*941, 1973.
58. Bryan, G. T. The pathogenesis of experimental bladder cancer. *Cancer Res. 37:*2813, 1977.
59. Boorman, G. A., Burek, J. D., Hollander, C. F. Carcinoma of the ureter and urinary bladder. *Am. J. Pathol. 88:*25, 1977.

60. Ertürk, E., Price, J. M., Morris, J. E., Cohen, S., Leith, R. S., Von Esch, A., Crovetti, A. J. The production of carcinoma of the urinary bladder in rats by feeding *N*-[4-(5-nitro-2-furyl)-2-thiazolyl]formamide.*Cancer Res. 27:*1998, 1967.

61. Erturk, E., Cohen, S. M., Bryan, G. T. Urinary bladder carcinogenicity of *N*-[4-(5-nitro-2-furyl)-2-thiazolyl]formamidein female Swiss mice. *Cancer Res. 30:*1309, 1970.

62. Erturk, E., Cohen, S. M., Price, I. M., Bryan, G. T. Pathogenesis, histology and transplantability of urinary bladder carcinomas induced in albino rats by oral administration of *N*-[4-(5-nitro-2-furyl)-2-thiazolyl]formamide. *Cancer Res. 29:*2219, 1969.

63. Soloway, M. S., Dekernoin, J. B., Rose, D., Persky, L. Effect of chemotherapeutic agents on bladder cancer: a new animal model. *Surg. Forum 24:*1973.

64. Soloway, M. S. Single and combination chemotherapy for primary murine bladder cancer. *Cancer 36:*333, 1975.

65. Soloway, M. S. Intravesical and systemic chemotherapy of murine bladder cancer. *Cancer Res. 37:*2918, 1977.

66. Magee, P. N., Barnes, J. M. The production of malignant primary hepatic tumors in the rat by feeding dimethylnitrosamine. *Br. J. Cancer 10:*114, 1956.

66a.Druckrey, H., Pressman, R., Ivanovic, S., Schmidt, C. H., Mennel, H. D., Stahl, K. W. Selektive Erzeugung von Blasenkrebs an Ratten durch Dibutyl und *N*-butyl-*N* butanol (4)-nitrosamine. *Z. Krebsforsch 66:*280, 1964.

67. Oyasu, R., Twasaki, T., Matsumoto, M., Hirao, Y., Tabuchi,Y. Induction of tumors in heterotrophic bladder by topical application of *N*-methyl-*N*-nitrosurea and *N*-butyl-*N*-(3-carboxypropyl)-nitrosamine.*Cancer Res. 38:*3019.

68. Toyoshima, K., Nobuyuki, I., Hiasa, Y., Kamamuto, Y., Makiura, S. Tissue culture of urinary bladder tumor induced in a rat by *N*-butyl-*N*(4-hydroxybutyl)-nitrosamine. Establishment of cell line tara bladder tumor II. *JNCI. 47:*979, 1971.

69. Bertram, J. S., Craig, A. W. Induction of bladder tumors in mice with dibutylnitrosamine. *Br. J. urol. 24:*352, 1970.

70. Bertram, J. S., Craig, A. W. Specific induction of bladder cancer in mice by butyl-(4-hydroxybutyl)-nitrosamine and the effects of hormonal modifications on the sex difference in response. *Eur. J. Cancer 8:*587, 1972.

71. Wood, M., Flaks, A., Clayson, D. B. The carcinogenic activity of dibutylnitrosamine in IF × C57 mice. *Eur. J. Cancer 6:*433, 1970.

72. Ito, N., Hiasa, Y., Tamai, A., Okajima, E., Kitamura, H. Histogenesis of urinary bladder tumors induced by *N*-butyl-*N*(4-hydroxybutyl)-nitrosamine in rats. *Gan 60:* 401, 1969.

73. Flaks, A., Flaks, B. Establishment and characterization of a transplantable dibutylnitrosamine-induced mouse bladder tumor line FCB. *Cancer Res. 33:*3285, 1973.

74. Cohen, A. E., Weisburger, E. K., Weisburger, J. H., Ward, J. M., Putnam, C. C. Cystoscopy of chemically induced bladder neoplasms in rabbits administered the carcinogen dibutylnitrosamine.*Invest. Urol. 12:*262, 1973.

75. Hicks, R. M., Wakefield, J. St.J. Rapid induction of bladder cancer in rats with *N*-methyl-*N*-nitrosurea.

76. Pamukca, A. M., Wattenberg, K. W., Price, J. M., Bryan, G. T. Pheothiaspin inhibition of intestinal and urinary bladder tumor induced in rats by bracken fern. *JNCI. 47:*155, 1971.

77. Pamukca, A. M., Yalciner, S., Price, J. M., Bryan, G. T. Effects of the co-administration of thiamine on the incidence of urinary bladder carcinomas in rats fed bracken fern. *Cancer Res. 30:*2671, 1970.

78. Pamukca, A. M., Price, J. M., Bryan, G. T. Naturally occurring and bracken fern induced bovine urinary bladder tumors. *Vet. Pathol. 13:*110, 1976.

79. Pamukca, A. M., Price, J. M., Bryan, G. T. Assay of fractions of bracken fern (*Pteris aquilina*) for carcinogenic activity. *Cancer Res. 30:*902, 1970.

80. Pamukca, A. M., Erturk, E., Yalciner, S., Milli, U., Bryan, G. T. Carcinogenic and mutagenic activities of milk from cows fed bracken fern (*Pteridium Aquilinum*). *Cancer Res. 38:*1556, 1978.

81. Pamukca, A. M., Gokso, S. G., Price, J. M. Urinary bladder neoplasms induced by feeding bracken germ (*Pteris aquilina*) to cows. *Cancer Res. 27:*917, 1967.

82. Pamukca, A. M., Erturk, E., Yalcimer, S., Bryan, G. T. Histogenesis of urinary bladder cancer induced in rats by bracken fern. *Invest. Urol. 14:*21, 1976.

83. Bogden, A. E., Esber, H. J. Predictive experimental animal tumor models: a concept. *Natl. Cancer Inst. Monogr. 49:*263, 1978.

84. Brendler, H. Experimental prostatic cancer: background of the problem. *Natl. Cancer Inst. Monogr. 12:*343, 1963.

85. Fingerhut, B., Veenema, R. B. An animal model for the study of prostatic adenocarcinoma. *Invest. Urol. 15:*42, 1977.

86. Holland, J. M. Prostatic hyperplasia and neoplasia in female praomy (mastomys) nataluisis. *JNCI. 45:*1229, 1970.

87. Leav, L., Ling, G. V. Adenocarcinoma of the canine prostate. *Cancer 72:*1329, 1968.

88. Scott, W. W., Coffey, D. S., Smolev, J. K. Experimental models for the study of prostatic carcinoma. *J. Urol. 118:*216, 1977.

89. Shain, S. A., McCullough, B., Segaloff, A. Spontaneous adenocarcinomas of the ventral prostate of aged A X C rats. *JNCI. 55:*177, 1975.

90. Snell, K. C., Stewart, H. L. Adenocarcinoma and proliferative hyperplasia of the prostate gland in female *Rattus* (mastomys) *natalensis. JNCI. 35:*7, 1965.

91. Engle, E. T., Stout, A. P. Spontaneous primary carcinoma of the prostate in a monkey (*Malaca mulatta*). *Am. J. Cancer 39:*334, 1940.

92. Dunning, W. F., Curtis, M. R., Segaloff, A. Methylcholanthrene squamous cell carcinoma of the rat prostate. *Cancer Res. 24:*256, 1963.

92a. Dunning, W. F. Prostate cancer in the rat. *Natl. Cancer Inst. Monogr. 12:*351, 1963.

93. Markland, F. S., Chopp, R. T., Cosgrove, M. D., Howard, E. B. Characterization of steroid hormone receptors in the Dunning R-3327 rat prostatic adenocarcinoma. *Cancer Res. 38:*2818, 1978.

94. Voight, W., Feldman, M., Dunning, W. F. 5-dihydroxy testosterone binding proteins and androgen sensitivity in prostatic cancers of the Copenhagen rat. *Cancer Res. 35:*1849, 1975.

95. Voight, W., Dunning, W. F. *In vivo* metabolism of testosterone-3H in R3327, an androgen sensitive rat prostatic adenocarcinoma. *Cancer Res. 34:*1447, 1974.

96. Isaacs, J. T., Heston, W. D. W., Weisman, R. M., Coffey, D. S. Animal models of the hormone sensitive and insensitive prostatic adenocarcinomas Dunning R3327H, R-3327HI and R-3327AT. *Cancer Res. 38:*4353, 1978.

97. Lubaroff, D. M., Canfield, L., Rasmussen, G. T., Reynolds, C. An animal model for the study of prostate carcinoma. *Natl. Cancer Inst. Monogr. 49:*275, 1978.

98. Smolev, J. K., Heston, W. D. W., Scott, W. W., Coffey, D. S. Characterization of the Dunning R3327H prostatic adenocarcinoma: an appropriate animal model for prostate cancer. *Cancer Treat. Rept. 62:*273, 1977.

99. Lopez, D. M., Voight, W. Adenocarcinoma R3327 of the Copenhagen rat as a suitable model for immunologic studies of prostate cancer. *Cancer Res. 37:*2057, 1977.

100. Voigt, W., Lopez, D. M. Characterization of prostate carcinoma lines in the Copenhagen rat. Workshop in GU Cancer, *JNCI. 49:*269, 1978.

101. Coffey, D. S., Smoler, J., Heston, W. D., Scott, W. Growth characteristics and immunogenicity of the R-3327 rat prostate carcinoma. *Natl. Inst. Cancer Monogr. 49:*289, 1978.

102. (Deleted in proof)

103. Lande, I. J., Feldbuth, T. L., Lubaroff, D. M., Bonney, W. W. Rat prostate carcinoma 11095-A: profile of organ and tumor-specific antigens. *Natl. Cancer Inst. Monogr. 49:*283, 1978.

104. Block, N. L., Camuzzi, F., Denefrio, J., Truner, M., Clafin, A., Stover, D., Politano, V. Chemotherapy of the transplantable adenocarcinoma (R3327) of the Copenhagen rat. *Oncology 34:*110, 1977.

105. (Deleted in proof)

106. Pollard, M. Spontaneous prostate adenocarcinoma in aged germ free Wistar rats. *JNCI. 51:*1235, 1973.

107. (Deleted in proof)

108. Chang, C. F., Pollard, M. *In vitro* propagation of prostate adenocarcinoma cells from rats. *Invest. Urol. 14:*331, 1977.

109. Pollard, M., Luckert, P. Patterns of spontaneous metastasis manifested by three rat prostatic adenocarcinomas. *J. Surg. Oncol. 12:*371, 1979.

110. Pollard, M., Luckert, P. H. Transplantable metastasizing prostate adenocarcinoma in rats. *JNCI. 54:*643, 1975.

111. Pollard, M., Burleson, G. R., Luckert, P. H. Factors that modify the rate and extent of spontaneous metastases of prostate tumors in rats. In *Cancer Invasion and Metastasis: Biologic Mechanisms and Therapy*, p. 357, edited by S. B. Day. Raven Press, New York, 1977.
112. Pollard, M., Luckert, P. H. Chemotherapy of metastatic prostate adenocarcinoma in germ free rats. 1. Effects of cyclophosphamide. *Cancer Treat. Rept. 60:*619, 1976.
113. Noble, R. L. The development of prostatic adenocarcinoma in Nb rats following prolonged sex hormone administration. *Cancer Res. 37:*1929, 1977.
114. Noble, R. L. Sex steroids as a cause of adenocarcinoma of the dorsal prostate in Nb rats, and their influence on the growth of transplants. *Oncology 34:*138, 1977.
115. Drago, J. R., Maurer, R. E., Gershwin, M. E., Eckels, D., Palmer, J. M. The effect of 5 FU and Adriamycin on heterotransplantation of Noble rat prostatic tumors in congenitally athymic (nude) mice. *Cancer 44:*424, 1979.
116. Drago, J. R., Ikeda, R. N., Maurer, R. E., Goldman, L. B., Tesluk, H. The Nb rate: prostatic adenocarcinoma model. *Invest. Urol. 16:*353, 1979.
117. Drago, J. R., Goldman, L. B., Maurer, R. E., Gershwin, M. E., Eckels, D. D. Therapeutic manipulation of Nb rat prostatic adenocarcinoma. *Invest. Urol. 17:*203, 1979.
118. Drago, J. R., Maurer, R. E., Gershwin, M. E. Immunobiology and therapeutic manipulation of heterotransplanted Nb rat prostatic adenocarcinoma. *Cancer Chemother. Pharmacol. 3:*167, 1979.
119. Drago, J. R., Gershwin, M. E., Maurer, R. E., Ikeda, R. M., Eckels, D. D. Immunobiology and therapeutic manipulation of heterotransplanted Nb rat prostate adenocarcinoma cells from rats. *Invest. Urol. 14:*331, 1977.
120. Drago, J. R., Maurer, R. E., Gershwin, M. E., Eckels, D. D., Goldman, L. B. chemotherapy of Nb rat adenocarcinoma of the prostate heterotransplanted into congenitally athymic (nude) mice: report of 5-fluorouracil and cyclophosphamide. *J. Surg. Res. 26:*400, 1979.
121. Mortofi, F. K., Price, E. B. Eds. *Tumors of the Male Genital System.* Armed Forces Institute of Pathology, Washington, DC, 1973.
122. Rivere, M., Chouronlinkov, J., Guerin, M. Production de tumeurs par injections intratesticulaires de chlorue de zinc chez la rat. *Bull. Assoc. Fr. Etude Cancer 47:*55, 1970.
123. Guthrie, J., Guthrie, O. T. Embryonal carcinomas in Syrian hamsters after intratesticular inoculation of zinc chloride during seasonal testicular growth. *Cancer Res. 34:* 2612, 1974.
124. Stevens, L. C., Little, C. C. Spontaneous testicular teratomas in an inbred strain of mice. *Proc. Natl. Acad. Sci. USA 40:*1080, 1954.
125. Stevens, L. C. A new subline of mice (129/ter Su) with a high incidence of spontaneous congenital testicular teratomas. *JNCI. 50:*235, 1973.
126. Solter, D., Dominis, M., Damjanov, I. Embryo-derived teratocarcinoma. II Teratoc ar-cinogenesis depends on the type of embryonic graft. *Int. J. Cancer 25:*341, 1980.
127. Jewett, M. A. S. Biology of testicular tumors. *Urol. Clin. North Am. 4:*495, 1977.
128. Kleinsmith, L. J., Pierce, G. B. Multipotentiality of a single embryonal carcinoma cell. *Cancer Res. 24:*1544, 1964.
129. Pierce, G. B., Wallace, D. Differentiation of malignant to benign cells. *Cancer Res. 31:* 127, 1971.
130. Strickland, S., Saway, M. J. Studies on the effect of retinoids on the differentiation of teratocarcinoma stem cells *in vitro* and *in vivo. Dev. Biol. 78:*76, 1980.
131. Knutson, J. C., Polahd, A. Keratinization of mouse teratoma cell line XB produced by 2, 3, 7, 8–128.
132. McBurney, M. W. Clonal lines of teratocarcinoma cells *in vitro*: differentiation and cytogenetic characteristics. *J. Cell. Physiol. 89:*441, 1976.
133. Smith, J. B., O'Neil, R. T. Alpha-fetoprotein: occurrence in germinal cell and liver malignancies. *Am. J. Med. 51:*767, 1971.
134. Teilum, G., Albrechtsen, R., Norgaard-Pederson, B. Immunofluorescent localization of alpha-fetoprotein synthesis in endodermal sinus tumor (yolk sac tumor). *Acta Pathol. Microbiol. Scand. A 82:*586, 1974.

135. Jewett, M.A. S. Personal communication.
136. Hall, J. D., Marsden, M., Rifkin, D., Teresky, A. K., Levine, A. J. In *Teratomas and Differentiation*, pp. 251–270, edited by M. I. Sherman and D. Solter. Academic Press, New York, 1975.
137. Kohler, G., Milstein, C. Derivation of specific antibody-producing tissue culture and tumor lines by cell fusion. *Eur. J. Immunol. 6:*511, 1976.
138. Solter, D., Knowles, B. B. Monoclonal antibody defining a stage-specific mouse embryonic antigen (SSEA-1). *Proc. Natl. Acad. Sci. USA 75:*5565, 1978.
139. Emanoil-Ravicovitch, R., Hojman-Montes-De-Orca, F., Robert, J., Garcette, M., Callahan, R., Peries, J., Boiron, M. Biochemical characterization of endogenous type C virus information in differentiated and undifferentiated murine teratocarcinoma-derived cell lines. *J. Virol. 34:*576, 1980.
140. Brinster, R. L. The effect of cells transferred into the mouse blastocyst on subsequent development. *J. Exp. Med. 140:*1049, 1974.
141. Papaioannou, V. E., Gardner, R. L., McBurney, M. W., Babinet, C., Evans, M. J. Participation of cultured teratocarcinoma cells in mouse embryogenesis. *J. Embryol. Exp. Morphol. 44:*93, 1978.

8

New Imaging Modalities in Genitourinary Cancer

The development and utilization of ultrasonography, computerized tomography, and radionuclide imaging has occurred rapidly during the last quarter century, and clinical application of these modalities has significantly modified and refined the diagnostic and therapeutic approach of many disease processes. No area in urology has felt the impact of these newer diagnostic modalities more than that of genitourinary cancer where structures previously inaccessible, or only accessible by more invasive techniques, can now be visualized with reasonable accuracy. These newer techniques are constantly being modified and improved and their role in diagnosis, staging, and treatment is constantly undergoing revision. Because of the development of these noninvasive techniques, the need for more invasive studies such as angiography, venography, and lymphanography is becoming less frequent and the indications for their use becoming more highly selective. It is now valid to ask questions such as: "Are renal angiograms necessary in the evaluation of every patient with a solid renal mass?"; "Are lymphangiograms necessary to assess para-aortic lymph nodes in all patients with testicular tumors?"; and "Can these noninvasive studies reduce the need for surgical staging?" Though the answers to these questions are varied and subject to much debate, all would agree that they are valid questions that deserve proper resolution.

PHYSICAL PRINCIPLES

Ultrasound

Medical ultrasound uses the principles of sound navigation and ranging (SONAR) to delineate the shape and consistency of internal body organs

NEW IMAGING MODALITIES IN GENITOURINARY CANCER   143

and structures.[1] The piezoelectric crystal which forms the ultrasound transducer is able to convert electrical energy into vibrational energy and electrical excitation of the crystal produces mechanical vibrations, the frequency of which is determined by the thickness of the transducer. The vibrations commonly of a frequency of a 1–20 mHz are transmitted into the body in short bursts lasting 10 ms. The sound waves are attenuated as they pass through the body and, when a tissue boundary is encountered resulting in a change in acoustic impedance, part of the energy is reflected. Reflection also depends on the size of the interface relative to the wave length, high frequency sound waves being reflected by smaller surfaces.[2] Since higher frequency sound transducers have greater resolution, but at the expense of depth of penetration, transducer selection becomes an important part of the ultrasound examination.

Except for the short period of sound emission (10 ms), transducers spend the time between emissions to receive reflected echoes and convert them back to electrical signals which, in turn, are displayed as images on a cathode ray tube or TV screen. The mode of display can be: single dimensional, A-mode (amplitude) which is useful for measuring distances of interfaces from each other; or two-dimensional B-mode (brightness) display which is obtained while the transducer is moved along an arc.[3] The advent of gray-scale convertors has greatly improved the image quality of B-mode scanners. More recently "real" time scanning has allowed a dynamic image to be viewed and, if desired, videotaped so that a permanent record may be obtained. These studies have been found to be particularly useful in assessing the vascular system, for example, determining inferior vena caval patency.

Computed Tomographic Scanning

Current fourth generation computed tomographic (CT) scanners consist basically of a system that rotates an x-ray tube 360° around the patient coupled with a ring of radiation detectors that also surround the patient. As the tube rotates, multiple readings of the transmitted radiation are taken by the detectors and from these the computer is able to reconstruct the internal body structures.[4,5] The picture one sees is composed of a matrix or grid of tiny squares called pixels (picture elements). Each pixel represents a small volume of the patient because the scan slices are of finite thickness. The computer calculates the amount of x-ray absorption for each volume element (voxel) in the patient. This amount of x-ray absorption is given a number of an arbitrary scale on which x-ray absorption of water has a value of 0. This number is called the Hounsfield, or CT-density, number and indicates in a relative fashion the amount of x-rays absorbed by the tissue. The scale runs from −1000 to +1000; thus, dense bone has a high CT number of approximately 800 to 1000, air has a low CT number of approximately −1000, and water has a CT number of 0. The computer assigns a shade of gray to each pixel corresponding to the CT number calculated for that pixel; thus, bone is assigned white, air is assigned black, and water is assigned a shade of mid-gray. The radiologist can vary the shades of gray assigned to any tissue density to optimize visual differentiation between similar tissue densities. The picture on the cathode ray screen is then photographed for a permanent record.

CT, therefore, has advantages over conventional radiological techniques. The first being the transaxial perspective which allows one to see the organs without superimposition of structures. Secondly, the high degree of density resolution allows differentiation between normal soft tissues. Fat, muscle, and fluid are easily differentiated and minute amounts of calcium are easily seen.

One technical problem with CT that should be understood by clinicians is the problem of partial volume averaging. Because the slice has a certain thickness, if two structures of different density occupy the slice thickness, the computer will average the CT numbers and give a false reading. For example, if a slice happens to fall on the interface between a renal cyst and normal kidney, the cyst will be seen but will appear to have higher CT numbers than one would expect from a fluid-filled structure. The same phenomenon will occur if a lesion fails to fill the CT slice thickness. The density of the lesion will be averaged with the surrounding tissue. This problem can be resolved by using thinner slice widths or by insuring that the lesion occupies the full thickness of the slice by taking several closely spaced cuts. Most renal studies will involve 10 to 16 slices at 1-cm intervals. In our unit, when investigating renal carcinoma, scans before and after the administration of intravenous contrast agent are taken. In addition, scans through the liver are always performed to evaluate for possible metastases.

Nuclear Imaging

The principles of radionuclide imaging involves the administration of a radioactively labeled material whose passage through the body can be measured quantitatively. By selecting specific substances to label with radioactivity, one can selectively study different body organs.[6]

ADRENAL GLANDS

Historically, the ability to image the small paired adrenal glands has lagged significantly behind our ability to biochemically determine disorders of these structures. Intravenous urography, anteriography, and retroperitoneal pneumography have all been used with uniformly poor results. Newer imaging modalities offer significant improvements in the assessment and diagnosis of disorders of these structures.

Ultrasound

Utilizing the liver as an acoustic window, the right adrenal gland can be imaged in most patients.[7-9] It is usually wedge shaped and lies between the right lobe of the liver and the right crus of the diaphragm posterior to the vena cava. The left adrenal is related to the left crus of the diaphragm, the anterosuperomedial aspect of the kidney, and the stomach or tail of the pancreas. It is more difficult to approach the left adrenal although it can be visualized in 80% of patients. Rib artifacts, the proximity of the left adrenal to the gas-filled stomach, the esophagogastric junction, or spleen are all potential pitfalls for the ultrasonographic viewing of the left adrenal, while the duodenum causes difficulties on the right side.

Adrenal masses can be detected reliably with modern ultrasonic examination and determinations made of solid, cystic, or complex-cystic masses. Prospective studies by Sample and Sarti[10, 11] indicate an overall accuracy of 90–95% with little difference in accuracy or specificity when comparing ultrasound to CT scanning. Most errors relate to attempts to detect hyperplastic glands while 10% of patients examined had nondiagnostic studies. Accuracy in evaluating adrenal medullary tumors is similar to that of cortical lesions and ultrasound does help in this regard. Sample and Sarti[10, 11] believe that CT is very reliable in delineating the anatomy surrounding the adrenal glands and the anatomy of the adrenal itself and, because CT is so easy to perform, it is probably the preferred initial modality once biochemical abnormalities have been established.

Computed Tomographic Scanning

Visualization of the adrenal gland by CT scanning relies on the presence of fat around the adrenal and therefore allows for reliable visualization of normal adrenal glands in all but the most asthenic patients (Fig. 8.1). Localization of unilateral adrenal masses (Figs. 8.2 and 8.3) is reliably achieved by CT. Occasionally, specific pathological diagnoses can be suggested by resolution of small amounts of calcification or fat within the tumor. Cystic lesions of the adrenal are reliably detected. Retroperitoneal CT scanning is an excellent method to search for pheochromocytomas and lesions greater than 1 cm can be detected with a great degree of accuracy.[12-15]

Radioisotope Scanning

Recently developed radionucleotide cholesterol scans have been used to outline functioning adrenal tissue (Fig. 8.4). ^{131}I-19-iodocholesterol or ^{131}I-6-iodomethyl-19 noncholesterol (NP-59) is administered intravenously and is localized in functioning adrenal tissue.[16] Although the radiation dose is high, it successfully localizes adrenal adenomas and areas of hyperplasia. Adrenal carcinomas and pheochromocytomas leave negative images and thus are diagnosed less accurately with this modality.

KIDNEY

Ultrasound's most extensive and earliest application in the field of urology applies to the evaluation of patients with renal masses. Being retroperitoneal structures, the kidneys are ideally suited to ultrasonographic or CT examination and both modalities are of great assistance in clarifying the nature of masses seen on a prior intravenous urogram.[17, 18] Each accurately distinguishes between a renal cyst and solid tumor while

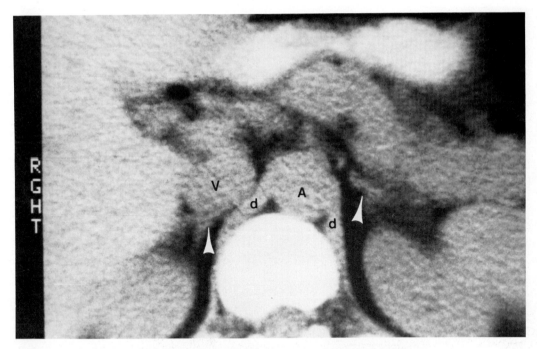

Figure 8.1. Normal adrenal glands (*white arrow heads*). The inverted Y-shaped right adrenal gland is lying in a classic location immediately posterior to the inferior vena cava (*V*). The somewhat triangular-shaped left adrenal gland is lying anterior to the upper pole of the left kidney, immediately lateral to the aorta (*A*) and crus of the diaphragm (*d*). The elongated soft tissue structure anterior to the left adrenal gland is the pancreas.

CT has an added advantage of, at times, providing insight into the nature of certain solid lesions. Radionucleotide imaging with ^{99}Tc-labeled glucoheptomate (GH) or dimercaptosuccinic acid (DMSA) is particularly useful in the patient in whom an intravenous urogram only suggests the presence of a renal mass. It distinguishes functioning from nonfunctioning tissue and, therefore, is the modality of choice for assessing pseudotumors such as Dromedary humps, hypertrophic columns of Bertin, or fetal lobulations.[19]

Renal Cyst

Both ultrasonography and CT-imaging examinations for visualizing renal cysts are highly reliable (Figs. 8.5 and 8.6). The overall accuracy of the sonic examination in conjunction with intravenous urography in predicting a renal cyst is reported to be 95% or better.[20-22] When this examination is supplemented by a renal cyst aspiration or by a CT examination, then the accuracy approaches 100%.

Because of the high number of renal cysts visualized incidentally at ultrasonography or CT, we no longer routinely perform renal cyst puncture for those lesions that satisfy all the criteria for a benign renal cyst. However, if the lesion does not satisfy all the criteria for a cyst, or if the

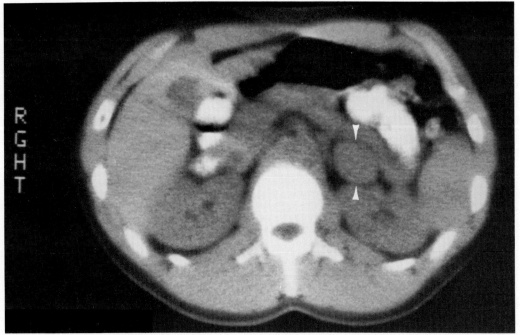

Figure 8.2. This 42-year-old man presented with biochemical evidence of a pheochromocytoma. A round tumor (*white arrow heads*) lying in the expected location of the left adrenal gland is identified. At surgery, a pheochromocytoma was removed. The right adrenal gland is not seen at this scan level.

patient has symptoms referable to the cysts, then renal cyst puncture should be performed under fluoroscopy or with an ultrasonically guided approach. A sample of fluid is routinely sent for cytology and biochemical analysis of LDH and cholesterol, both of which are low in the fluid from a benign cyst. Injection of contrast medium through the needle provides an excellent method of viewing the walls of a cyst, and may occasionally be useful in problem cases.

Methods of evaluating patients with renal masses have undergone considerable change in recent years. If the lesion appears to be a renal cyst on intravenous urography then renal ultrasound is the next appropriate investigation and all subsequent investigations are dictated by its results. Computerized tomography is utilized if the ultrasonic examination was unsuccessful or indefinite (Fig. 8.7).

Solid Renal Mass

Solid tumors can be detected by ultrasound with almost the same accuracy as cystic ones (Fig. 8.8). It must be determined whether or not the mass is of the same consistency as surrounding parenchyma and whether or not it is homogeneous.[20–25]

Ultrasound provides assistance in staging patients with renal cancer. An assessment can be made of the para-aortic lymph nodes but it is particularly useful in assessing the status of the renal vein and vena

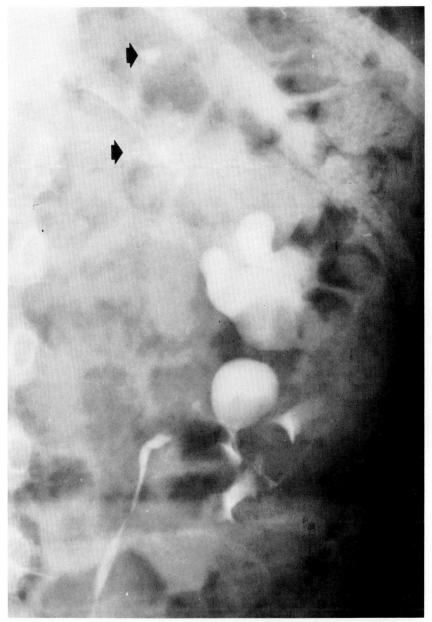

Figure 8.3. Neuroblastoma in a 3-year-old girl. Note the stippled calcification (*arrows*) in a supermedial location to the kidney. The left renal axis is more vertical than normal. The marrowing of the renal pelvis and obstructive uropathy in the upper pole calyces was due to invasion of the renal pelvis by the tumor.

cava.[26, 27] With the advent of "real-time" ultrasonic studies, dynamic views of these structures can be obtained and an accurate assessment of vein patency made. It has replaced the need for inferior venacavography in many patients.

CT is also excellent in assessing solid renal masses[28–30] and offers the

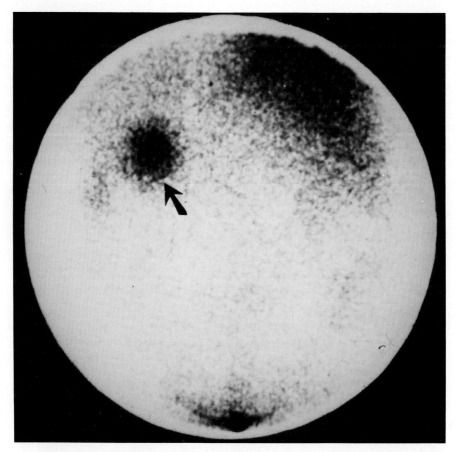

Figure 8.4. A posterior nuclear medicine scan with the radiopharmaceutical NP-59, showing a left adrenal adenoma (*arrow*) in a patient with Cushing's disease. The right adrenal is not identified due to suppression of the gland by the adenoma.

additional advantage of being the most sensitive method available to detect invasion of the perirenal structures (Fig. 8.9). The perirenal fat and Gerota's fascia can be visualized and invasion into and through these structures can be accurately detected. CT will reliably detect enlarged para-aortic lymph nodes and can also be used to detect the presence of liver metastases. A recent analysis of 70 cases of renal carcinoma studied by CT suggests that CT is as accurate as high dose arteriography in evaluating renal vein and inferior vena cava involvement, and more accurate than high dose arteriography in evaluating perirenal and nodal involvement.[31] If this work is confirmed, the use of CT for staging prior to angiography would have the advantage of reducing the complexity, time, and contrast medium dosage required at angiography. In some cases, if the surgeon believed that knowledge of the number of renal arteries was not of critical importance, the use of CT prior to angiography has the added advantage of providing an evaluation that helps in assessing the need for angiographic embolization.

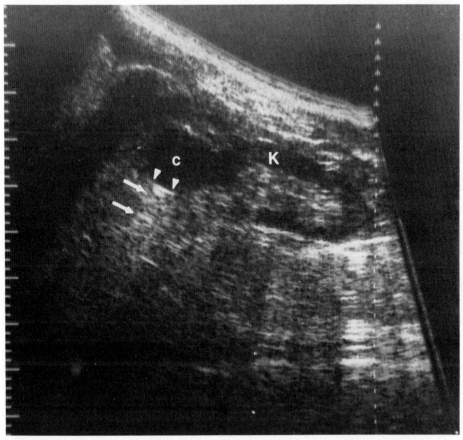

Figure 8.5. A typical renal cyst (*c*) involving the upper pole of the kidney (*K*) is seen on this longitudinal ultrasound scan. Note the sharp back wall (*arrow heads*) and the zone of increased sound transmission (*arrows*) which characterize a simple cyst.

Both CT and ultrasound have been used with success in evaluating the renal bed following surgery, in searching for recurrent or persistent disease.[32, 33] Occasionally, bowel loops lying in the renal bed may cause confusion in ultrasound images and these loops are easily identified on CT scanning.

Other Solid Lesions

COMPLEX CYSTIC OR INDETERMINATE RENAL MASSES

In both the CT and sonic examination of renal masses, not all studies fulfill all the criteria of being either a solid or cystic lesion. Typical examples of such masses include tumors with necrosis or hemorrhage or inflammatory lesions (Fig. 8.7). Classically, the size of the "cyst"-like area is smaller than the size of the total mass as determined by intravenous urography, thus suggesting the presence of a solid component surrounding a cystic structure.[34]

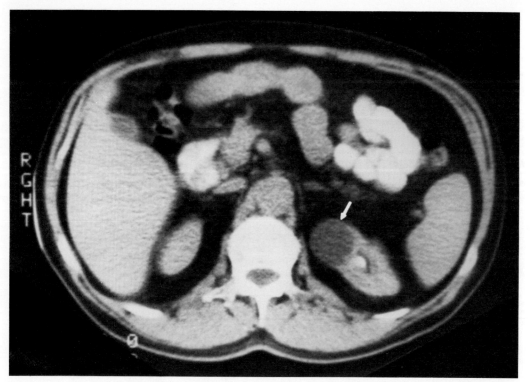

Figure 8.6.   A typical renal cyst on CT scan (*arrow*). Note the sharp margin with the contrast-enhanced renal tissue, the imperceptible wall of the cyst, and the fact that the cyst does not enhance with contrast medium. These are all criteria for diagnosis of renal cyst by CT.

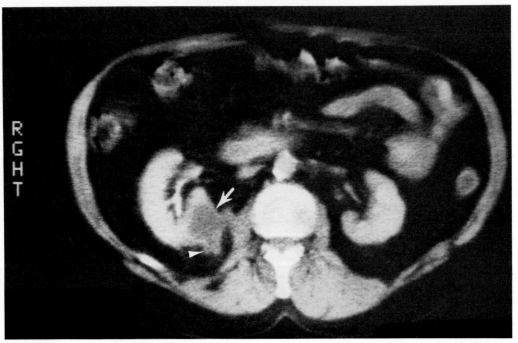

Figure 8.7.   This cystic lesion of the kidney does not demonstrate the criteria for a simple cyst. Note the thick wall (*arrow*) and the irregular extension of soft tissue into the perinephric fat (*arrow head*). This would be an indeterminate lesion by CT criteria. Clinical history and needle aspiration under ultrasound guidance proved that this was a renal abscess.

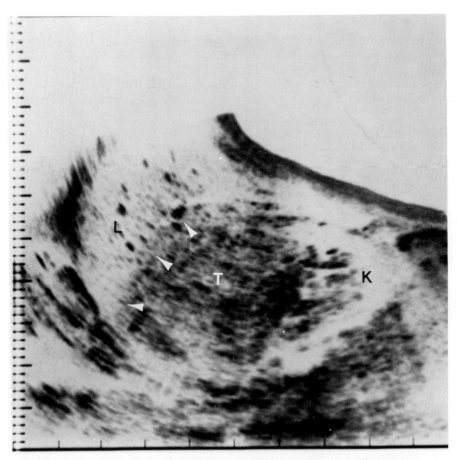

Figure 8.8. A large right hypernephroma extending out of the kidney and invading the psoas and quadratus lumborum muscles is identified. (Longitudinal ultrasound). The echogenic tumor (*T*) is seen to invade the liver (*L*). The zone of invasion is identified by the *white arrowheads*. The normal appearing lower pole of the kidney is labelled *K*.

METASTASES

Metastatic renal lesions from a primary lesion in the lung or breast are not uncommonly found.[35, 36] Many metastatic carcinomas are homogeneous and therefore sonoluscent but, being solid, will not have increased through transmission as seen in the true cyst. Metastatic lesions tend to be spherical in shape.

TRANSITIONAL CELL TUMORS

None of the newer modalities replace retrograde pyelography, pelvic brushing, and urinary cytology in the diagnosis of transitional cell tumors of the renal pelvis and ureter, but they are helpful in assessing renal parenchymal invasion in more aggressive lesions. Accurate staging can be performed with both CT and sonography.

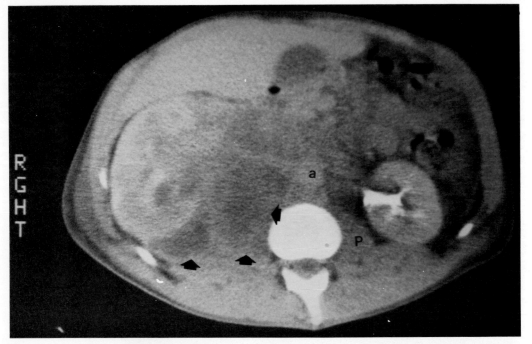

Figure 8.9. CT scan of same patient as in Fig. 8.8 (invading tumor, *arrows*). In this postcontrast scan, the tumor is of somewhat lower density than the renal tissue. The tumor extends up to the aorta (*a*) and anteriorly towards the liver. The left psoas muscle (*P*) is labeled for comparison.

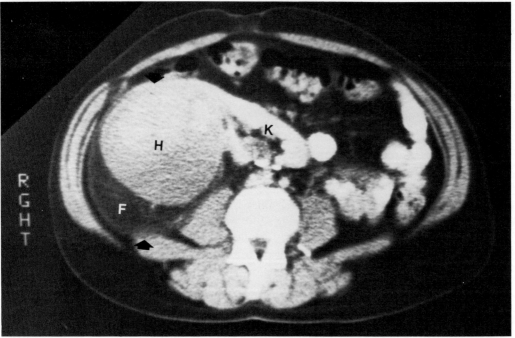

Figure 8.10. A large 16-cm angiomyolipoma (*arrows*) is seen to displace the kidney (*K*) inferiorly and across the midline. The tumor is composed of two densities. The high density (*H*) represents bleeding into the tumor, a well known complication of large angiomyolipomas. The low density component (*F*) represents fat in the tumor.

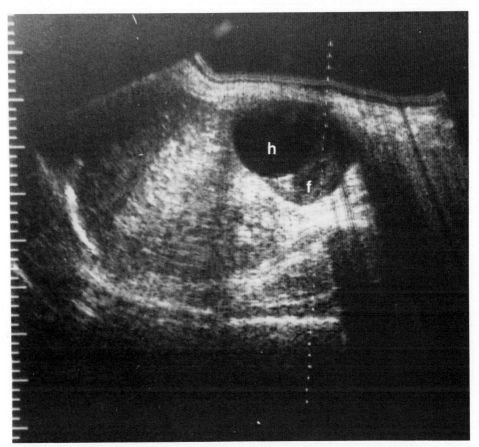

Figure 8.11. An ultrasound scan through the same patient as in Figure 8.10. The kidney is not present on this scan slice which is taken solely through the upper part of the tumor. The hemorrhage is seen as an anechoic area (*h*). Sonographically, the fat is shown as an area of high level echoes (*f*).

ANGIOMYOLIPOMA

Angiographic accuracy in the preoperative diagnosis of angiomyolipoma has been unreliable and its differentiation from hypernephroma is unpredictable.[37] Both sonography and CT have been useful in both diagnosing angiomyolipomas and in screening of patients with von Hippel-Lindau syndrome for the development of renal cell carcinoma[38, 39] (Figs. 8.10 and 8.11). The fat content of the tumor gives a characteristic sonic pattern with a high level of internal echos at low gain, unlike renal cell carcinoma which are sonoluscent at low gain levels. Computerized tomography is also quite sensitive in detecting fat content of masses and is the best method of screening patients with von Hippel-Lindau syndrome.[40]

PEDIATRIC RENAL MASSES

The most common renal tumor in the pediatric age group is Wilms'

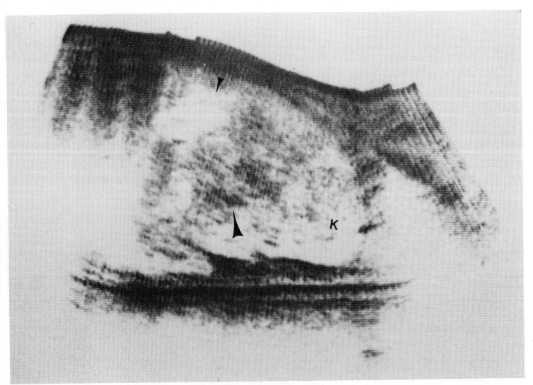

Figure 8.12. A longitudinal ultrasound scan through the kidney in a 4-year-old child with Wilm's tumor. Only the lower pole of the kidney (*K*) can be demonstrated. The remainder of the kidney is replaced by tumor with a complex echo pattern, some areas demonstrating high level echoes (*large arrow head*), while others demonstrate relative echo lucency (*small arrow head*).

tumor. The sonic appearance varies from that of an entirely solid mass to one with a complex cystic pattern due to the presence of internal hemorrhage and/or tissue necrosis[41] (Fig. 8.12). Ultrasound has been helpful in the evaluation of these patients and particularly helpful in separating renal from adrenal masses. The lack of fat in the retroperitoneal area in many young children makes computerized tomography less reliable in assessing the para-aortic nodes than in the adult population.

Although neuroblastoma can be found in many locations, the most common is in the adrenal gland. Because of varying therapeutic approaches, it is imperative that this mass be differentiated from Wilms' tumor. Much help can be gained by knowing the age of the patient and by obtaining a plain abdominal radiograph to demonstrate the stippled calcification often associated with neuroblastomas (Fig. 8.3). As with intravenous urography, ultrasound has been useful alone or in combination with CT in providing valuable clinical information regarding the solid or cystic nature of the lesion and defining whether it is adrenal or renal in origin. These studies also can provide information regarding hepatic metastases and lymph node involvement. CT compliments the ultrasound examination by readily visualizing the areas obscured by bowel gas.

BLADDER

Although cystoscopy is the most accurate method of diagnosing a bladder tumor, methods of assessing extent or stage of disease have previously been either invasive or unreliable. Examination under anesthesia and full thickness biopsies are cornerstones for preoperative staging protocols but, recently, the addition of sonography and CT have greatly helped in the planning of appropriate therapy.

Ultrasonic examination of the pelvis can be achieved by transabdominal, transrectal, transuretheral, or perineal methods of scanning. Sonic examinations of the bladder allows reliable assessment of stage A and C lesions although partial thickness muscle invasion cannot be reliably differentiated[42,43] (Fig. 8.13). For assessment of the bladder base, transrectal examinations have also produced accurate results. With the selective use of preoperative radiation therapy, accurate reproducible staging systems are necessary not only to select candidates for preoperative radiation but also to assess response.

The pelvis with its well developed fat planes is also well suited for external CT examination. The bladder is distended with 150 ml of CO_2

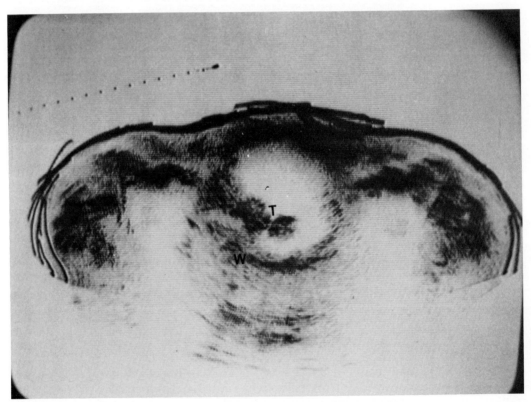

Figure 8.13. Abdominal ultrasound examination of urinary bladder in patient with infiltrative bladder tumor (*T*). Tumor invasion of the bladder wall (*W*) can be detected but extent of involvement is difficult to differentiate. Surgical exploration revealed a stage C lesion.

NEW IMAGING MODALITIES IN GENITOURINARY CANCER   157

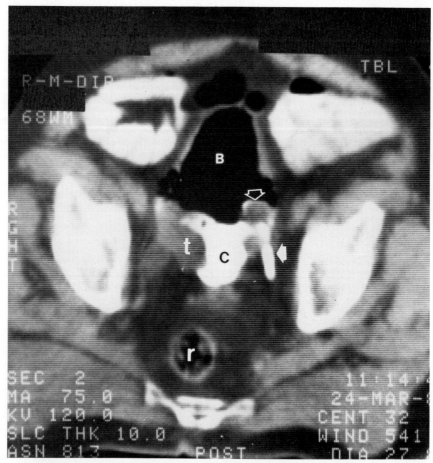

Figure 8.14. Scan through the area of the trigone in a 68-year-old man with bladder tumors. The air-filled bladder (*B*) with positive contrast agent (*C*) lying posteriorly is identified. A small tumor (*open arrow*) partially obstructs the left ureter (*closed arrow*). A second larger tumor (*t*) is seen on the right. Neither tumor was shown to extend beyond the bladder wall. The rectum (*r*) is labeled for identification. Cystectomy was performed and histological examination revealed the presence of a stage B_2 transitional cell carcinoma.

and administration of an intravenous contrast agent allows detection of the lower ureters and ureterovesical junction.[44] Excellent visualization of the bladder wall and perivesicle tissues is obtained in a reproducible fashion. Several series have shown a very high degree of staging accuracy with CT scanning when compared to surgical finding.[45-48] Not only can it detect stage A, B, and C lesions, but it can at times assess the pelvic lymph nodes as well (Fig. 8.14). It is an extremely valuable noninvasive method for the planning of and assessing response to preoperative radiation therapy. Unfortunately, like ultrasound, this modality does not allow the consistent separation of B_1 and B_2 tumors.

PROSTATE

Standard methods of visualizing the prostate have, until recently, been unrewarding but both CT and sonography have greatly expanded our imaging capacity. Ultrasonic examination of the prostate can be achieved by transabdominal, transurethral, and transrectal techniques.[49-53] Transrectal ultrasound has been shown to be accurate in determining prostate size and in detecting the presence or absence of internal irregularities such as calculi, infection, infarction, and carcinoma (Figs. 8.15 and 8.16). Unfortunately, currently available instruments do not allow for the consistent differentiation between prostatic carcinoma, calculi, and chronic inflammation. When physical examination and prostate ultrasound suggest benign prostatic hyperplasia, the chance of malignancy is very low. Problems occur, however, in patients with diffuse unsuspected tumors (stage A_2). Ultrasonic procedures have yet to allow for the early detection of these lesions with any degree of reliability.[43] Prostatic ultrasound is particularly accurate in assessing the local extent of the disease and has been helpful in localizing highly suspicious areas within the gland that require biopsy. Additionally, transrectal ultrasound provides an objective method of following patients with carcinoma of the prostate and in assessing local response to nonsurgical therapy (endocrine radiation). General response to endocrine therapy can be monitored; however, evidence of reactivation often goes undetected which greatly limits this technique in an effort to detect early disease recurrence.

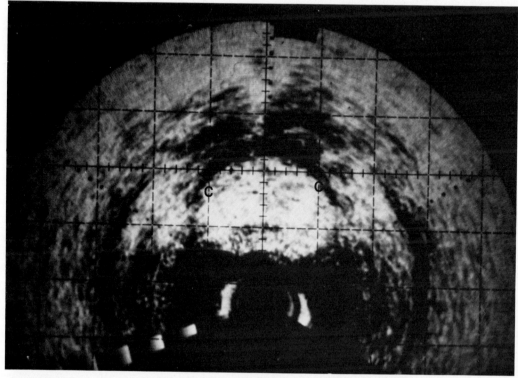

Figure 8.15. Transrectal prostate ultrasonic scan of 65-year-old patient with clinical and surgically confirmed benign prostatic hyperplasia. Prostatic capsule (*C*) is continuous and well demarcated.

NEW IMAGING MODALITIES IN GENITOURINARY CANCER   159

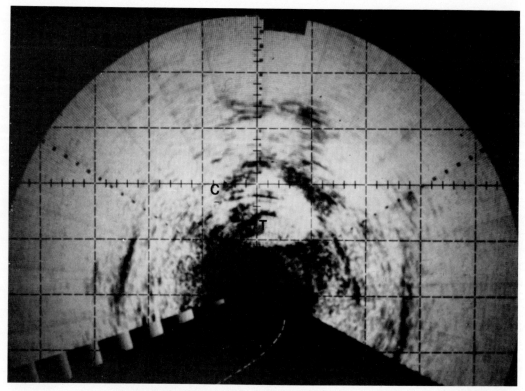

Figure 8.16. Transrectal prostatic ultrasonic scan of 72-year-old patient with prostatic carcinoma. The tumor (*T*) involves the right lobe and irregularity of the prostatic capsule (*C*) indicates invasion.

The role of CT in the diagnosis of early carcinoma of the prostate is not as well defined as that of transrectal ultrasound but it appears to have no major advantage.[54] It is very useful in visualizing transcapsular spread and involvement of the seminal vesicles. The use of intravenous contrast agents to assess ureteric encasement can at times also be helpful. Pelvic lymph node involvement has been detected by both CT and abdominal ultrasound studies. As with ultrasound, CT has been used in measuring response to nonsurgical therapy and in planning radiation therapy. This technique also has a unique place in the patient with an absent rectum secondary to prior surgery or injury.

TESTICULAR TUMORS

The role of the newer imaging modalities has made significant contribution to the diagnosis, staging, and treatment of testicular tumors. Ultrasound has been used to accurately determine the location, origin and consistency of intrascrotal masses.[55–57] It also has been used to assess testicular consistency when a hydrocele precludes adequate physical examination. Clearly, nothing will replace an inguinal surgical exploration for the suspicious lesion.

CT is well suited for retroperitoneal examination in that the large amount of low density fat provides an excellent contrast for visualizing the para-aortic lymph nodes (Fig. 8.17). Enlarged nodes are clearly seen and many produce the floating aorta sign. This occurs when a calcified aorta is seen entirely surrounded by enlarged lymph nodes; the calcified aortic wall appears to be suspended in a sea of soft tissue mass. Comparison of CT with lymphangiography shows that CT is at least as accurate as lymphangiography in detecting para-aortic node enlargement and provides a better method of assessing the true extent of the disease.[58]

Retroperitoneal ultrasound also has been used to stage patients with testicular tumors.[59, 60] Para-aortic lymph node enlargement can be accurately detected if bowel gas does not obscure the retroperitoneum. Unlike lymphangiography, it cannot detect the internal histopathology of an enlarged lymph node but it can often visualize renal hilar and high para-aortic nodes which are poorly, if ever, seen on lymphangiography.

Although both CT and ultrasound can visualize the retroperitoneum, we feel that CT is the preferred method because there will be occasions when abdominal gas will obscure the retroperitoneal area to the ultrasound beam. However, ultrasound is an easily repeatable, noninvasive examination and can be successfully used if CT scanning is not available.

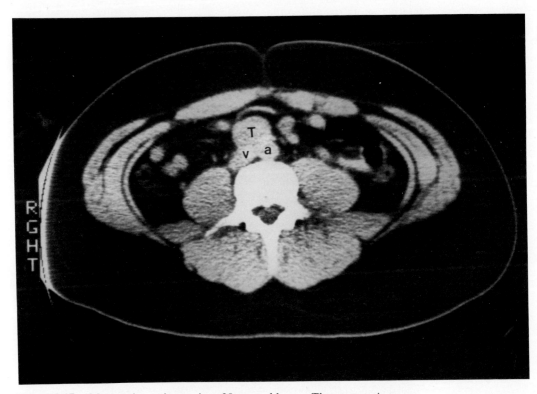

Figure 8.17. Metastatic seminoma in a 28-year-old man. The metastatic tumor (*T*) lies immediately anterior to the inferior vena cava (*v*) and aorta (*a*). This is a slightly unusual location for this solitary metastasis, as it lies below the level of the kidneys.

The role of each is similar in both seminomatous and nonseminomatous lesions.[61] We feel that the role of retroperitoneal lymphangiography is in doubt in the assessment of patients with testicular tumors and is no longer routinely performed in our unit.

Nuclear Imaging

It has been shown clearly that the most sensitive method of assessing nonseminomatous tumor recurrences is by following tumor markers.[62] It also has been shown that a negative computerized tomographic scan in the presence of elevated markers does not obviate the surgeon from retroperitoneal lymph node exploration. Javadpour and others[64] have recently reported using radioimmunodetection methods to determine the site of metastatic nonseminomatous tumors. They report the detection and localization of metastases of extra metastatic germ cell cancer-producing human chorionic gonadotropin (HCG) after patients were administered an intravenous injection of 1.0 mCi of radioactive-labeled goat antibodies to human chorionic somatomammotropin (HCS). Total body photoscans of the chest and abdomen performed 24 and 48 hours following injection revealed pulmonary metastases that were visualized on chest x-ray, as well as the presence of retroperitoneal tumor not detected by lymphangiogram, abdominal computer tomogram, or inferior venacavagram. The diagnostic and staging potential of this noninvasive method of radioimmunodetection of testicular cancer is in its experimental stages, but is likely to have significant impact not only on this disease but in others as well.

REFERENCES

1. Russell, J. M., Resnick, M. I. Ultrasound in urology. *Urol. Clin. North Am. 6:*445, 1979.
2. Baddemeyer, E. The physics of diagnostic ultrasound. *Radiol. Clin. North Am. 8:*391, 1975.
3. Barnett, E., and Morley, P. In *Ultrasound in Scientific Foundations of Urology*, Vol. II, p. 446. Edited by D. I. Williams, and G. D. Chisolm. Yearbook Medical, Chicago 1976.
4. McClennan, B. L., and Fair, W. R. CT scanning in urology. *Urol. Clin. North Am. 6:* 343, 1979.
5. Hattery, R. R., Williamson, B., Jr., and Hartman, G. W. Computed tomography of genitourinary tract and retroperitoneum. In *Clinical Urography*, p. 339. Edited by D. M. Witten, G. H. Myers, Jr., D. C. Utz, W. B. Saunders, Philadelphia, 1977.
6. Ball, J. D., and Maynard, C. D. Nuclear imaging in urology. *Urol. Clin. North Am. 6:* 327.
7. Sample, W. F. Ultrasonography of the Adrenal Gland in Ultrasound in Urology, p. 73. Edited by M. I. Resnick, and R. G. Sanders. Williams & Wilkins, Baltimore, 1979.
8. Sample, W. F. A new technique for evaluation of the adrenal gland with gray scale ultrasonography. *Radiology 124:*463, 1977.
9. Sample, W. F. Adrenal ultrasonography. Radiology *127:*461, 1978.
10. Sample, E. F., and Sarti, D. A. Computed tomography and gray scale ultrasonography anatomic correlations and pitfalls in upper abdomen. *Gastrointest. Radiol. 3:*243, 1978.
11. Sample, W. F., and Sarti, D. A. Computed tomography and gray scale ultrasonography of the adrenal gland: a Comparative Study. *Radiology 128:*377, 1978.
12. Stewart, B. H., Bravo, E. L., Aaga, J., Meaney, T. F., and Tarazi, R. Localization of pheochromocytoma by computed tomography. *N. Engl. J. Med. 299:*4601, 1977.
13. Epstein, A. F., Patel, S. K., and Petasnick, J. P. Computed tomography of adrenal gland. *JAMA 242:*2791, 1979.

14. Karstaedt, N., Sagel, S. S., and Stanley, R. J., *et al.* Computed tomography of the adrenal gland. *Radiology 129:*723, 1978.
15. Korobkin, M., White, E. A., and Kressel, H. Y., *et al.* Computed tomography in diagnosis of adrenal disease. AJR *132:*231, 1979.
16. Parthasarathy, K. L., Bakshi, J., Ackenhalt, R., Villa, M., and Dial, R. Adrenal scintigraphy utilizing [131]I-19-iodocholesterol. *Clin. Nucl. Med. 1:*150, 1976.
17. Goldberg, B. B. *Diagnostic Ultrasound in Clinical Medicine*, p. 45. Medcon Press, New York. 1973.
18. Green, W. M., and King, D. L. Diagnostic ultrasound of the urinary tract. *J. Clin. Ultrasound 4:*55, 1976.
19. Dunnick, N. R. Radiologic diagnosis in urologic cancer. In *Principals and Management of Urologic Cancer*, p. 127. Edited by N. Javadpour. Williams & Wilkins, Baltimore, 1976.
20. Sherwood, T. Renal masses and ultrasound. *Br. Med. J. 4:*682, 1975.
21. Lingard, D. A., and Lawson, T. L. Accuracy of ultrasound in predicting the nature of renal masses. *J. Urol. 122:*724, 1979.
22. Green, W. M., King, D. L., and Gasarella, W. J. A re-appraisal of sonolucent renal masses. *Radiology 121:*163, 1973.
23. Goldberg, B. B. *Abdominal Ultrasonography: Intraperitoneal Structures in Diagnostic Uses of Ultrasound*, p. 286. Edited by B. B. Goldberg, N. M., Kotler, M. C. Ziskin, and R. D. Waxham, Grune & Stratton, New York, 1975.
24. Hassani, M. *Retroperitoneal Tomography in Ultrasound of the Abdomen.* Springer-Verlag, New York, 1976.
25. Cunningham, J. J. *Renal Tumors and Pseudotumors in Ultrasound in Urology*, p. 122. Edited by M. I. Resnick, and R. C., Sanders, Williams & Wilkins, Baltimore, 1979.
26. Gosnik, B. B. The inferior vena cava: mass effects. *AJR 130:*533, 1978.
27. Goldstein, H. M., Green, B., and Weaver, R. M. Ultrasonic detection of renal tumor extension into the inferior vena cava. *AJR 130:*1083, 1978.
28. Hattery, R. R., Williamson, B., and Stephen, S. H., *et al.* Computed tomography of renal abnormalities. *Radiol. Clin. North Am. 15:*401, 1977.
29. Magilner, A. D., and Ostrum, B. J. Computed tomography in the diagnosis of renal masses. *Radiology 126:*715, 1978.
30. Lagergren, C. Evaluation of tumor extension by whole body scans. *Urol. Res. 6:*191, 1978.
31. Weyman, P. J., McClennan, B. L., and Stanley, R. J., *et al.* Comparison of computed tomography and angiography in the evaluation of renal carcinoma. *Radiology 137:*417, 1980.
32. Bernadino, M. E., Green, B., and Goldstein, H. M. Ultrasonography evaluation of post nephrectomy renal cancer patients. *Radiology 128:*455, 1978.
33. Bernadino, M. E., deSantos, S. A., Johnson, E., and Brachen, R. B. Computed tomography—evaluation of post nephrectomy patients. *Radiology 130:*183, 1979.
34. Goldberg, B. B., and Pollock, H. H. Differentiation of renal masses using a mode ultrasound. *J. Urol. 105:*765, 1971.
35. Olsson, C. A., Mozen, J. D., and Laverte, R. O. Pulmonary cancer metastatic to kidney—a common renal neoplasm. *J. Urol. 105:*492, 1971.
36. Wentzell, R. A., and Benkeiser, S. W. Malignant lymphomatosis of the kidney. *J. Urol. 74:*177, 1955.
37. Baron, M., Keiter, F., and Brendler, H. Preoperative diagnosis of renal angiomyoplipoma. *J. Urol. 117:*701, 1977.
38. Lee, T. G., Henderson, S. C., Freeny, P. C., Raskin, M. M., Benson, E. P., and Pearse, H. D. Ultrasonic findings of renal angiomyoplipoma. *J. Clin. Ultrasound 6:*150, 1978.
39. Scheible, W., Ellenbogen, P. H., Leopold, G. R., and Stao, N. T. Lipomatous tumors of the kidney and adrenal: apparent echographic specificity. *Radiology 129:*153, 1978.
40. Levine, E., Lee, K. R., Weigel, J. W., and Farber, B. Computed tomography in the diagnosis of renal carcinoma complicating Hippel-Lindau syndrome. *Radiology 130:*703, 1979.
41. Sumner, T. E. *Pediatric Ultrasonography in Ultrasound in Urology*, p. 275. Edited by M. I. Resnick, and R. C. Sanders. Williams & Wilkins, Baltimore, 1979.

42. Harada, K., Igari, D., and Tanhaski, Y., *et al.* Staging of bladder tumors by means of transrectal ultrasonography. *J. Clin. Ultrasound 5:*388, 1977.

43. Resnick, M. I., and Boyce, W. H. *Ultrasonography of the Urinary Bladder, Seminal Vesicles and Prostate in Ultrasound in Urology*, p. 220. Edited by M. I. Resnick, and R. C. Sanders. Williams & Wilkins, Baltimore, 1979.

44. Seidelman, F. E., Cohen, W. N., and Bryan, P. J. Computed tomographic staging of bladder neoplasms. *Radiol. Clin. North Am. 15:*419, 1977.

45. Yu, W. S., Sagerman, R. H., King, G. A., Chung, C. T., and Yu, Y. W. The value of computed tomography in the management of bladder cancer. *Int. J. Radiat. Oncol. Biol. Phys. 5:*135, 1979.

46. Seidelman, F. E., Temes, S. P., Cohen, W. N., Bryan, P. J., Patic, U., and Sherry, R. G. Computed tomography of gas filled bladder. *Urology 9:*337, 1977.

47. Seidelman, F. E., Cohen, W. N., Bryan, P. T., Temes, S. P., Kraus, D., and Scheonrock, G. Accuracy of CT staging of bladder neoplasms using the gas-filled method: report of 21 patients with surgical confirmations. *AJR 130:*435, 1978.

48. Hamlin, D. J., and Cockett, A. T. K. Computed tomography of bladder: staging of bladder cancer using low density opacification technique. *Urology 13:*331, 1979.

49. Watanabe, H., Igari, D., Tanahaski, Y., Harada, K., and Saithoh, M. Development and application of the new equipment for transrectal ultrasonography. *J. Clin. Ultrasound, 2:*91, 1974.

50. Watanabe, H., Igari, D., Tanahaski, Y., Harada, K., and Saithoh, M. Measurement of size and weight of prostate by means of transrectal ultrasonotomography. *Tohoku J. Exp. Med. 114:*277, 1974.

51. Watanabe, H., Igari, D., and Tanahaski, Y., *et al.* Transrectal ultrasonotomography of the prostate. *J. Urol. 114:*734, 1975.

52. Resnick, M. I., Willard, J., and Boyce, W. H. Ultrasonic evaluation of the prostatic nodule. *J. Urol. 120:*86, 1978.

53. Resnick, M. I., Willard, J., and Boyce, W. H. Recent progress in ultrasonography of bladder and prostate. *J. Urol. 117:*44, 1977.

54. Paquette, F. R., Ahuja, A. S., Carson, P. L., Mack, L. A., Ibbott, G. S., and Johnson, M. L. A comparative study of computerized tomography and ultrasound for treatment planning of prostate cancer. *Int. J. Radiat. Oncol. Biol. Phys. 5:*289, 1979.

55. Gottesman, J. E., Sample, W. F., and Skinner, D. G., *et al:* Diagnostic ultrasound in the evaluation of scrotal masses. *J. Urol. 118:*601, 1977.

56. Sample, W. F. *Ultrasonography of the Scrotum in Ultrasound in Urology*, p. 251. Edited by M. I. Resnick, and R. C. Sanders. Williams & Wilkins, Baltimore, 1979.

57. Leopold, G. R., Woo, V. L., Scheible, F. W., Nachtsheim, D., and Gosnick, R. High resolution ultrasonography of scrotal pathology. *Radiology 131:*719, 1979.

58. Hutschenreiter, G., Alken, P., and Schneider, H. M. The value of sonography and lymphography in the detection of retroperitoneal metastases in the testicular tumor. *J. Urol. 122:*766, 1979.

59. Goldberg, B. B., Pollack, H. M., and Nicolas, H. B. *Retroperitoneum in Ultrasound in Urology*, p. 188. Edited by M. I. Resnick, and R. C. Sanders. Williams & Wilkins, Baltimore, 1979.

60. Skinner, D. G. Management of Nonseminomatous Tumors of the Testes in Genitourinary Cancer, p. 470. Edited by D. G. Skinner, and J. B. de Kernion, W. B. Saunders, Philadelphia, 1978.

61. Zelch, M. G., and Haaga, J. R. Clinical comparison of computed tomography and lymphangiography for detection of retroperitoneal adenopathy. *Radiol. Clin. North Am. 17:*157, 1979.

62. Lange, P. H., McIntire, K. R., Waldmann, T. A., *et al.* Serum alpha-fetoprotein and human chorionic gonadotropin in the diagnosis and management of nonseminomatous germ-cell testicular cancer. *N. Engl. J. Med. 295:*1237, 1976.

63. Javadpour, N., Doppman, J. L., Bergman, S. M., *et al.* Correlation of computed tomography and serum tumor markers in metastatic retroperitoneal testicular tumor. *J. Comput. Assist. Tomogr. 2:*176, 1978.

64. Javadpour, N., Kim, E., Primus, F. J., Deland, F., and Goldenberg, D. M. Radioimmuno detection of metastatic testicular cancer with radioactive antibodies to HCG. Presented to AIA annual meeting, San Francisco, Calif., 1980.

9

Diagnostic and Interventional Radiology

Rapid technological improvements have resulted in dramatic changes in the radiology of urologic cancer. Since its introduction in 1973, computed tomography (CT) has been adapted to whole body scanning. Scan times have been reduced to as little as 2 seconds and various options have been added to allow rapid sequential scanning. Tilting gantrys enable radiologists to select the most appropriate angle to scan any specific area, and reconstructed images may be generated in coronal or sagittal planes in addition to the standard transverse projection.

Diagnostic ultrasound has progressed from bistable scanning, in which images were produced by the repetitious addition of multiple scans, to gray-scale scanning where superior images are obtained with a single pass of the transducer. Analog scan converters have been replaced by digital converters which allow postsignal processing and maintain a consistent image. The improvement in real-time imaging now allows its use as a rapid screening examination for many problems. Currently, patterns of sound reflection are being examined to identify potentially tissue specific ultrasonographic signatures.[1]

CT and ultrasound are often complementary examinations. While the presence of fat improves CT images by providing the contrast to identify normal structures, fat is relatively echogenic and hampers examination by ultrasound. Conversely, thin patients are difficult to examine with CT but are nearly ideal for ultrasound. Gas inhibits sound transmission to such an extent that ultrasound examinations must occasionally be aborted due to overlying bowel gas. Although some artifact may be produced by gas, CT images do not suffer significant degradation when gas is present.

While CT and ultrasound have enabled radiologists to detect and define morphologic abnormalities, new interventional techniques allow radiolo-

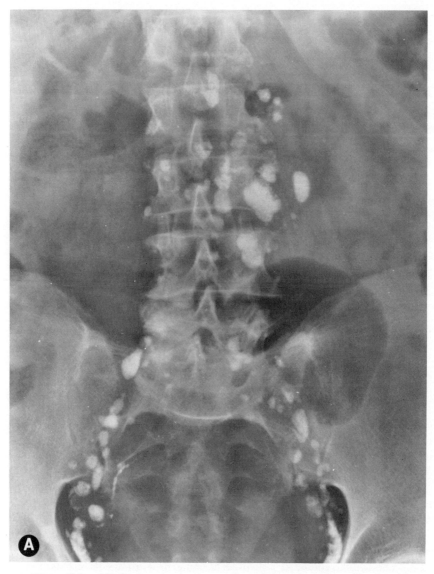

Figure 9.1. (*A*) Percutaneous retroperitoneal lymph node aspiration biopsy. Normal staging lymphogram in patient with transitional cell carcinoma of bladder.

gists to obtain tissue for cytologic or histologic evaluation and to participate directly in patient treatment. Transcatheter vascular occlusion may be therapeutic when a bleeding vessel can be identified. Embolization of tumors may make subsequent surgery much easier and safer. In other cases, tumor embolization can provide palliation or relief of pain. The application of vascular techniques to problems of nonresectable ureteral obstruction has resulted in the development of percutaneous nephrostomy techniques which decompress the collecting system and preserve renal function.

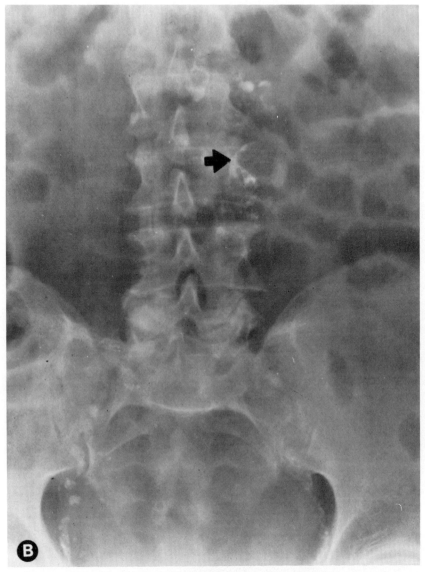

Figure 9.1. (*B*) Percutaneous retroperitoneal lymph node aspiration biopsy. Four months later than Fig. 9.1*A*, a surveillance abdominal film demonstrated enlargement of left paraaortic lymph nodes (*arrow*) indicating tumor metastases.

PERCUTANEOUS BIOPSY

Percutaneous aspiration biopsy using a thin walled 22- or 23-gauge needle has proven to be a safe and accurate procedure. Using these fine needles, virtually any tissue which can be imaged is susceptible to a directed aspiration biopsy (Fig. 9.1). Fluoroscopy and ultrasound are the most convenient modalities for directing percutaneous biopsies[2, 3] but CT also may be useful, particularly with the faster scan times.[4] A skilled cytologist, however, is essential to maximize the yield of this procedure.

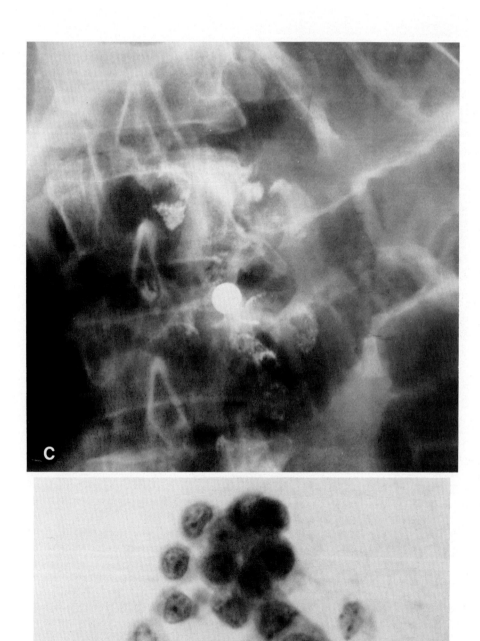

Figure 9.1. (*C* and *D*) Percutaneous retroperitoneal lymph node aspiration biopsy. (*C*) Percutaneous aspiration of the expanded lymph node was performed under fluoroscopic guidance. (*D*) The aspirated cells are malignant displaying prominent nucleoli, clumped chromatin, and a high nucleus to cytoplasm ratio.

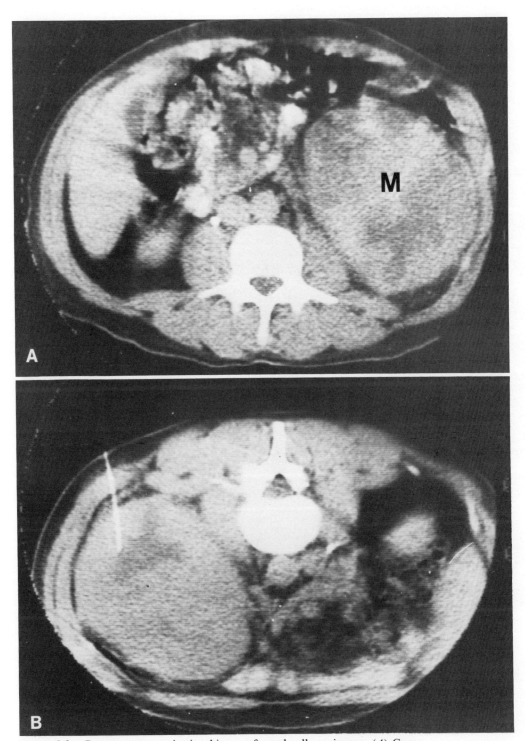

Figure 9.2. Percutaneous aspiration biopsy of renal cell carcinoma. (*A*) Computed tomography examination with patient supine demonstrates a large left renal mass (*M*). (*B*) Percutaneous aspiration biopsy with patient prone revealed malignant cells.

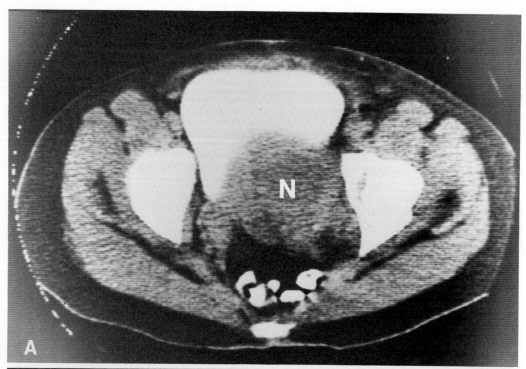

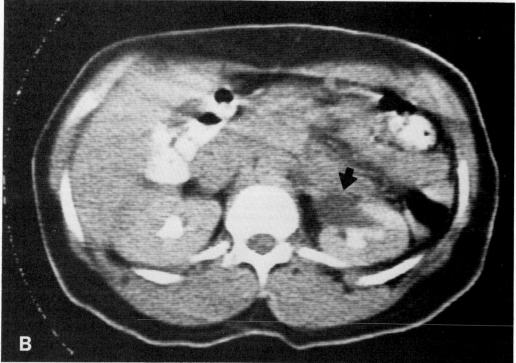

Figure 9.3. (*A* and *B*) Percutaneous nephrostomy. (*A*) A large neurofibrosarcoma (*N*) in the left pelvis indenting the posterior bladder was present on computed tomography. (*B*) Higher sections demonstrated left hydronephrosis (*arrow*).

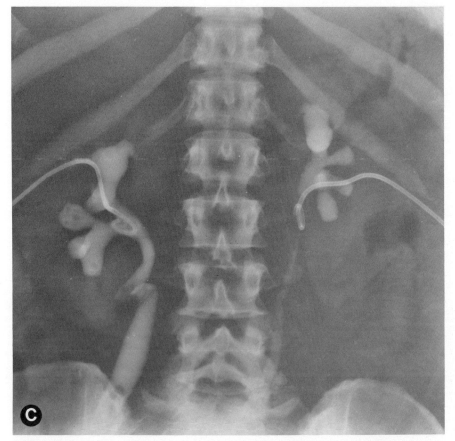

Figure 9.3. (*C*) Percutaneous nephrostomy. Subsequently, both ureters became obstructed and bilateral draining nephrostomies were placed.

A diagnosis of malignancy may be made by percutaneous aspiration biopsy in a patient with abnormal tissue but no known underlying cancer. This may be helpful in caring for a patient in certain clinical settings, but a more formal biopsy is often required to identify the histologic subtype of the tumor.

A more common use of percutaneous aspiration biopsy is during the staging of previously diagnosed tumors. In such cases, cytologic interpretation is easier as the primary tumor is known. Aspiration biopsy of abnormal areas may be performed to confirm the existence of metastatic tumor. After therapy has been initiated, tissues which harbor metastases may return toward normal. It is radiographically difficult, however, to determine if a persistent abnormality is due to scarring of the treated tumor or to residual disease. Percutaneous aspiration biopsy may be useful in documenting that the persistent abnormality harbors malignant tumor.[5]

Fine needle aspiration biopsies are less satisfactory in cases when the tumor has undergone central necrosis or when the tumor is sufficiently well differentiated that cytology is not diagnostic. In this situation, a

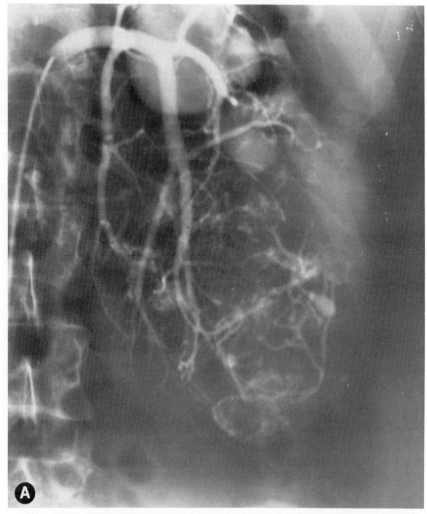

Figure 9.4. (*A*) Renal cell carcinoma. Renal arteriogram opacifies a vascular left renal mass. Presurgical vascular occlusion was performed with steel coils.

biopsy using a larger cutting needle may be warranted. Biopsy specimens 1 mm wide and 15 to 20 mm long are obtained and are suitable for histologic evaluation. The use of cutting needles, however, significantly increases the likelihood of complication. An aspiration needle may be passed through overlying structures such as bowel or blood vessels without causing clinically detectable damage, but great care must be taken to precisely position the entire biopsy segment of a cutting needle in the tumor. The segment of tissue removed by the cutting needle is much larger and thus the chance of removing a portion of adjacent normal tissue is increased. If medium or large vessels either near or within the tumor are included in the biopsy, the patient may develop severe hemorrhage. The risks of other complications depend upon the area biopsied. Although cutting needle biopsies provide much better specimens for

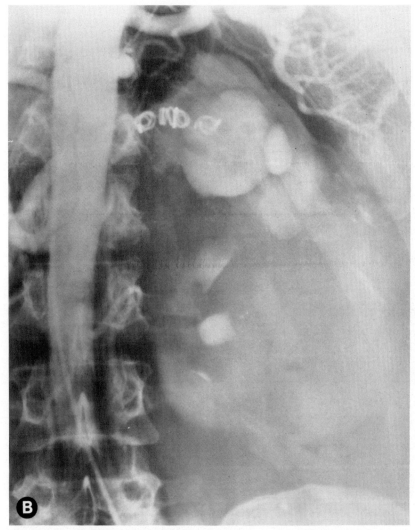

Figure 9.4. (*B*) Renal cell carcinoma. Repeat aortogram demonstrates the complete occlusion of the renal artery. (Case courtesy of Dr. David R. Buck, National Naval Medical Center, Bethesda, Md.)

pathologic examination than aspiration biopsies, the benefits of this procedure must be weighed against the increased risks to the patient.

Directed percutaneous biopsies may be obtained from any area which can be radiologically imaged. The kidney is well suited to directed biopsy (Fig. 9.2) as it can be readily imaged by CT, ultrasound, or fluoroscopy after the injection of intravenous contrast material. Masses in the adrenal gland can be biopsied under CT guidance, while lesions in the wall of the bladder can be approached with CT, ultrasound, or fluoroscopic control. The prostate is imaged with both CT and ultrasound although differentiation of malignant from nonmalignant tissue within the gland is more difficult. Although mass lesions of the ureter are rare, adjacent masses may cause ureteral obstruction. These masses may be directly imaged and

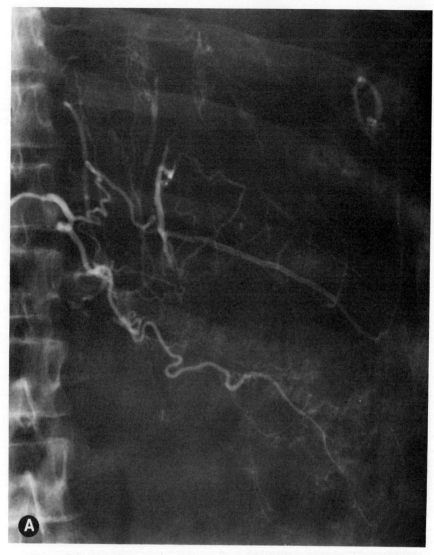

Figure 9.5. (*A*) Transcatheter vascular occlusion of adrenal carcinoma. The arterial supply of this large left adrenal carcinoma arose from several vessels but most prominently from (*A*) the T11 intercostal and (*B*, *see below*) L3 lumbar arteries.

biopsied using either CT or ultrasound localization. Indirectly obstructing mass lesions can be localized by opacifying the ureter and directing the biopsy to the adjacent tissue.

PERCUTANEOUS NEPHROSTOMY

Ureteral obstruction, if unrelieved, will progress to renal failure and uremia. This is particularly unfortunate when the kidneys are otherwise

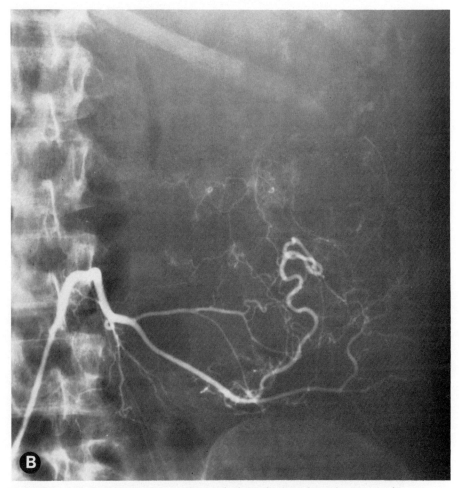

Figure 9.5 (*B*) Transcatheter vascular occlusion of adrenal carcinoma. A significant portion of the arterial supply of this large left adrenal carcinoma arose from the L3 lumbar artery.

normal. Percutaneous nephrostomy offers a nonsurgical method of urinary diversion which decompresses the collecting system and preserves renal function.[6-9] External drainage systems are easily cared for and may enable the patient to maintain an acceptable life style. In some cases, a ureteral stent may be left in place to bypass the obstruction and the external drainage catheter removed.

Percutaneous nephrostomies may be placed with either ultrasound or CT guidance but are usually done under fluoroscopic control. If there is renal function, a small amount of contrast material may be injected intravenously to opacify the renal pelvis. Otherwise, a 22-gauge fine needle is used to puncture the renal pelvis (from a posterior approach through the renal parenchyma) and contrast material is injected directly into the collecting system. Once the target is identified, a larger needle and catheter is passed through the kidney into the renal pelvis. A more

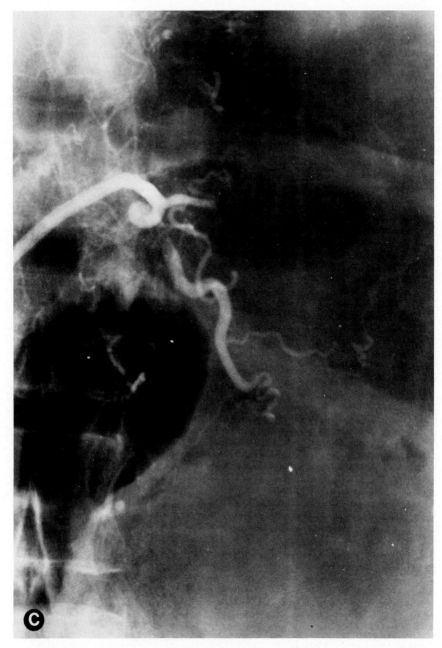

Figure 9.5. (*C*) Transcatheter vascular occlusion of adrenal carcinoma. Repeat injection of vessels shown in Fig. 9.5*A* after embolization with Gelfoam Sterile Sponge demonstrates the vascular occlusion.

posterolateral approach is used so the patient will be comfortable in the supine position. A variety of catheters are available but the use of one with a tightly curved end and multiple side holes is preferable. This catheter is left in place, with the curved portion in the renal pelvis and draining to a reservoir outside the patient (Fig. 9.3).

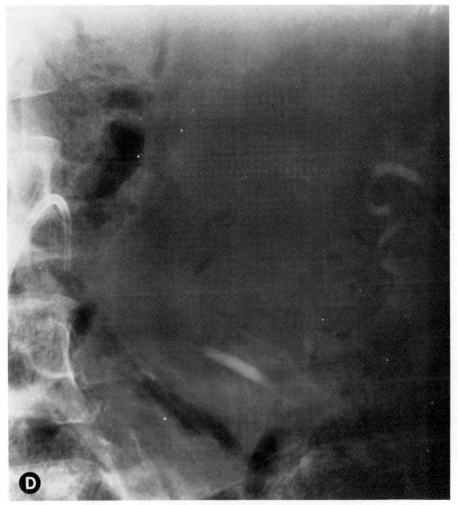

Figure 9.5. (*D*) Transcatheter vascular occlusion of adrenal carcinoma. Repeat injection of vessel shown in Fig. 9.5*B* after embolization with Gelfoam Sterile Sponge demonstrates the vascular occlusion.

If a ureteral obstruction can be passed, a catheter can be used to provide passage of urine into the bladder. A variety of catheters are available including a detachable catheter which can be left in the ureter as an indwelling ureteral stent, in which event the external portion of the catheter is removed. If the ureteral stent becomes unnecessary, it may be removed from the bladder by cystoscopy.

VASCULAR OCCLUSION

Transcatheter vascular occlusion has been used to stop hemorrhage from a variety of sites such as bowel, liver, kidney, and bladder.[10–12] Temporary vascular occlusion may be obtained by injecting autologous clot or Gelfoam Sterile Sponge through the catheter into the bleeding

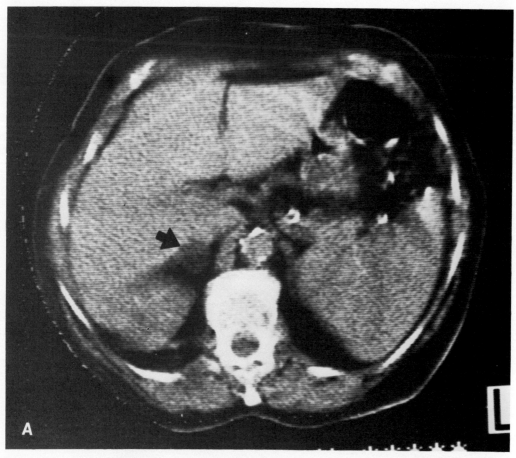

Figure 9.6. (*A*) Right adrenal adenoma. Computed tomography demonstrates a low density right adrenal mass (*arrow*) in a patient with primary aldosteronism.

vessel. This will frequently stop the hemorrhage which does not recur even after the clot has been resorbed.

Patients with urologic cancer may benefit from vascular occlusion to: (1) decrease tumor vascularity prior to surgery (Fig. 9.4); (2) provide palliation for an unresectable tumor (Fig. 9.5); or (3) relieve pain arising from a tumor. When permanent arterial occlusion is desired, nonresorbable materials such as steel pellets or coils are appropriate. The straightened coil is passed through a catheter into the vessel to be occluded. When the coil exits from the catheter, it resumes the coiled shape. Wool threads attached to the coil aid in the thrombogenicity. Other materials such as cyanoacrylate which can be injected into the vascular tree of the tumor are currently being evaluated.[13]

ADRENAL TUMORS

Tumors of the adrenal gland may present either as a result of local

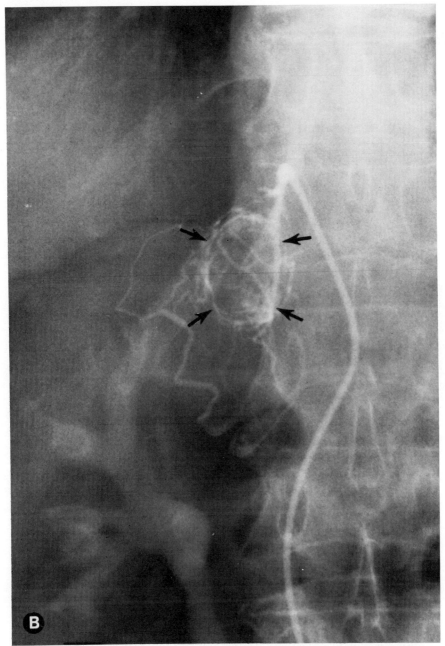

Figure 9.6. (*B*) Right adrenal adenoma. Venous sampling confirmed the presence of a right adrenal aldosteronoma which was also seen (*arrows*) on the adrenal venogram.

tumor bulk or as a manifestation of hormones produced by the tumor. Approximately one half of adrenal cortical carcinomas are functional and most of these present as either Cushing's or virilization syndrome.[14-16]

Among patients presenting with functional adrenal cortical tumors, the

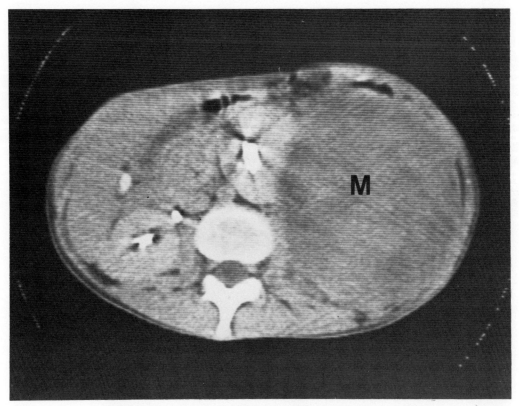

Figure 9.7. Adrenal carcinoma. A huge retroperitoneal mass (*M*) is displacing the kidney anteromedially.

benign adenomas tend to be smaller than 4 cm in diameter, while the adrenal carcinomas are usually larger than 5 cm in diameter. Malignant adrenal tumors frequently extend along the adrenal vein into the inferior vena cava.[17] When either large size or intravenous extension is noted, malignancy is more likely. Patients with nonfunctional adrenal carcinomas usually present with pain, a palpable mass, or with metastatic disease. They also may be found during the investigation of an unrelated problem.

The patient who presents with manifestations of overproduction of an adrenal hormone must be evaluated to determine if this is due to a primary adrenal tumor or bilateral adrenal hyperplasia.[18] The radiographic evaluation depends primarily upon CT, which can often make this distinction (Fig. 9.6). If the CT examination is not diagnostic, however, adrenal venous sampling is indicated.

Bilateral adrenal venous samples are obtained and two adrenal cortical hormones measured: the hormone responsible for the clinical syndrome and a second hormone unaffected by overproduction of the first.[19] Thus, when a patient with Conn's syndrome is being studied, both aldosterone and cortisol are measured in the samples obtained. The ratio of aldosterone to cortisol is calculated to correct for the dilution in the sample by blood obtained from the renal or phrenic veins or inferior vena cava.

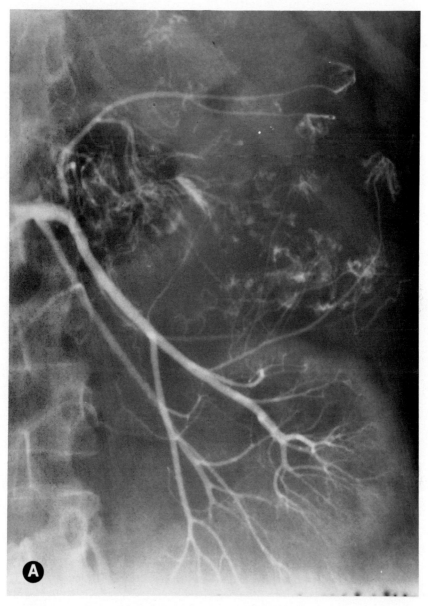

Figure 9.8. (*A*) Left adrenal carcinoma. Arterial phases of left renal arteriogram demonstrate a large suprarenal mass with tumor vascularity.

A large adrenal tumor (Fig. 9.7) or evidence of extension into the inferior vena cava suggests malignancy. In such cases, the CT examination should be followed by venography (Fig. 9.8) to precisely define the extent of the venous invasion. Arteriography also will be useful to identify the degree of vascularity as well as the major supplying vessels. If the patient is a surgical candidate, preoperative tumor embolization may be performed to diminish tumor vascularity. Tumor embolization may be

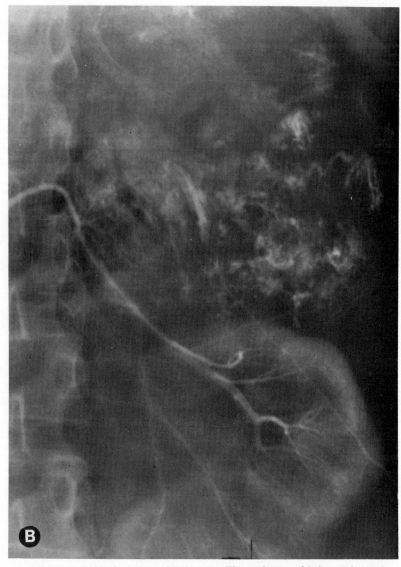

Figure 9.8. (*B*) Left adrenal carcinoma. Capillary phases of left renal arteriogram demonstrate a large suprarenal mass with tumor vascularity.

employed in nonsurgical patients as a palliative effort to relieve pain or to treat a local complication such as hemorrhage (Fig. 9.5).

Pheochromocytomas may be diagnosed by measuring elevated serum levels of catecholamines. The problem for the radiologist is localization. CT usually permits identification of the tumor, whether it is located in one of the adrenal glands or the paraaortic tissues (Fig. 9.9). If CT reveals normal adrenal glands, the examination should be carried down to the pelvis to look for an ectopic tumor. Arteriography is often useful to confirm the vascular nature of the suspected pheochromocytoma and to clarify the arterial supply.

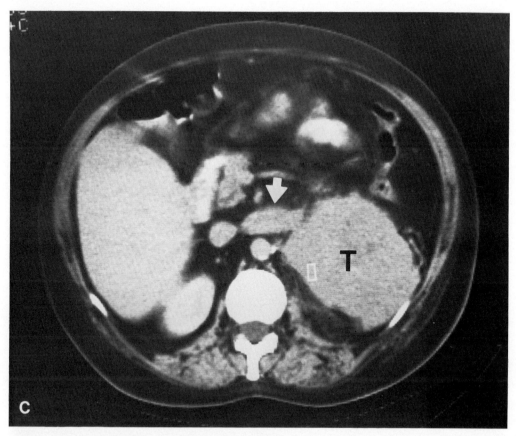

Figure 9.8. (*C*) Left adrenal carcinoma. The tumor mass (*T*) as well as intravenous extension (*arrow*) is seen on computed tomography.

In patients with pheochromocytoma, venous sampling is reserved for diagnostic problems such as inability to localize the primary tumor or for recurrent or metastatic tumor. In such cases, either epinephrine or norepinephrine may be measured. Venous samples are obtained from the most likely sites and further diagnostic efforts can be concentrated on the area of elevated hormone levels. One must also remember that patients with pheochromocytoma may belong to the multiple endocrine neoplasia syndrome (MEN) in which other endocrine tumors may be present or develop later. In addition these patients with the MEN syndrome have a higher incidence of bilateral pheochromocytomas.[20]

RENAL CELL CARCINOMA

Patients with renal cell carcinoma commonly present with flank pain, a palpable mass, hematuria, or anemia. The intravenous pyelogram (IVP) is the initial screening radiographic procedure. Primary renal tumors distort the pyelocalyceal system, have poorly defined margins, and are

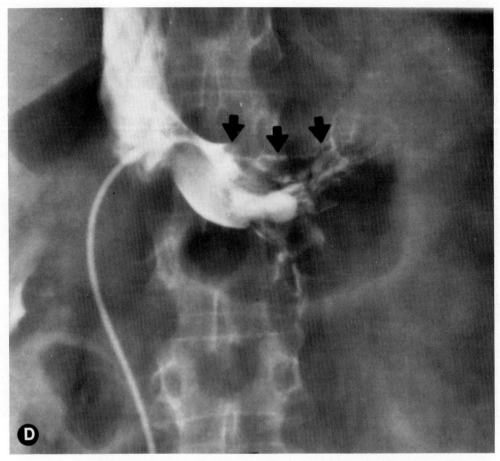

Figure 9.8. (*D*) Left adrenal carcinoma. A selective venogram confirms the extension of the carcinoma down the adrenal vein into the left renal vein (*arrows*). (Case courtesy of Dr. John A. Long, Jr., Arlington Hospital, Arlington, Va.)

occasionally calcified. Ultrasound is useful for confirming the solid nature of such masses.

If the renal mass has features suggesting a renal cyst, aspiration may be warranted. This may be guided either by fluoroscopy after the injection of intravenous contrast material or with ultrasound. Fluid withdrawn from benign cysts is clear, contains no fat, and has a negative cytology. If these criteria are not met, the nature of the cyst must be considered indeterminant and further studies obtained. The increased use of CT and ultrasound has demonstrated many more cysts than were identified on excretory urograms and, although cyst puncture has become a safe and accurate procedure, it is difficult to justify the aspiration of every renal cyst discovered.

Computed tomography may provide a clue as to the etiology of a renal mass lesion by providing density measurements. Angiomyolipomas characteristically appear as a localized area of fat density on CT and increased

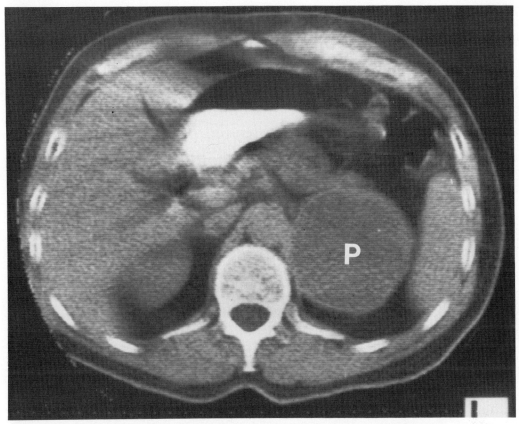

Figure 9.9. Pheochromocytoma. A large left adrenal pheochromocytoma (*P*) is well demonstrated on computed tomography.

echogenicity on ultrasound.[21] The CT appearance of renal cell carcinoma is sufficiently varied, however, that biopsy may be required to confirm the diagnosis.

CT contributes to the staging evaluation of renal cell carcinoma by demonstrating local tumor extension.[22, 23] Involvement of the inferior vena cava and left renal vein are often demonstrated on CT.[24] Tumor growth is more difficult to detect on the right due to the shorter and more oblique course of the right renal vein. Regional lymph node metastases as well as invasion of Gerota's fascia and involvement of adjacent muscles or the liver also may be identified. Although intravascular tumor extension can be demonstrated with either angiography or ultrasound, involvement of adjacent organs or muscles can be shown only with CT.

Selective renal arteriography is helpful preoperatively as it defines the degree of vascularity of the renal tumor, and demonstrates any anomalies in the arterial supply to the involved kidney. Identifying renal venous and inferior vena caval extension is also useful to the urologist.[25, 26] Although the arterial supply to intravenous extension of a renal carcinoma can often be seen on the arteriogram, inferior vena cavography or renal venography are indicated to define the extent of venous invasion.

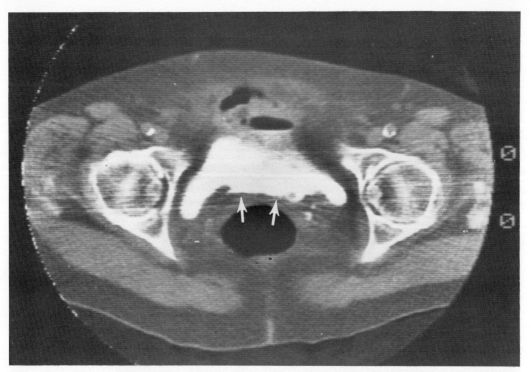

Figure 9.10. Bladder cancer. Computed tomography demonstrates the irregular posterior wall (*arrows*) of transitional cell carcinoma of the bladder.

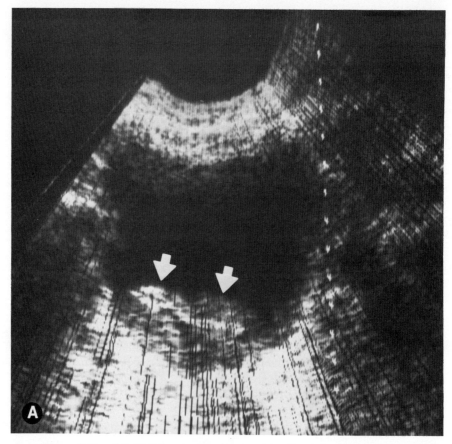

Figure 9.11. (*A*) Bladder cancer. A mass extending into the bladder lumen is well visualized (*arrows*) by ultrasound in a transverse view.

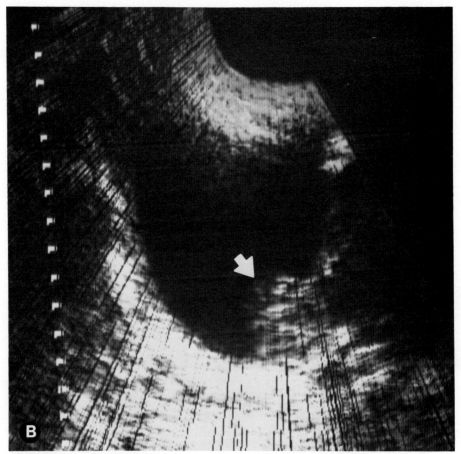

Figure 9.11. (*B*) Bladder cancer. A mass extending into the bladder lumen in well visualized (*arrow*) by ultrasound in a longitudinal view.

The treatment of renal cell carcinoma is surgical excision. If metastases are present, nephrectomy may still result in regression of metastases. Not all patients are adequate surgical candidates and transcatheter vascular occlusion may provide palliation. Vascular occlusion also has been used to diminish tumor vascular supply prior to surgery (Fig. 9.4) or to treat complications of the tumor such as hematuria or high output cardiac failure.

BLADDER CANCER

The diagnosis of bladder cancer is usually made at cystoscopy. An IVP should precede cystoscopy to alert the urologist to upper tract pathology such as ureteral obstruction or renal pelvic filling defects which suggest a transitional cell carcinoma.

The radiographic staging evaluation of bladder cancer includes bipedal lymphography,[27] arteriography,[28] CT[29-31] (Fig. 9.10), and ultrasound[32]

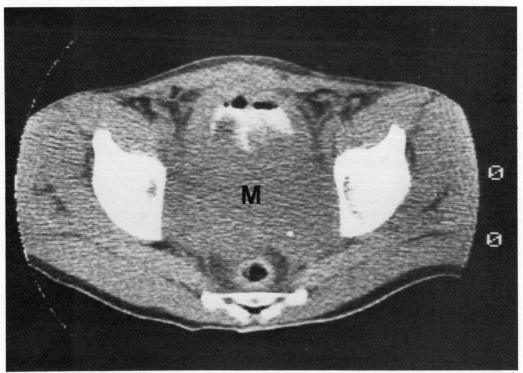

Figure 9.12. Rhabdomyosarcoma of the prostate. A huge mass (*M*) distorts the prostate and is invading the posterior wall of the bladder. Seen by computed tomography.

(Fig. 9.11). The lymphatic drainage of the bladder is to the hypogastric or internal iliac lymph nodes which are not routinely opacified with pedal lymphography. Thus, metastases must reach the common iliac or paraaortic lymph node chains before they can be recognized. This inherent limitation in lymphography has prevented its widespread acceptance as a staging tool. However, ability to monitor opacified lymph nodes with surveillance abdominal films[27] and the development of fine needle aspiration techniques has provided a resurgance of interest in lymphography for bladder cancer (Fig. 9.1).

Arteriography has been advocated as a method of detecting local pelvic extension[28] but is being replaced by noninvasive modalities such as CT and ultrasound.[29-32] When adequate pelvic fat is present, CT can be used to detect local tumor extension.

PROSTATE CANCER

The diagnosis of prostatic cancer is made by biopsy. Although cystography and excretory urography can detect enlargement of the prostate gland, this is a nonspecific finding most commonly due to benign prostatic hypertrophy.

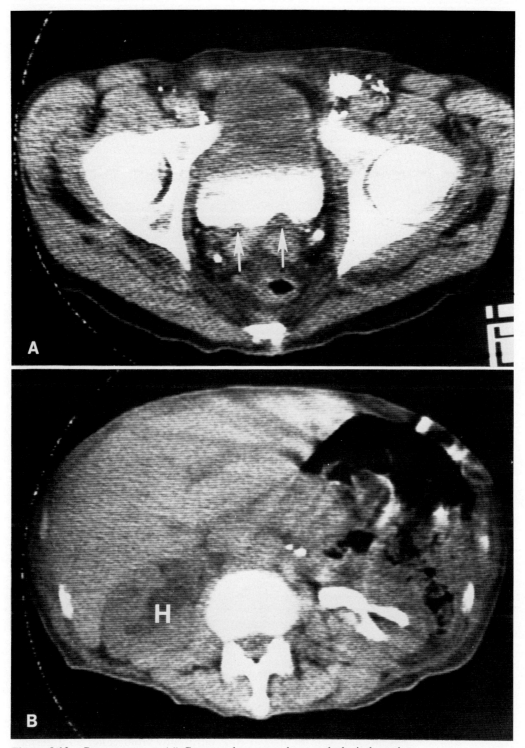

Figure 9.13. Prostate cancer. (*A*) Computed tomography reveals the indentation upon the posterior surface of the bladder by the prostate carcinoma (*arrows*). (*B*) Higher sections demonstrate hydronephrosis of the right renal collecting system (*H*).

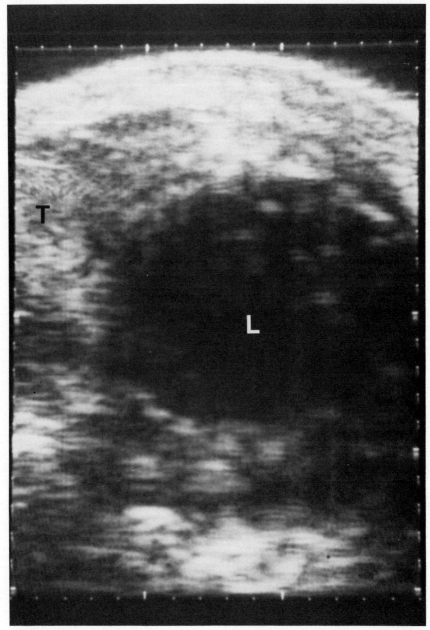

Figure 9.14. Testicular mass. Transverse ultrasound scan of the testis revealed an echolucent lymphomatous mass (*L*) within the more echogenic normal testicular tissue (*T*). (Case courtesy of Dr. F. William Scheible, San Diego University Hospital, San Diego, Calif.)

The prostate can be imaged with ultrasound from either an anterior approach through the bladder or posteriorly from a transducer in the rectum.[33] The anterior approach is limited by the pubic bone which prevents optimal examination. The transrectal approach has been used

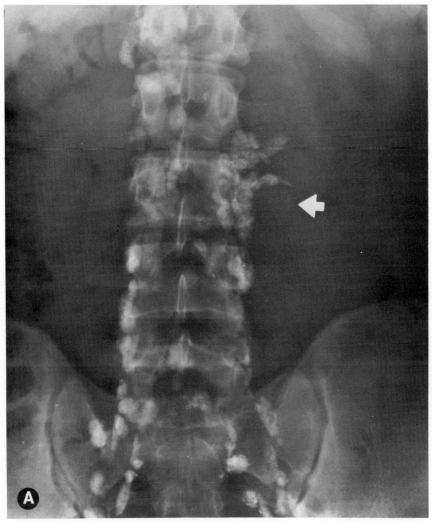

Figure 9.15. (*A*) Testicular carcinoma. Metastases to the paraaortic lymph nodes (*arrow*) from embryonal carcinoma of the left testis are demonstrated by lymphography.

successfully with excellent results[34] but is not yet widely used in the United States. While the prostate gland enlarges symmetrically in benign prostatic hypertrophy, cancer produces a more focal enlargement which produces irregular internal echoes.

Bipedal lymphography continues to be a useful modality in staging prostate cancer.[35, 36] The application of fine needle aspiration biopsy techniques to uncertain cases has improved the accuracy of the lymphographic interpretation.[37, 38]

Computed tomography demonstrates local pelvic extension of prostate cancer as it does with bladder tumors.[39–40] Invasion of the bladder wall (Fig. 9.12), involvement of local lymph nodes or the pelvic sidewall, and

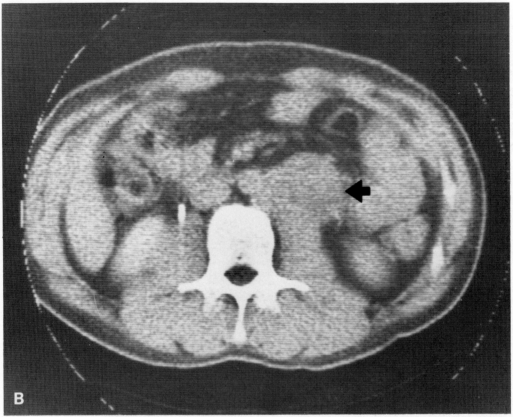

Figure 9.15. (*B*) Testicular carcinoma. Metastases to the paraaortic lymph nodes (*arrow*) from embryonal carcinoma of the left testis are demonstrated by computed tomography.

ureteral obstruction (Fig. 9.13) can all be appreciated. This information can be used directly for CT simulation of radiation therapy treatment ports.

TESTICULAR CANCER

Due to the risk of tumor dissemination, testicular masses are not biopsied and radical orchiectomy with histologic evaluation is the procedure of choice. The development of a high resolution, high frequency, transducer for use in superficial tissues such as the testis now allows a noninvasive method of evaluating scrotal masses.[41] An ultrasound examination with a small parts scanner can differentiate nontesticular scrotal masses such as hydroceles, spermatoceles, or chronic epididymitis.[42] True testicular masses also can be identified (Fig. 9.14). Testicular carcinoma appears as a region of decreased echogenicity within the more echogenic normal testis. Further evaluation in larger series of patients must be undertaken before small-parts scanning can replace orchiectomy, how-

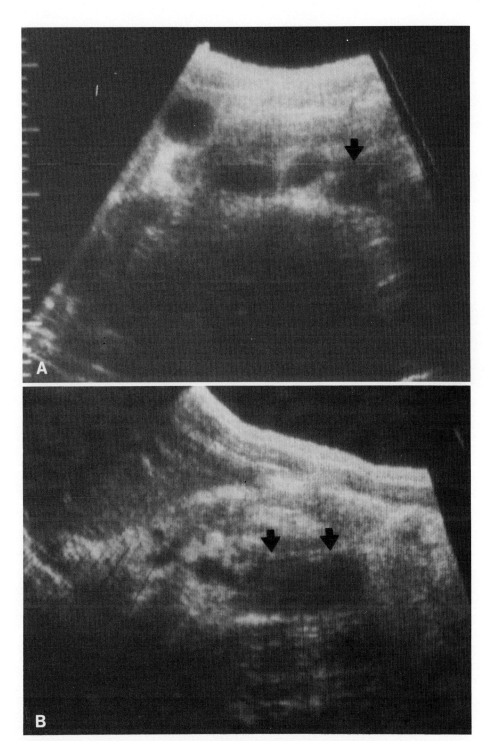

Figure 9.16. Testicular carcinoma. Large echolucent areas (*arrows*) on ultrasound examination in (*A*) transverse and (*B*) longitudinal projections of the abdomen indicate paraaortic lymph node metastases.

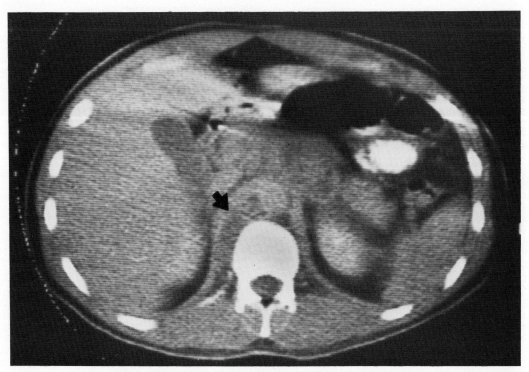

Figure 9.17. Retrocrural metastases. Computed tomography identifies metastases from testicular carcinoma in the retrocrural space (*arrow*).

ever, this technique is particularly attractive in those patients with a single functioning testis.

The staging evaluation of testicular cancer includes lymphangiography and CT (Fig. 9.15), ultrasound (Fig. 9.16), and CT of the abdomen and full lung tomography. The accuracy of lymphography for detecting retroperitoneal lymph node metastases is approximately 85%.[43, 44] Lymphography has several advantages over either CT or ultrasound. (1) Since resolution is better on abdominal radiographs, smaller lymph node metastases can be detected with lymphography; (2) the opacified lymph nodes provide convenient targets for percutaneous fine needle aspiration to clarify equivocal studies or provide cytologic proof when needed; and (3) once the lymph nodes are opacified, surveillance abdominal radiographs may be easily obtained to monitor disease progression.

The precise extent of bulky disease is, however, much better appreciated by either CT or ultrasound.[44-46] In addition, neither of these modalities is limited to visualization of the paraaortic lymph nodes as is the lymphogram and other frequently involved areas such as renal hila and retrocrural regions (Fig. 9.17) may be evaluated. Large studies are currently underway to assess the proper role of these examinations in the staging of testicular cancer.

REFERENCES

1. Price, R. R., Jones, T. B., Goddard, J. and James, A. E., Jr. Basic concepts of ultrasonic tissue characterization. *Radiol. Clin. North. Am. 18:*21, 1980.
2. Zornoza, J., Wallace, S., Goldstein, H. M., Lukeman, J. M. and Jing, B. S. Transperitoneal percutaneous retroperitoneal lymph node aspiration biopsy. *Radiology 122:*111, 1977.
3. Ferrucci, J. T., Jr., Wittenberg, J., Mueller, P. R., Simeone, J. F., Harbin, W. P., Kirkpatrick, R. H., and Taft, P. D. Diagnosis of abdominal malignancy by radiologic fine needle aspiration biopsy. *AJR 134:*323, 1980.
4. Haaga, J. R., and Alfidi, R. J. Precise biopsy localization by computed tomography. Radiology 118:603, 1976.
5. Dunnick, N. R., Fisher, R. I., Chu, E. W., and Young, R. C. Percutaneous aspiration of retroperitoneal lymph nodes in ovarian cancer. *AJR 135:*109, 1980.
6. Pfister, R. C., and Newhouse, J. H. Interventional percutaneous pyeloureteral techniques: I Antegrade pyelography and ureteral perfusion. *Radiol. Clin. North Am. 17:* 341, 1979.
7. Pfister, R. C., and Newhouse, J. H. Interventional percutaneous pyeloureteral techniques. II Percutaneous nephrostomy and other procedures. *Radiol. Clin. North Am. 17:* 351, 1979.
8. Barbaric, Z. L. Interventional radiology. *Radiol. Clin. North Am. 17:*413, 1979.
9. Stables, D. P., and Johnson, M. Percutaneous nephrostomy: the role of ultrasound. *Clin. Diagn. Ultrasound. 2:*73, 1979.
10. White, R. I., Jr. Arterial embolization for control of renal hemorrhage. *J. Urol. 115:*121, 1976.
11. Mitchell, M. E., Waltman, A. C., Athanasoulis, C. A., Kerr, W. S., Jr., and Deetler, S. P. Control of massive prostatic bleeding with angiographic techniques. *J. Urol. 115:*692, 1976.
12. Athanasoulis, C. A. Therapeutic applications of angiography. *N. Engl. J. Med. 302:* 1117, 1980.
13. Goldin, A. R., Barnes, D. R., and Jacobsen, I. Percutaneous infarction of renal tumors. Comparison between gelatin sponge embolization and cyanoacrylate occlusion. *Urology 11:*197, 1978.
14. Lipsett, M. B., Hertz, R., and Ross, G. T. Clinical and pathophysiological aspects of adrenocortical carcinoma. *Am. J. Med. 35:*374, 1963.
15. Hutter, A. M., and Kayhoe, D. E. Adrenal cortical carcinoma. Clinical features of 138 patients. *Am. J. Med. 41:*572, 1966.
16. Sullivan, M., Boileau, M., and Hodges, C. V. Adrenal cortical carcinoma. *J. Urol. 120:* 660, 1978.
17. Dunnick, N. R., Doppman, J. L., and Geelhoed, G. W. Intravenous extension of endocrine tumors. *AJR 135:*471, 1980.
18. Dunnick, N. R., Schaner, E. G., Doppman, J. L., Strott, C. A., Gill, J. R., Jr., and Javadpour, N. Computed tomography in adrenal tumors. *AJR 132:*43, 1979.
19. Dunnick, N. R., Doppman, J. L., Mills, S. R., and Gill, J. R., Jr. Preoperative diagnosis and localization of aldosteronomas by measurement of corticosteroids in adrenal venous blood. *Radiology 133:*331, 1979.
20. Cho, K. J., Freier, D. T., McCormick, T. L., Nishiyama, R. H., Forrest, M. E., Kaufman, A., and Borlaza, G. S. Adrenal medullary disease in multiple endocrine neoplasia type II. *AJR 134:*23, 1980.
21. Shawker, T. H., Horvath, K.L., Dunnick, N. R., and Javadpour, N. Renal angiomyolipoma: diagnosis by combined ultrasound and computed tomography. *J. Urol. 121:*675, 1979.
22. Love, L., Churchill, R., Reynes, C., Schuster, G. A., Moncada, R., and Berkow, A. Computed tomography staging of renal carcinoma. *Urol. Radiol. 1:*3, 1979.
23. Levine, E., Lee, K. R., and Weigel, J. Preoperative determination of abdominal extent of renal cell carcinoma by computed tomography. *Radiology 132:*395, 1979.
24. Marks, W. M., Korobkin, M., Callen, P. W., and Kaiser, J. A. CT diagnosis of tumor thrombosis of the renal vein and inferior vena cava. *AJR 131:*843, 1978.

DIAGNOSTIC AND INTERVENTIONAL RADIOLOGY   195

25. Madayag, M. A., Ambos, M. A., Lefleur, R. S., and Bosniak, M. A. Involvement of the inferior vena cava in patients with renal cell carcinoma. *Radiology 133:*321, 1979.
26. Goncharenko, V., Gerlock, A. J., Kadir, S., and Turner, B. Incidence and distribution of venous extension in 70 hypernephromas. *AJR 133:*263, 1979.
27. Johnson, D. E., Kaesler, K. E., Kaminsky, S., Jing, B. S., and Wallace, S. Lymphangiography as an aid in staging bladder carcinoma. *South. Med. J. 69:*28, 1976.
28. Lang, E. K. Angiography in the diagnosis and staging of pelvic neoplasms. *Radiology 134:*353, 1980.
29. Seidelmann, F. E., Cohen, W. N., Bryan, P. J., Temes, S. P., Kraus, D., and Schoenrock, G. Accuracy of CT staging of balldder neoplasms using the gas filled method: report of 21 patients with surgical confirmation. *AJR 130:*735, 1978.
30. McClennan, B. L., and Fair, W. R. CT Scanning in Urology. *Urol. Clin. North Am. 6:* 343, 1979.
31. Schlager, B., Asbel, S. O., Baker, A. S., Sklaroff, D. M., Seydel, H. G., and Ostrum, B. J. The use of computed tomography scanning in treatment planning for bladder cancer. *Int. J. Radiat. Oncol. Biol. Phys. 5:*99, 1979.
32. McLaughlin, I. S., Morley, P., Deane, R. F., Barnett, E., Graham, A. G., and Kyle, K. F. Ultrasound in the staging of bladder tumors. *Br. J. Urol. 47:*51, 1975.
33. Watanabe, H. Prostatic ultrasound. *Clin. Diagn. Ultrasound. 2:*125, 1979.
34. Kazuya, H., Dairoku, I., and Yoshikatsu, T. Gray scale transrectal ultrasonography of the prostate. *J. Clin. Ultrasound. 7:*45, 1979.
35. Spellman, M. C., Castellino, R. A., Ray, G. R., Pistenma, D. A., and Bagshaw, M. D. An evaluation of lymphography in localized carcinoma of the prostate. *Radiology 125:* 637, 1977.
36. Prando, A., Wallace, S., VonEschenback, A. C., Jing, B. S., Rosengren, J. E., and Hussey, D. H. Lymphangiography in staging of carcinoma of the prostate. *Radiology 131:*641, 1979.
37. Efremidis, S. C., Pagliarulo, A., Dan, S. J., Wever, H. N., Dillon, R. N., Nieburgs, H., and Mitty, H. A. Post-lymphangiographic fine needle aspiration biopsy in staging carcinoma of the prostate: preliminary report. *J. Urol. 122:*495, 1979.
38. MacIntosh, P. K., Thomson, K. R., and Barbaric, Z. L. Percutaneous transperitoneal lymph node biopsy as a means of improving lymphographic diagnosis. *Radiology 131:* 647, 1979.
39. Korobkin, M., Callen, P. W., and Fisch, A. E. Computed tomography of the pelvis and retroperitoneum. *Radiol. Clin. North Am. 17:*301, 1979.
40. Price, J. M., and Davidson, A. J. Computed tomography in the evaluation of the suspected carcinomatous prostate. *Urol. Radiol. 1:*39, 1979.
41. Leopold, G. R., Woo, V. L., Scheible, F. W., Nachtsheim, D., and Gosink, B. B. High resolution ultrasonography of scrotal pathology. *Radiology 131:*719, 1979.
42. Sample, W. F., Gottesman, J. E., Skinner, D. G., and Ehrlich, R. M. Gray scale ultrasound of the scrotum. *Radiology 127:*225, 1978.
43. Kademian, M., and Wirtanen, G. Accuracy of bipedal lymphography in testicular tumors. *Urology 9:*218, 1977.
44. Dunnick, N. R., and Javadpour, N. The value of computed tomography and lymphography in detecting retroperitoneal metastases from non-seminomatous testicular tumors. *AJR 136:*1093, 1981
45. Lee, J. K. T., McClennan, B. L., Stanley, R. J., and Sagel, S. S. Computed tomography in the staging of testicular neoplasms. *Radiology 130:*387, 1979.
46. Burney, B. T., and Klatte, E. C. Ultrasound and computed tomography of the abdomen in the staging and management of testicular carcinoma. *Radiology 132:*415, 1979.

10

Advances in Surgery of Urologic Cancer

Improved diagnostic and therapeutic procedures have led to earlier diagnosis and more accurate surgical treatment of certain urologic cancers. These improved diagnostic and therapeutic procedures include sonography, computed tomography, tumor markers, and interventional percutaneous techniques. The percutaneous techniques include transcatheter embolization, nephrostomy, biopsy, perfusion of therapeutic agents, and/or control of bleeding[1, 2] (Table 10.1). Percutaneous angiographic procedures may serve to reduce blood flow or ablate the function of an organ. Percutaneous antegrade pyelographic procedures may also serve as a temporary or permanent drainage of an obstructed kidney or for aspiration biopsy and instillation of chemotherapeutic agents to the tumor. The applications of these techniques will be discussed under the specific organs. Although the primary treatment of urologic cancer still remains surgical management, the limitations of surgery alone also has been defined more accurately. Improved surgical techniques, defining their indications, and combining them with efficatious chemotherapy and radiotherapy have prolonged the survival of certain urologic cancers including testicular cancer, Wilms' tumor, and embryonal rhabdomyosarcomas. The objectives of this chapter are to review the recent advances in surgical management and its limitations as applied to urologic cancer.

ADRENAL CANCER

The recent advances in management of adrenal neoplasms have been mainly in the basic adrenal function, localization techniques by venous sampling, hormonal markers, and computed tomography. Although some progress has been made in physiology and localization of adrenal tumors, many problems, including the need for adjuvant therapy, remain unresolved. Adrenal carcinoma, a slow growing tumor with relative low

Table 10.1
Interventional radiology in certain urologic cancer

Embolization of tumors
  Adrenal tumors
  Renal cell carcinoma
Control of bleeding
  Selective occlusion of the artery
  Ablation of function of the organ
Intraarterial infusion
  Renal cancer
  Bladder cancer
  Transcatheter brush biopsy of intravenous tumor thrombi
    for histologic diagnosis

propensity to metastasize, is one of the surgical diseases of the adrenal gland. The majority of the adrenal carcinomas are functional and most commonly produce 17-ketosteroids (17-Ks) or 17-hydroxycorticosteroids (17-OHCS). There the recurrent tumor may be detected by following these hormonal markers. Due to the lack of chemotherapeutic or other modalities or therapy, surgery has played an important role in the management of these patients.[3] In general, the treatment of choice of the adrenal neoplasms are surgical resection including their isolated resectable metastases. We also have gained the impression that patients with bulky localized tumor have prolonged survival and live more comfortably after cytoreductive surgery. However, the limited number of such patients had prevented a prospective randomized study of the role of cytoreductive surgery in this tumor. We have occasionally undertaken an en bloc removal of the mass, including the spleen and/or kidney involved in invasion. Also, in following a given patient after resection of primary tumor, we have removed the inferior vena caval tumor followed by liver and/or pulmonary resection of isolated tumor. We have utilized a combined thoracoabdominal and sternal splitting incisions to remove a large primary tumor with invasion into the suprarenal portion of the inferior vena cava (IVC) extending to the entrance of the left atrium with good results in selected cases[3] (Fig. 10.1). The actual value of this kind of surgery is not completely clear due to lack of controlled clinical trials. However, in the absence of other effective modalities, it appears that these efforts are justified in selected cases. Although the transabdominal incision remains the approach of choice for the majority of adrenal tumors, posterior and lateral approaches have been utilized in selected cases, especially in benign tumors that are well localized preoperatively.

KIDNEY

Percutaneous needle aspiration and cytology of renal cystic masses have made renal exploration unnecessary for most of these lesions. They also have helped the diagnosis of a necrotic tumor by aspiration of the necrotic materials and pathologic examination; therefore, the surgeon can

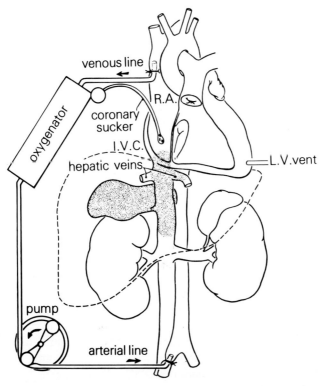

Figure 10.1. Extracorporeal technique for resection of a primary adrenal cancer with extension to the *hepatic veins* and right atrium (*R.A.*).

perform a radical nephrectomy without further exposure and manipulation of the mass during surgery.

Embolization

In search of an effective method for treatment of patients who present with disseminated renal cell carcinoma, a number of investigators have advocated embolization techniques. A number of techniques have been developed utilizing blood clot, muscle, silicone, microspheres, coil, glass beads, stainless steel pellets, and Gelfoam by transcatheter embolization. Embolization is accomplished by Swan Ganz catheter under the fluoroscopic control. The postinfarction problems include pain, fever, and gastrointestinal manifestations depending on the degree of infarction. Although these symptoms can be controlled by medications, more permanent and disturbing complications such as embolism of peripheral vessels with gangrene of the extremities and paraplegia have been reported. As far as the results of such treatment is concerned, there is no controlled clinical trial to substantiate the efficacy of this technique. Since some investigators stated that patient selection is necessary for this technique in terms of less tumor burden and dissemination, one wonders if improved survivals are due to the natural history of the tumor rather than any therapeutic effect of embolization. Due to the lack of controlled data at the present time, it is not possible to assess the efficacy of renal artery embolism in the treatment of disseminated renal cell carcinoma. We have utilized renal artery embolism in patients with disseminated renal cancer or metastases to the kidneys with severe intractable pain or hematuria. In conclusion, the angioocclusive techniques have been advocated for inoperable primary renal cell carcinoma in order to stop intractable hematuria. Also, this technique has been utilized prior to nephrectomy for renal cell carcinoma to "facilitate" the operation, "prevent" the theoretical spreading of tumor cells, "enhance" immunologic response of the host and, therefore, "prolong" the survival. Although these theoretical assumptions are attractive, the value of renal artery occlusion prior to nephrectomy for renal cell carcinoma should be investigated in controlled studies before one can justify the inconvenience, cost, and risk of this technique to patients.

Another area of controversy in the management of renal cancer is the application of lymphadenectomy. The major problems in evaluating the survival of patients with or without lymphadenectomy has been lack of prospective randomized studies. Some urologic surgeons have indicated that the lack of effective chemotherapeutic agents and lack of a stepwise lymphatic spread limits the efficacy of lymphadenectomy. However, other urologists prefer a radical nephrectomy and regional lymphadenectomy. This includes removal of the cancer, perinephritic fat and ipsilateral adrenal gland, en bloc or separately, with adjacent perinephritic and periaortic or pericaval lymph nodes. Although there is no randomized clinical trial available, Robson[4] in a retrospective study has shown an overall 10-year survival rate of 66% with radical nephrectomy *versus* 22% with simple nephrectomy.

As far as the surgical approach is concerned, in our hands, the transabdominal and thoracoabdominal approaches have been satisfactory in radical nephrectomy for renal cell carcinoma. Thoracoabdominal approach is especially suitable for a large tumor in the upper pole of the kidney. Simultaneous excision of the primary tumor and ipsilateral lung metastases may be accomplished by a thoracoabdominal incision. Also, simultaneous removal of extensive tumor thrombus from the inferior vena cava may be accomplished through combined abdominal and thoracic incisions including a sternal splitting incision.

Extracorporeal Surgery

Extracorporeal surgery has been utilized in the management of unilateral or bilateral renal cell carcinoma, Wilms' tumor, and transitional carcinoma of the calyx and renal pelvis. Since the first reported case of extracorporeal surgery of a cancer in a solitary kidney, a number of cases have been reported and they cite the advantages of extracorporeal surgery for renal cancer. These include better visualization, a wider margin of resection, and decreased likelihood of wound contamination with tumor cells. Although extracorporeal renal surgery may have some indications in selected cases, such as when a large tumor is in the middle portion of a solitary kidney, we reserve extracorporeal surgery for cases in which

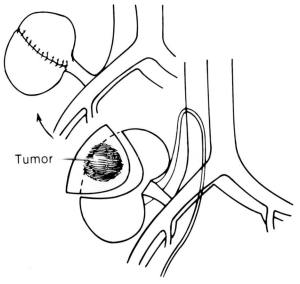

Figure 10.2. Schematic demonstration of *tumor* resection from the middle of a solitary kidney.

resection of the tumor by conventional *in situ* surgery is not feasible (Fig. 10.2).

Certain authors report bilateral nephrectomy for these problems with subsequent dialysis and renal transplantation. However, it should be noted that patients with primary neoplasm are poor candidates for allotransplantation and immunosuppression due to the possible risk of promoting tumor recurrence.

URETERS AND BLADDER

Urinary Diversion

The increasing rate of exenterative pelvic surgery for malignancy has increased the need of searching for a better urinary conduit. There is no perfect substitute for bladder function. Options for urinary diversion includes diversion of urine directly into the intact colon, isolated rectum, isolated cecum, or a continent ileal pouch. Although all these procedures have their indications in selected cases, the major techniques of urinary diversion have been urinary conduit utilizing an isolated segment of small intestine or colon to an external appliance. To avoid the effects and complications of radiation, a segment of midileum, jejunum, sigmoid, or transverse colon has been used with no significant anatomic or physiologic problems.[5-7] Although the ileal loop has been a widely utilized method of urinary diversion in patients undergoing pelvic surgery in malignancy, most series report a 30 to 70% incidence of complications including urinary tract infections, stones, stomal stenosis, and deterioration of renal function. Since open ureters anastomose to the ileal segment, free reflux can carry infection and pressure to the kidneys. Of the 296 pelvic exenterations performed in patients with pelvic malignancies at the Surgery Branch of the National Cancer Institute, incidence of ileal conduit complications also was similar. In a number of cases, a slow developing fibrosis developed in the ileal loop segment rendering the conduit afunctional and obstructed, resulting in bilateral hydronephrosis. These changes were thought to be due to pelvic radiation, ischemic ureteritis with fibrosis, and scarring of the ileal segment. Major revision of the ileal conduit in these patients has been technically difficult due to pelvic fibrosis and adhesion secondary to multiple pelvic surgical procedures and/or pelvic radiation, causing the small intestine to be matted and bound into a conglomerate in the pelvis. In these patients, we have chosen to avoid the pelvis and perform a proximal bypass procedure as previously reported[6] (Fig. 10.3). The experience with antireflux ureterointestinal anastomosis has been gained from ureterosigmoidostomy. The utilization of ureterosigmoidostomy declined due to the frequent incidence of pyelonephritis and electrolyte imbalance. These complications may minimize utilization of a segment of colon in an antireflux anastomosis to an isolated colon segment that can be redirected from skin to the intact colon or that remains as a permanent diversion with external appliance. The exact technique has been described by a number of authors utilizing a meticulous ureteral mucosa to colonic mucosa and creating a nonobstructive antireflux submucosal tunnel. We have previously reported our results of sigmoid conduit as an alternative to the ileal conduit. An update of previously reported series of over 300 cases of pelvic exenteration at the National Cancer Institute has shown that the results of colonic conduit are superior to those of ileal conduit in terms of preservation of renal function. In these patients undergoing total pelvic exenteration with

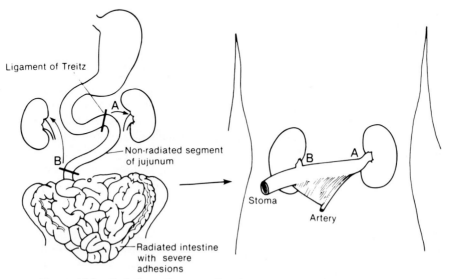

Figure 10.3. Isolation of a nonradiated proximal jejunal segment to perform a pyelo-jejuno-cutaneous diversion in patients with failure of previous ileal conduit.

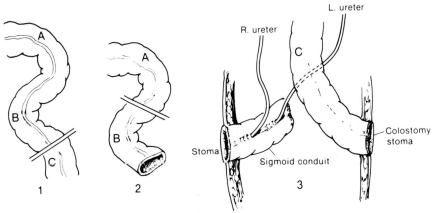

Figure 10.4. Technique of sigmoid conduit in a patient undergoing total pelvic exeneration for pelvic malignancy.

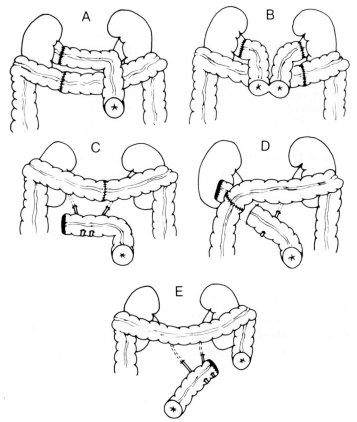

Figure 10.5. (*A–E*) Various techniques of colonic urinary diversions with, or without, colostomies.

creation of a colostomy, a sigmoid conduit has been utilized when possible, which obviates an additional small bowel anastomosis (Figs. 10.4 and 10.5).

In conclusion, urinary diversion has improved utilizing an antireflux ureterocolonic anastomosis, that avoids the radiated segment of the bowel and ureters in the construction of the conduit. Although there is no perfect substitute for the bladder, nonrefluxing, short, straight, and well constructed sigmoid or transverse colonic conduit is the operation of choice for urinary diversion at the time of this writing. Nevertheless, the fate of antireflux colonic conduit is not clear due to the short follow-up of these cases. We have seen progressive hydronephrosis in patients 5 years after this operation without any apparent obstruction.

Role of Surgery in Carcinoma *In Situ*

Over the past decade it has become apparent that a flat carcinoma *in situ* of the bladder may lead to invasive cancer. Also, the other important achievement was the realization that urinary cytology is the most accurate screening test in this cancer when properly performed and interpreted. This type of cancer is often multicentric and may involve the urothelial coverage of the ureters, bladder, and prostatic urethra. Predicting the ultimate fate of such tumor has been difficult, however utilization of ABO isoantigens are under intense investigations as a possible predictor. The treatment of a flat carcinoma *in situ* of the bladder is controversial, but accumulated results indicate that perhaps cystectomy is the treatment of choice in the lesions that are multifocal or diffuse.

Recurrent Vesicovaginal Fistula After Pelvic Surgery and Radiation for Malignancies

Although a number of conservative and surgical modalities have been used to treat such recurrent vesicovaginal fistulas, some patients undergo repeated operations without cure. We have utilized the following technique that also has been utilized by other authors with certain modifications.[8]

SURGICAL TECHNIQUE

The bladder is exposed through a suprapubic midline or transverse incision, and bivalved in such a manner as to bisect the fistula also. Ureteral catheters are inserted into the ureteral orifices to avoid injury to the ureters. The vaginal stump is then freed distally about 2 to 4 cm from the fistula. The scar or inflammatory tissue of the vagina must be completely removed. The vaginal stump, which is usually frozen in place, is dissected free and the defect closed in two layers; the first layer is sutured with a continuous 2-0 chromic catgut suture, and the second layer is sutured with interrupted 2-0 chromic catgut sutures. Both are sutured in a transverse manner. Care must be taken to mobilize the vaginal stump, so it will not lie close to the trigonal area near the site of the fistula; otherwise, the fistula may reform. The vesical part of the fistula is excised completely from both edges of the bivalved bladder, and the bladder

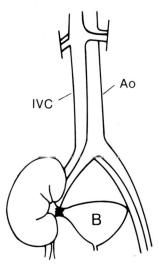

Figure 10.6. Pyelovesical anastomosis and autotransplantation of the right kidney.

closed in three layers with nonabsorbable sutures. The first layer is a continuous suture, while the second and third are interrupted sutures. A pouch of peritoneum is also interposed between the closed bladder and the vaginal stump. The ureteral catheters are removed, and a 32 Fr Malecot catheter is inserted suprapubically just before the bladder is closed. An indwelling urethral catheter is avoided to prevent constant irritation of the trigonal area and possible recurrence of the fistula. Postoperatively, the patient is kept in a prone position as much as possible. The suprapubic tube is connected to a vented suction to avoid constant accumulation of urine at the site of the fistula. The advantages of this technique include: (1) direct access to the vaginal and vesical sides of the fistula, (2) complete resection of the fistula with adjacent areas, (3) direct observation of ureteral orifices, and (4) separation of the vaginal stump and the trigone with interposition of the peritoneum.

Another recent surgical technique is pyelovesical anastomosis and renal autotransplantation. This technique may be utilized for certain severe diseases of the ureter with a solitary kidney (Fig. 10.6).

PROSTATIC CANCER

The improvements in the understanding of prostatic cancer have been mainly in the realization that most of the time-honored principles were not based on clinical trials that were carefully controlled. Also, the fact that carcinoma of the prostate occurs in an older population with life-threatening diseases have made evaluations of survival and quality of life difficult. Furthermore, the availability of different treatment modalities and lack of controlled comparison of these modalities in a randomized fashion have made the management of prostatic cancer controversial.

Substantial progress has been made through the National Prostatic Cancer Project. However, it appears that the treatment of choice for stage A_1 prostatic cancer with well differentiated prostatic cancer is simply observation, and the treatment of choice for stage B_1 is a retropubic radical prostatectomy with close attention to the pelvic lymph nodes for accurate staging.[9, 10, 11] The treatment of stage A_2, B_2, C, D_1, and D_2 are more controversial. Although the techniques of pelvic lymphadenectomy and radical retropubic prostatectomy have been refined, the exact role of these operations are not clear.

The technique of iodine-125 implantation has brought some hope for treatment of localized prostatic cancers. However, it is not clear if achievement of local control is permanent, or simply protracted. Due to the lack of controlled studies, it is also not clear whether, this form of therapy prolongs the survival of patients with localized disease when compared with other forms of therapy.

TESTICULAR CANCER

Recent advances in the diagnosis and management of testicular cancer have increased its potential curability. The majority of these advances have been in the development of accurate testicular tumor markers and highly effective chemotherapeutic agents. The application of computed tomography and meticulous regional lymphadenectomy also have played an important role in accurate staging and in designing appropriate therapeutic strategies.

Epidemiologic and case studies have suggested the role of genetics in the etiology of testicular cancer. Epidemiologically, testicular cancer is extremely rare in the black population when compared to the nonblack population in the United States. The incidence of testicular cancer in Uganda is 0.09/100,000 male subjects, compared to 2.5/100,000 male subjects in England. The fact that migration of the black population from Africa (incidence of 0.09/100,000 male subjects) and the white population (about 2.5/100,000 male subjects) to the United States (incidence of 2.1 to 2.2/100,000 male subjects) does not change the incidence of testicular cancer in these populations strongly favors the role of genetic rather than environmental factors in the etiology of testicular cancer. The main treatment of stage I and nonbulky stage II (stage II, A, B, and C) is retroperitoneal lymphadenectomy.

The staging of testicular tumors must accurately reflect both the extent and the natural progression of the disease. Only then can the physician assess the cancer, select the appropriate treatment, and estimate the patient's prognosis. Although the conventional method of staging testicular tumors reflects tumor extent to some degree, and thus has some predictive value, it does not provide a precise evaluation of the extent of dissemination, or of tumor volume and resectability. The major problem with this staging method is its lack of discrimination between varying degrees of local and metastatic spread within the category of stage I disease. Nor does the stage II designation adequately reflect the variable

Table 10.2
Surgicopathologic staging for testicular cancer

Stage I	Local spread
	A. Confined to testis
	B. Involves testicular adnexa
	C. Involves scrotal wall
Stage II	Confined to retroperitoneal lymphatics
	A. Microscopic
	B. Gross involvement without capsular invasion
	C. Gross involvement with capsular invasion
	D. Massive involvement of retroperitoneal structures
Stage III	Beyond the retroperitoneum
	A. Solitary metastasis
	B. Multiple metastases

degree of regional lymphatic involvement; it combines patients with minimal, potentially surgically curable disease with patients who have massive, surgically incurable disease. The stage III category does not differentiate between single and multiple metastases and does not distinguish between pulmonary and other sites of parenchymal dissemination. Because of these shortcomings, we have utilized a staging classification (Table 10.2). Although somewhat more complex, it more accurately defines the extent of disease, aids in determining appropriate therapy, and improves prognostic capabilities. Also, it more fully considers other factors that are essential to modern therapy and accurate prognosis of these diseases.[12]

Retroperitoneal Lymphadenectomy

At the National Cancer Institute, we perform a bilateral lymphadenectomy, including renal, aortic, caval, ipsilateral iliac, and obturator lymphatics. The abdomen of the patients undergoing retroperitoneal lymph node dissection are explored through a midline vertical incision extending from the xiphoid process to the pubis. An incision is made over the posterior peritoneum from the ligament of Treitz to the aortic bifurcation and then extended over the common iliac arteries. The inferior mesenteric artery is clamped with a noncrushing vascular clamp before it is ligated, to ensure the adequacy of collateral circulation to the sigmoid colon and rectum. Both gonadal arteries and veins are ligated and included in the specimens. The lateral borders of the dissection are the ureters. The superior border is the superior mesenteric artery; inferiorly, the border is the proximal portion of the common iliac artery on the contralateral side and the distal part of the external iliac artery on the ipsilateral side. However, in bulky stage II or III, we have shown in a randomized clinical trial that patients should receive initial chemotherapy followed by resection of residual disease.

SURGICAL TECHNIQUE

The surgical technique of cytoreductive surgery is hereby discussed in detail. Patients undergoing cytoreductive surgery receive a midline vertical incision from the xiphoid process to the pubis. On entering the peritoneal cavity, a thorough exploration is performed. The kidneys and ureters are identified and dissected free and usually represent the lateral margins of the dissection. Control of the vena cava and aorta is gained distally at a convenient site, and control proximally is achieved at a level just beneath the renal vessels. The mass of retroperitoneal tumor and vena cava are resected en bloc, with great care taken around the aorta. The lumbar veins are ligated individually. By resecting the vena cava, we have been able to remove much more tumor that otherwise would have been inaccessible.[9] The major risk of surgery is uncontrollable hemorrhage from injury to either the inferior vena cava or aorta which is encased in tumor. The surgery itself, because of the extensive nature and presence of large collateral vessels, may be associated with a considerable amount of intraoperative blood loss. En bloc resection of the vena cava eliminates the IVC as a source of hemorrhage and, by allowing greater access around the aorta, diminishes the likelihood of injury to this structure. Intraluminal clot or tumor is frequently documented on preoperative inferior venacavography.

The feasibility of resecting the IVC has been demonstrated in the management of renal cell carcinoma, trauma, and rare primary tumors of IVC. Much experience with acute interruption of the IVC and its complications has been gained from ligation of the IVC for thromboembolic problems. Most patients experience varying degrees of postoperative leg edema, which has been well controlled with conservative measures. We attribute this lack of significant postoperative edema to the gradual development of extensive collateral vessels forming as a result of the tumor encroaching on the IVC.

The management of testicular cancer is still evolving. Our current management at the NCI is as follows. Because a number of cases of testicular germ cell tumors are first seen by the primary physician, it is important to take the appropriate clinical approach to a scrotal mass. Initially, unless the clinical history indicates otherwise, any scrotal mass in a young male patient is suspect. A radical inguinal orchiectomy is usually the initial therapy and also serves as a specimen for the pathologist. The subsequent therapy depends on the cell type of the tumor. In patients with stage I and nonbulky stage II seminoma, radiotherapy is the treatment of choice. In pure choriocarcinoma, it appears that chemotherapy alone is the treatment of choice since these patients almost always present with stage III cancer. However, treatment for stage I and nonbulky stage II testicular cancer is retroperitoneal lymphadenectomy. It is important to reiterate the subject of inadequate orchiectomy. Some investigators[13] have advocated ilioinguinal lymphadenectomy with en bloc removal of the remaining spermatic cord, together with an inguinal lymphadenectomy to "prevent" local recurrence. However, Johnson and Babaian[14] have reported 16 cases with inadequate orchiectomy who subsequently underwent en bloc partial scrotectomy and removal of the remaining spermatic cord through two incisions without any recurrence in follow-up. Our experience also supports this conservative approach since the majority of the patients are referred for definite therapy shortly after "contaminated" orchiectomy. Moreover, these patients are being followed carefully for their recurrent cancer elsewhere. In case of recurrent tumor in the ilioinguinal area, surgical removal of the nodes and/or chemotherapy may be used.

CARCINOMA OF PENIS

The major problem in treatment of penile carcinoma is whether ilioin guinal lymphadenectomy or radiotherapy is the most effective modality. The natural history of penile cancer indicates the propensity of this cancer to metastasize to the ilioinguinal lymph nodes and become localized in the sentinel inguinal lymph node. This finding of metastases staying localized to the lymph nodes have attracted the attention of urologic surgeons and radiotherapists to the importance of regional lymphatics in the treatment of penile cancer. However, about 20% of patients with clinically negative nodes have microscopic metastases. On the other hand, 50% with clinically positive nodes have no histologically detectable tumor after lymphadenectomy. Furthermore, the complications of inguinal lymphadenectomy for carcinoma of the penis have been reported to be 20 to 50%. Therefore, several clinicians have expressed certain reservations in performing lymphadenectomy in all patients with penile carcinoma due to the high rate of false negative and false positive results. However, the recent advances in technical and supportive measures have contributed in reducing the mortality and morbidity of inguinal lymphadenectomy in penile cancer.[15, 16] These improvements include: (1) resolution of infection in inguinal lymph node by antibiotic; (2) utilization of a midline incision to remove the deep iliac lymphatics and an incision parallel to the inguinal ligament to reduce the chance of aseptic necrosis of the flap; (3) protection of the femoral vessels by transferring the sartorious muscle; (4) development of a thick flap to prevent flap necrosis; and (5) proper drainage, anticoagulation, and early immobilization of the extremities. It should be emphasized that due to the lack of controlled studies the following questions remain: (1) does erradication of microscopic metastases reduce the rate of local recurrence and prolong the survival in relation to the complication? and (2) if so, can we accomplish this by radiotherapy? These questions should be answered in controlled clinical trials.

REFERENCES

1. Athanasoulis, C. A. Therapeutic applications of angiography. *N. Engl. J. Med. 302:* 1174, 1980.
2. Barbaric, Z. L. Interventional uroradiology. *Radiol. Clin. North Am. 17:*413,1979.
3. Javadpour, N., Woltering, E., and Brennan, M. F. Adrenal neoplasms. *Curr. Prob. Surg. 17:*1, 1980.
4. Robson, C. J., Churchill, B., and Anderson, W. Radical nephrectomy for renal cell carcinoma. *J. Urol. 101:*297, 1969.
5. Bricker, E. M. Current status of urinary diversion. *Cancer 45:*2986, 1980.
6. Norton, J. A., and Javadpour, N. Jejunal loop interposition in patients with ileal conduit failure after pelvic exenteration. *Am. J. Surg. 134:*404, 1977.

7. Sullivan, J. W., Grabstald, H., and Whitmore, W. F. Complications of ureteroileal conduit with radical cystectomy: review of 336 cases. *J. Urol. 124:*797, 1980.
8. Javadpour, N., John, T., Wilson, M. R., *et al.* Transperitoneal vesical bivalve in repair of recurrent vesicovaginal fistula. *Obstet. Gynecol. 41:*469, 1973.
9. Morales, P., and Golimbu, M. The therapeutic role of pelvic lymphadenectomy in prostatic cancer. *Urol. Clin. North Am. 7:*623, 1980.
10. Paulson, P. F. The prognostic role of lymphadenectomy in adenocarcinoma of the prostate. *Urol. Clin. North Am. 7:*615, 1980.
11. Walsh, P. C., and Jewett, H. J. Radical surgery for prostatic cancer. *Cancer 45:*1906, 1980.
12. Javadpour, N. Staging procedures and the role of surgery in testicular cancer. *Cancer Treat. Rept. 63:*1637, 1979.
13. Markland, C., Kedia, K., and Fraley, E. E. Inadequate orchiectomy for patients with testicular tumor. *JAMA 224:*1025, 1973.
14. Johnson, D. E., and Babian, R. J. The case for conservative surgical management of the ilio-inguinal region after inadequate orchiectomy. *J. Urol. 123:*44, 1980.
15. Catalona, W. J. Role of lymphadenectomy in carcinoma of the penis. *Urol. Clin. North Am. 7:*783, 1980.
16. Grabstald, H. Controversies concerning lymph node dissection for cancer of the penis. *Urol. Clin. North Am. 7:*793, 1980.

11

Advances in Chemotherapy

Until recently, chemotherapy for patients with metastatic urologic malignancies, except for germ cell tumors of the testis, was administered as a "last resort" after curative attempts with surgery and irradiation had failed. A resurgent interest in the use of cytotoxic drugs developed because of new, effective diamminedichloroplatinum(II) (*cis*-platin, or DDP) regimens employed in the management of patients with nonseminomatous germ cell tumors, and the efficacy of both old and new agents for metastatic bladder carcinoma. Various studies in urological malignancies utilizing combination regimens have not always been carefully controlled and, in most instances, randomized trials, which could establish an enhanced efficacy of such combinations over the best single agent, have not been performed.

Clinical drug studies in patients with prostatic, renal, and even bladder cancer are only at the stage of establishing antitumor activity and defining appropriate response criteria. While measuring regression of tumor is not a major issue in most patients with renal cancer, it is with prostatic cancer because of the lack of *objective*, (bidimensional) criteria.[1]

Advances in the management of patients with urological cancers have not depended solely upon drug studies. New methodologies now allow *in vitro* and *in vivo* animal studies. The techniques for culturing human tumor stem cells *in vitro* now exist, not only for acute leukemia but for solid tumors as well.[2] Presently, such techniques are being evaluated in order to develop an *in vitro* drug sensitivity assay similar to that available for antimicrobial therapy.[2] In addition, human tumor xenografting into nude mice is another clinically useful method of establishing tumor growth for drug sensitivity testing. Although major technical problems still remain, hopefully, "tailor-made" therapies for individual cases can be developed in the future. An innovative new approach is the administration of large doses of chemotherapeutic agents previously considered to be lethal.[3] Bone marrow transplantation, a technique in patients with solid tumors which has had limited trials because of marginally effective cytotoxic drugs,[4] is now an established treatment modality of management for acute leukemia. Since the bone marrow in patients with germ cell tumors is often not involved, chemotherapy with autologous stem cell transplantation (ASCT) in selected patients with seminoma,[5] mediastinal,[6] and primary lung[7,8] germ cell tumors would be ideal; remissions already have been documented with this technique.[4] While the role for ASCT in the management of patients with cancer remains conjectural, early pilot studies have demonstrated the ability of cryopreserved bone marrow stem cells obtained from marrow, as well as from peripheral blood, to re-populate the marrow and reduce the anticipated period of pancytopenia. The theoretical implementation of such programs in other genitourinary malignancies are obvious, particularly as adjuvant therapy in so called "poor risk" cases.

Of major importance in the management of all cancer patients has been the experience gained by clinical investigators such as surgeons, medical oncologists, radiotherapists, and immunologists in developing a composite, initial, multimodality therapy for patients with genitourinary tumors. The effectiveness of such a multidisciplinary approach is evidenced by cooperation of various investigators in protocols for patients with nonseminomatous germ cell tumors.

This chapter will attempt to outline the progress already made, the future direction for future clinical studies, the areas of successful multimodality therapies, and the need for an honest appraisal of the present status of the art in patients with urological malignancies.

METASTATIC GERM CELL TUMORS OF TESTIS

The treatment of patients with germ cell tumors of the testis has changed substantially during the past 5 years. Several recent comprehensive reviews summarize the current understanding of embryogenesis, animal models, and *in vitro* and *in vivo* culture systems and discuss histopathologic, surgical, and radiotherapeutic controversies.[9-11] However, the cure of metastatic disease is dependent on the proper use of biologic markers, the administration of intensive chemotherapy, and the proper timing of surgical removal of remaining disease.

Biologic Markers

The cardinal role of serial determinations of serum biologic markers in management of patients with germ cell tumors has become firmly established. Presently three markers—α-fetoprotein (AFP), human chorionic gonadotropin (β subunit) (hCG) and lactate dehydrogenase isoenzyme (LDH)—have been identified as essential components for diagnosis, staging, and management of germ cell tumors. Carcinoembryonic antigen (CEA) which has been of some use clinically in the management of patients with gastrointestinal and other malignancies is of marginal significance as a good marker for germ cell tumors. The value of other potential markers such as a pregnancy-specific protein (SP-1) and 3′,3′,5′-triiodothyronine (reverse T_3).[12, 12a] Placental protein 5 (PP5) still need to be defined.

hCG, consisting of an α and a β subunit, is normally a product of the placenta. Although excretion of hCG in the urine of patients with germ cell tumors was recognized several decades ago, serum assay techniques for their measurement have been insensitive. Development of the double-antibody radioimmunoassay made possible the measurement of nanogram quantities of protein in the serum, and it was rapidly applied to tumor marker proteins. Vaitukitis[13] recognized the immunological specificity of the β subunit of hCG and developed a radioimmunoassay to it. Subsequent studies confirmed its presence in patients with germ cell tumor and other selected cancers.[14] About 50% of cases with metastatic nonseminomatous germ cell tumors will have elevated serum levels of hCG as measured by the assay for the β subunit. Occasionally, patients with seminoma also will exhibit elevated levels of hCG without demonstrable nonseminomatous disease; in such cases, immunoperoxidase studies have localized the production to syncytiotrophoblast giant cells.[15] An assay for the α subunit of hCG recently has been developed which may be useful in tumor localization *via* percutaneous intravenous sampling because of its short half-life of 15 min.[11] In contrast, β hCG has a half-life of 16 to 24 hours. Since the α subunit is common to several pituitary hormones, its role in the overall management of patients with these tumors is undefined.

AFP, a product of the fetal liver, yolk sac, and gastrointestinal tract, is present in the developing fetus[10] and generally disappears from serum in the neonatal period. In 1967, Abelev[16] described AFP in the sera of many patients with cancer, including some patients with germ cell tumors. Waldmann and McIntire[17] developed a radioimmunoassay for AFP and noted elevated serum levels in patients with germ cell tumors. The overall incidence is between 50 to 75% in patients with nonseminomatous disease, particularly in those cases with endodermal sinus tumor components. Patients with elevated levels of AFP should always be considered to have a nonseminomatous tumor.

Up to 90% of patients will have elevated levels of either hCG or AFP or both[10] and, because the assays are highly sensitive and the values obtained are very specific for the disease, determining AFP and hCG is mandatory both prior to, and after, therapy. The levels of AFP and hCG obtained prior to treatment seem to correlate with prognosis, and their rate of change after therapy may be an early indicator of adequacy of treatment and completeness of response.[3, 18-20]

Interpretation of elevations and declines in serum marker values requires knowledge of the half-life clearance of these proteins. The half-life in serum of AFP is approximately 5 days; that of hCG is between 16 and 24 hours.[11, 21, 22] Levels which fall at a rate predicted by the half-life indicate a good response to therapy. Levels which decline more slowly than predicted, even if they eventually become undetectable, generally imply inadequate therapy and the presence of residual disease. In contrast, when serum markers decline at a predictable rate and clinical evidence for residual pulmonary or retroperitoneal disease persists, the remaining tissue may simply be teratoma (benign) or necrotic tumor masses. In such circumstances, a biopsy is needed to exclude the presence of malignant tumor. When levels of either or both proteins are persistently elevated or increasing, the presence of active tumor is confirmed even in the absence of clinical or radiologic evidence for disease. Therefore, *serial* marker values are indispensible aides in treatment planning at all phases of this disease.[23]

Evaluations of marker values do not correlate with disease activity in specific circumstances. Marker levels occasionally increase abruptly following systemic chemotherapy, possibly due either to tumor destruction and/or to a transient release of marker proteins into the serum.[24, 25] Men with elevated levels of luteinizing hormone as a result of bilateral orchiectomy or suppression of testicular function by chemotherapy may have slightly elevated levels of hCG by radioimmunoassay. These *stable*, slight elevations of hCG are detected because of cross-reactivity between the assays for luteinizing hormone and hCG.[11] Recently, transient elevations of hCG, β subunit, have been noted in patients who use marijuana.[26] Elevated AFP levels in the absence of germinal tumors have been noted with massive hepatic regeneration or a coexistent hepatoma or other malignancy. Nevertheless, persistent elevations of hCG or AFP nearly always mean residual or recurrent tumor.

LDH is the common name for a group of isoenzymes found in most body tissues. Levels of LDH are abnormally increased in about 50% of patients with germ cell tumors and can be elevated when both AFP and hCG levels are normal. Elevation of LDH does not correlate with liver metastases but does correlate with the extent of disease.[27, 28] Isoenzyme determinations usually reveal elevations of the most cathodic fraction ("LDH-1").[12a, 28, 29] Since LDH is ubiquitous in body tissue, it lacks the specificity of AFP and hCG; isoenzyme determinations are generally more useful. Elevated LDH levels, particularly LDH-1 in a patient with a germ cell tumor, even in the absence of elevations of hCG and AFP, should prompt a thorough search for disease. However, without corroborating clinical documentation, thereapy should be withheld. LDH-X, an isoenzyme specific to mature spermatozoa, has not been studied in patients with germ cell tumors.[30] Recently, LDH-Z has been described in a patient with choriocarcinoma, but the clinical significance of this observation is obscure.[31]

CEA, which has been studied by several investigators, was found to be elevated in approximately 10% of cases. No clear cut association with disease activity has been demonstrated.[32–34]

Several normally-occurring human placental proteins have been sought in the sera of patients with germ cell tumors.[35] SP-1, which is a product of the syncytiotrophoblast, is found in the serum during pregnancy and can be detected in approximately 25 to 50% of patients with germ cell tumors. Although levels of SP-1 generally parallel levels of hCG, occasional discordance from hCG levels has been noted: normal hCG levels with elevated SP-1 levels. PP-5 is also a product of the syncytiotrophoblast but serum levels are generally low.[36] Whether these or other placental proteins will be clinically useful remains to be determined.

Advanced Disease

Complete remission (CR) and long disease-free survival in patients with metastatic testicular cancer were first described by Li *et al.*[37] and Kennedy.[38] In 1970, Samuels and Howe[39] reported efficacy with vinblastine used singly and, after the antitumor activity of bleomycin was established,[40] clinical trials of vinblastine or vincristine with intermittent or continuous infusion schedules of bleomycin resulted in an increase in the number of complete and partial remissions. Such responses also produced prolonged disease-free survival.[40–43]

The current era in chemotherapy of germ cell tumors began with DDP.[44] Doses of DDP less than 60 mg/m^2 were used in combination with other agents. Although response rates improved, toxicity was increased and cure rates were similar to regimens with vinblastine and continuous infusion bleomycin administration.[45, 46] Einhorn and Donohue[47] reported the substantial activity of a high dose of DDP (100 mg/m^2) divided into five daily doses, combined with vinblastine and intermittent bleomycin (VBP). Most patients achieved CR status with drugs alone and disease-free survivors were frequent. Cvitkovic *et al.*[48] and Hayes *et al.*[49] established the activity of high single dose DDP (120 mg/m^2) against germ cell tumors when hydration and mannitol diuresis were used to prevent nephrotoxicity. Investigators at Memorial Sloan-Kettering Cancer Center (Memorial Hospital) then combined single high dose DDP with cyclophosphamide,[50] actinomycin D,[51] vinblastine, and continuous infusion bleomycin to form the VAB-III and subsequent regimens.[52–56]

Concurrent with evolution of these treatment plans, changes in the surgical management of metastases from germ cell tumors occurred. Hong *et al.*[57] reported benign teratomas in 12 patients with previous histologic evidence of tumor. The residual masses in some patients were found to have only necrotic tumor when such lesions were removed.[3] Since persistent clinical evidence of tumor could be benign, malignant or necrotic, surgical excision of residual disease after chemotherapy, both in the abdomen and in the lung, has become indispensable. Although long-term follow-up will be required to assess survival, patients with necrotic tumor or benign teratoma may survive longer than patients with residual malignant disease.[58, 59] Of note, some investigators have claimed that rapid tumor growth after an operative procedure has occurred in patients with preoperatively elevated levels of serum biological markers.[60]

Many investigators have employed the VBP or VAB regimens, either as originally conceived or in a modified form, and results of such studies are summarized in Table 11.1 In most trials, the CR rate after chemotherapy and surgical excision of residual disease is between 50 to 82% with approximately 60% survivors at 2 or more years. In patients having only necrotic tissue found at operation, the surgical procedure has served as a "second look" to insure a disease-free state. At this time, any comparison of the efficacy of various regimens must take into account

Table 11.1
Response rates and survival of patients with metastatic testicular cancer

Drugs Used	Number Patients	CR[a]		NED	References
		Drug	Drug & Surgery		
		%	%	%	
CVAP	25		44	36	61
VBP	28	71	82	79	3
VBP	47	70	81	60	47
VBP Ad	79	67	80	71	62
CVABP (VAB III)	89	62		45	53
CVABP (VAB IV)	55	53	73	60	53
VBP	126	51		45	63
CVABP (VAB VI)	25	64	92		54, 56

[a] The abbreviations used are: CR, complete remission; NED, No evidence of disease; V, vinblastine; B, bleomycin; P, cisplatin (DDP); C, cyclophosphamide; A, actinomycin-D; and Ad, adriamycin.

variability in patient selection and study requirements. Such factors include the number of previously treated cases, the accuracy of biological markers, the extent of the initial diagnostic work-up and subsequent restaging procedures, the number of patients with elevated levels of biologic markers as the only evidence of disease *versus* minimal measurable disease *versus* bulky disease, the definitions employed to define the extent of disease and, lastly, the extent of pathologic examination and the type and completeness of the radical node dissection. It appears that the presently effective combination drug regimens which include high doses of DDP will cure most cases which initially present with only elevations in biologic markers or with minimal tumor bulk. Only a very large randomized study would be able to detect a small difference in response rates in patients treated by different protocols.

Other drugs have been added to the present regimens, either during induction or during maintenance therapy, and the doses often have been modified. The addition of doxorubicin to VBP has been studied in a randomized prospective fashion and was found not to improve response rates.[62, 64] The same study also demonstrated that a smaller dose of vinblastine (0.3 mg/kg) was as effective and less toxic than a larger dose (0.4 mg/kg).[62, 64]

Although most investigators administer DDP during the induction period, Samuels *et al.*[65] believe that a regimen with continuous infusion of bleomycin and high doses of vinblastine without DDP is as efficacious as regimens containing high dose DDP. A CR rate of 65%, with 47% of patients surviving free of disease, compares favorably with other regimens. However, total doses of vinblastine have been escalated to 0.6 mg/kg and most patients are continuously hospitalized in the first two courses of therapy because of severe pancytopenia. This is in sharp contrast to the relatively short hospitalizations generally required for treatment in patients given VBP or VAB regimens.

Seminoma

Most patients with seminoma have low stage disease and thus are cured by radiotherapy.[10] An important question which will be difficult to answer is whether radiation therapy is needed for patients with stage I tumors. Since survival rates with the present modalities approach 100% and radiation doses are minimal, it is doubtful that a prospective randomized study could be initiated to appropriately answer this question.

Approximately 10% of cases present with disseminated disease or relapse after irradiation. Occasionally, patients will have elevated serum levels of hCG which may imply hidden nonseminomatous disease. Approximately one-fourth of cases with advanced seminoma, with or without elevated hCG levels, will be found either after repeated biopsies or at autopsy, or clinically with elevated AFP levels, to have nonseminomatous germ cell tumor elements.[66] The rare patient with seminoma and a palpable abdominal mass also does poorly.[67] Such patients should be treated with protocols for nonseminomatous germ cell tumor (NSGCT).

Metastatic seminoma is uncommon. Results of chemotherapy are understandably meager. No one single institution has been able to gather sufficient numbers of cases to evaluate alkylating agents in phase II disease-oriented trials. Yagoda and Vugrin[68] reviewed single agent chemotherapy data for seminoma and reported the experience at Memorial Hospital with high dose cyclophosphamide and DDP. Three of 9 patients with advanced seminoma achieved CR status and 2 additional patients achieved a partial remission (PR). Samuels et al.[69] reported that 13 of 15 patients with advanced seminoma responded to DDP alone or with cyclophosphamide when both drugs were administered weekly. Because of the appearance of nonseminomatous metastases in some patients, most investigators have begun to use the protocols employed for nonseminomatous germ cell tumors. In patients receiving VBP, a 63% CR rate has been reported in 11 of 12 patients, most of whom have remained alive and free of disease.[70] At Memorial Hospital, the VAB protocol also has been employed in such patients. Thus, patients with advanced seminoma treated with standard regimens seem to respond in a fashion similar to those with advanced nonseminomatous disease. As these patients are treated in a more consistent fashion, more reliable data should become available.

Adjuvant Chemotherapy

Pooled data from several reports on the primary management of patients with stages I and II testicular cancer with radiation therapy, retroperitoneal lymph node dissection (RLND), or both, indicate approximately 85% and 50% survive with stage I and II disease, respectively (Table 11.2). Because of the high relapse rate in patients with stage II disease, adjuvant chemotherapy after RLND is reasonable. It is difficult to support the use of adjuvant chemotherapy for stage I disease since only 15% of patients may benefit. Such therapy should be considered only for stage II cases because of the high relapse rate.

Table 11.2
Pooled survival data of patients treated for stage I and stage II nonger-minomatous testicular tumors[71-82]

Therapy	Emb.[a]		Terato.		Pooled	
		%		%		%
			Stage I			
RT					124/146	85
RLND	77/88	88	117/145	81	194/233	83
RLND & RT	20/25	75	37/48	77	90/107	84
Total	97/113	86	154/193	80	408/486	84
			Stage II			
RT					39/75	52
RLND	19/27	70	6/11	55	42/62	68
RLND & RT	30/71	42	40/85	47	98/213	46
Total	49/98	50	46/96	48	179/350	51

[a] The abbreviations used are Emb., embryonal carcinoma; Terato., teratocarcinoma; RT, radiation therapy; and RLND, retroperitoneal lymph node dissection.

The first adjuvant chemotherapy trial in patients with stage II disease used a treatment regimen consisting of vinblastine, bleomycin, and actinomycin D (mini-VAB). The overall results of mini-VAB therapy indicated some benefit but a retrospective analysis of the data revealed no benefit to the subset of patients with greater retroperitoneal disease. Patients were retrospectively divided into good- and bad-risk groups, based on biologic marker levels, number and size of involved retroperitoneal lymph nodes, and presence or absence of extranodal invasion. Although no "good risk" patients relapsed, tumors recurred in 10 of 29 "bad risk" cases. A subsequent trial which employed a more intensive chemotherapeutic regimen (VAB-III) resulted in no relapses in the "bad risk" patient.[83, 84] Similar data has now been reported by other investigators with VBP as adjuvant therapy.[85, 86] It is evident that even in an adjuvant setting intensive chemotherapy must be given if cure is to be achieved. Such data strongly suggests that adjuvant chemotherapy can be effective in preventing relapse. However, with a better understanding of the natural history of the disease, appropriate patient selection becomes important. There is no question that chemotherapy for advanced disease is curative; however, physicians must now ask whether adjuvant chemotherapy is necessary for all patients with stage II disease. If pooled data are taken at face value and patients are not stratified for extent of retroperitoneal disease, up to 50% of stage II cases may receive chemotheraphy unnecessarily. A retrospective analysis at the University of Indiana of a small number of patients who relapsed after stage I and stage II disease has revealed nearly 100% survival when intensive chemotherapy was initiated at the first evidence of relapse. Similar data has been found at Memorial Hospital. Only prospective randomized trials can objectively determine the benefit, if any, of immediate adjuvant chemotherapy *versus* careful follow-up and treatment at relapse. Such a study with Memorial Hospital, the University of Indiana, and other cancer centers and cooperative groups has been initiated to answer the question of adjuvant *versus* delayed chemotherapy.[87] It is unique to this tumor that results of treatment at the time of relapse may be equivalent to the results obtained with adjuvant therapy.

Extragonadal Tumors

Germ cell tumors also arise in the retroperitoneum, mediastinum, and pineal gland. The frequency is very low when compared to testicular primaries and the experience with their management is therefore limited. Although there is some debate concerning the prognosis of patients with retroperitoneal and mediastinal tumors, most patients with this presentation have bulky disease, and therapy has not been as successful as in patients with advanced testicular cancer. Nevertheless, the approach to therapy is similar: intensive chemotherapy with VAB or VBP followed by surgical excision of residual disease.[6, 88] While a "hilar scar" is occasionally found in some testes specimens and is thought to represent an area of spontaneous NSGCT regression, the primary site of origin in these patients is assumed to be extragonadal. Some diagnostic, noninvasive tests used to evaluate the testis include thermography, computerized transaxial tomography, and soft tissue x-ray techniques.

Atypical Presentations

Since therapy for metastatic germ cell tumors is potentially curative, it is imperative that physicians adequately evaluate patients for such tumors. Fox *et al.*[7] in 1979 and Greco *et al.*[8] in 1980 reported an atypical germ cell tumor syndrome. These patients are generally young men who present with a malignant neoplasm in the lungs, mediastinum, and/or other midline structures without a testicular mass and the histopathology is often not diagnostic of a germ cell tumor. Serum levels of AFP or hCG, or both, are infrequently elevated, but elevated serum levels or positive immunocytochemical tissue stains for AFP and hCG indicate a germ cell origin in approximately 65% of cases.[8] Of major consequence, many patients with this type of "undifferentiated carcinoma" will achieve a complete remission when intensive chemotherapy regimens used for germ cell tumors are promptly initiated.

Toxicity

The acute and chronic toxicities of VAB and VBP are summarized in Table 11.3. While mucositis is probably more common in patients given VAB, myelosuppression seems to be greater with the VBP regimen. Recently, smaller doses of vinblastine have been used in the CVB regimen which has resulted in a diminished risk of nadir sepsis without sacrificing efficacy.[3, 62] Significant nephrotoxicity is uncommon with proper attention to adequate hydration with or without mannitol diuresis. However, with

Table 11.3
Acute and chronic toxicities in patients receiving VAB or VBP

Acute	Chronic
Nausea and vomiting	Renal dysfunction
Alopecia	Pulmonary fibrosis
Renal failure	Auditory dysfunction
Myelosuppression	Hyperpigmentation
Mucositis	Hypogonadism
Skin rash	

both regimens, gastrointestinal toxicity, particularly nausea and vomiting, and alopecia are universal. Disabling pulmonary toxicity is minimized with cessation of bleomycin when serially monitored changes are noted in the vital capacity or the diffusion capacity of carbon dioxide (DLCO). Patients requiring surgical procedures after bleomycin should receive an F_IO_2 of 21% during the operation because of reports of severe pulmonary toxicity resulting from the use of high F_IO_2 after bleomycin.[89] Auditory and severe cutaneous toxicities are rare. Hyperpigmentation, myalgias, and peripheral neuropathy are common but rarely of clinical significance. Hypogonadism may be more frequent than previously recognized.[90]

With the present success in treating patients with germ cell tumors, increased survival may lead to delayed toxicities of chemotherapy or irradiation, or both. Alkylating agents, bleomycin, and other drugs can induce major chromosomal abnormalities[91] and may lead to a higher incidence of leukemia and other neoplasms. Such sequelae after successful treatment for Hodgkin's disease and ovarian cancer already have been described.[92-94] No current data suggests that secondary malignancies occur with unusual frequency after chemotherapy in patients with germ cell tumors, but the fear of such sequelae have led most investigators to shorten the overall duration of treatment.

Other delayed toxicities may be as severe as second malignancy. Case reports of myocardial infarction and Raynaud's phenomenon have appeared.[95-97] Raynaud's phenomenon was noted in 37% of patients treated at the University of Minnesota, and the authors reported two additional cases of myocardial infarction.[98] Such reports suggest that vascular damage may result from regimens containing vinblastine, bleomycin, and DDP. Such patients with germ cell tumors are young and will require careful prospective follow-up to determine the potential sequelae of present therapies.

Future Directions

Improvement in major response rates already in excess of 90% will be difficult to achieve. Alteration in induction or elimination of maintenance schedules, establishment of effective salvage regimens, individualized treatment of patients with good and bad prognoses, and earlier detection are areas of continued interest relative to improving cure rates.

The duration and frequency of induction have varied considerably. Higher relapse rates are observed with long intervals between induction cycles, implying that the treatment schedule may be extremely important (Table 11.4). In addition, the number of induction cycles may be important in eliminating microscopic foci of residual disease.[3] Currently, three to six cycles of either VBP or VAB are administered at 3 to 4 week intervals, and then residual disease is surgically excised. Further induction or salvage chemotherapy is indicated when persistent residual malignant tumor is found.

Maintenance therapy in patients with germ cell tumors achieving CR is of unproven value. In 13 patients who had achieved CR status after treatment with mithramycin and who were unmaintained thereafter, 11 remained free of disease.[99] Two additional studies demonstrated no survival advantage in patients who had received maintenance chemotherapy.[100,101] Only a randomized trial can adequately clarify this issue; one such study of patients given VBP is near completion and preliminary data indicate no survival advantage to patients administered maintenance therapy.[102]

Proven effective salvage therapy for patients who have relapsed or who never achieved CR status is needed. Several small studies have indicated that VP-16-213 is an active agent singly. Radice et al.[103] collected reports of 21 patients given VP-16-213 and noted PR in 8 cases. Williams et al.[104] noted PRs in 3 patients and Cavalli et al.[105] in a phase II trial of VP-16-213 described 5 PRs in 28 evaluable patients. Lastly, Fitzharris et al.[106] noted major responses with VP-16-213 in 12 of 26 patients. Williams et al.[104] who used combinations including VDP, VP-16-213, doxorubicin, and bleomycin described 14 complete responders in 33 previously treated patients with 12 patients alive and free of disease. Another combination including VP-16-213 plus DDP plus bleomycin plus doxorubicin, with a different schedule, has resulted in 4 complete responders in 7 patients, with 2 long survivors.[107] These results support the murine evidence for synergism between VP-16-213 and DDP.[108]

Intensive "lethal" chemotherapy with autologous stem cell transplan-

Table 11.4
Number of and interval between induction cycles of various regimens used to treat patients with metastatic testicular cancer

Drugs Used	No. Cycles	Intervals Between Cycles (wk)	CR[a]	Relapse	References
			%	%	
VBP (UMH)	4–6	3–4	82	10	3
VBP	3	3–4	85	30	47
VBP ± Ad	4	3–4	82	12	62
VAB III	2	24–32	62	27	53
VAB IV	3	12–16	73	18	53
VBP (SWOG)	4	3–4	51	11	63
VAB VI	3–5	4	92		54, 56

[a] The abbreviations used are: CR, complete remission; V, vinblastine; B, bleomycin; P, cis-plantin (DDP); A, actinomycin-D; Ad, adriamycin; UMH, University of Minnesota Hospital; and SWOG, Southwest Oncology Group.

tation (ASCT) is another form of salvage therapy entering clinical trials. NSGCT rarely invades the bone marrow and thus marrow stem cells (colony-forming units) can be obtained by repeated aspiration, cryopreserved, and later infused after potentially lethal chemotherapy has been administered. Obviously, meticulous care is required to minimize the toxicity which is substantial and nutritional and blood product support is necessary. Other problems include infections, and fluid and electrolyte abnormalities. The use of ASCT has resulted in remissions in previously treated cases but at considerable cost, substantial toxicity, and prolonged hospitalization.[4] Its role in the management of selected patients is limited at this time.

A distinction must be made between patients with "good" and "poor" prognoses. Variables such as bulk of disease, histopathology, marker values, symptomatic interval, prior RLND, prior chemotherapy, and prior radiotherapy need to be statistically evaluated through multivariate analysis to distinguish between interdependence and independence of variables. Distinct subsets of patients at high risk for recurrence after CR or at high risk for not achieving a CR, would allow investigation of new therapeutic stratagems (e.g. ASCT) while not exposing patients with a good prognosis to unneeded complications. A preliminary report of such a multivariate analysis showed only three independent variables: the number of extra-abdominal organ sites of metastasis, the presence or absence of abdominal disease, and levels of AFP.[109] The potential value of such a model in planning clinical trials is obvious.

Approximately 30% of patients with metastatic testicular cancer eventually succumb to their disease. New agents will be necessary to improve the therapeutic index and limit toxicity. Relatively few agents have been studied in formal phase II studies in patients with germ cell tumors. With fewer patients to enter in such studies—a result of effective chemotherapy—cooperative trials will be necessary to evaluate the efficacy of new agents. Of note, many currently available agents have not yet been studied singly (i.e. the nitrosoureas, purine, and pyrimidine antagonists). New agents of interest include new platinum complexes[110] and anthracycline analogs.[111]

Mature, benign NSGCT elements are generally resistant to chemotherapy but fortunately, in many instances, these tumors can be surgically removed or, because of a very small growth fraction and long doubling time, may not significantly shorten survival. One of the more novel possibilities of tumor manipulation is the use of retinoids (i.e. cis-retinoic acid) or other, as yet undefined, "maturation factors" to induce differentiation.[112]

Lastly, it is evident to all who care for these patients with germ cell tumors that some have a considerable delay prior to diagnosis. Both patients and physicians are responsible for this delay and the duration from symptom to diagnosis correlates with the clinical stage at the time of diagnosis.[113] Since the testicle is available for easy examination, self-examination by young men should be encouraged in educational programs sponsored by institutions and public agencies, and proper diagnostic suspicions should be inculcated in physicians through lectures and seminars.[114]

Conclusion

Germ cell tumors of the testis are curable. Future investigations should lead to earlier diagnosis, more successful therapy, less toxicity and chemotherapeutic and surgical interventions, and cure for almost all patients with this tumor.

PROSTATIC CANCER

Cytotoxic antineoplastic agents for treatment of adenocarcinoma of the prostate have been studied systematically only for the past 5 to 6 years.[115-118] Prior to 1973, chemotherapy data were limited and consisted mostly of small numbers of cases from multiple phase I-phase II studies.[1] Patients referred to medical oncologists and selected for chemotherapy trials basically represent a nonhomogenous group whose prior therapy often has varied: orchiectomy, hormonal manipulation, combinations of estrogens and orchiectomy, extensive prior irradiation, and at times, prior chemotherapy. In addition, extensive prior irradiation to marrow-producing areas sometimes precluded adequate dosages of antineoplastic agents. Thus, many clinical studies in the past have concluded that cytotoxic chemotherapy was ineffective.[1]

Prospective disease-oriented phase II and randomized phase III trials have been difficult to initiate because of the variable "natural history" of the disease and the absence of standard parameters to measure response.[119-125] Most patients lack bidimensionally measurable lesions: a necessary prerequisite to estimate objectively the value of any therapeutic intervention. Many past and present studies have entered patients with unidimensional, or only evaluable parameters such as changes in pelvic masses, pleural effusions, peripheral edema, lymphangiograms, intravenous pyelograms, radionuclide bone scans, and skeletal surveys.[126, 127] Attempts to circumvent the inadequacies inherent in evaluating such "weak" parameters have resulted in utilization of secondary response criteria such as improvements in abnormal laboratory values (serum acid and alkaline phosphatase, carcinoembryonic antigen, lactic dehydrogenase, and hemoglobin levels), and in subjective symptoms (changes in analgesic requirements, weight, and performance status).[122, 123, 126, 128] Various combinations of such objective and subjective parameters have been incorporated into many categories of response.[119, 129-131] The incertitude of truly defining response and the inability to objectively evaluate such changes is evidenced by the numbers of response criteria employed in clinical trials, and by the increasing number of patients assigned to the category, stabilization of disease (STAB)—a designation which may simply indicate the present difficulties in adequately documenting active progression (PROG) of disease.[118, 132, 133]

In some studies, clinical response criteria have been so varied and, at times, so poorly defined,[134] that complete remission (CR), partial remission (PR), minor response (MR), and STAB may only represent minor changes in abnormal laboratory parameters and/or improvement in performance status.[123, 134–136] Yet, worsening of such parameters may be minimized or even excluded in defining subsequent PROG. When all else fails, response has been justified statistically by relating such criteria to (minor) increases in survival.[126, 137] However, patient selection—the unknown variable in prostatic cancer—coupled with conscientious management of medical problems in patients with prostatic cancer can profoundly affect overall survival.[117, 129, 132]

Osseous metastases, the most frequent form of tumor dissemination in prostatic cancer, are particularly difficult to evaluate.[130, 138] New areas of activity in a radionuclide scan do not necessarily denote PROG; rather, they may represent healing.[130, 139] Changes on skeletal surveys may take several months to occur, and the inability to document PROG in the interval between tests may lead to the erroneous assignment of a patient to a response category. Although the incidence of objectively measurable tumor regression in osseous sites is frequently low, the duration of an apparent STAB of boney metastases may be significant.[117, 118] In addition, there is evidence that the subgroup of patients whose disease is limited to osseous sites may have a better long-term prognosis than patients with soft tissue or visceral metastases.[140]

The category STAB becomes more difficult to interpret because of the heterogenous cell population in prostatic tumors.[141] Not only could one ascribe tumor heterogeneity to account for drug resistance but for hormonal resistance too. There is little doubt that prostatic tumor cells are composed of androgen-sensitive and insensitive cells.[142] The growth of androgen-insensitive cells following castration is probably indicative of an adaptation response—an altered cellular environment or, possibly, a multifocal origin with cells insensitive to hormonal and/or chemotherapeutic maneuvers (? rapidly growing) overgrowing other sensitive clones.[143] In addition, relapse to a previous hormonal manipulation such as orchiectomy, may select a resistant population of cells which Paulson et al.[132] believes hinders the effectiveness of chemotherapy. Obviously, a mixed response also represents tumor heterogeneity and, while this response category may be of importance, until such time that adequate parameters are available to truly document the extent of tumor destruction, the overall conclusion must be that such patient should be excluded from the overall "objective" response rates.[118]

The time interval from initial hormonal therapy to start of chemotherapy ("lead time") may significantly influence response and survival.[118, 129, 144] Patients whose interval from diagnosis to chemotherapy is long may have a slow growing or relatively dormant tumor population that is less responsive to cytotoxic therapy while those with a shortened lead time may skew a population toward (apparent) responders because they are seen earlier in their illness and survive for a longer period of time from protocol.[118]

The importance of the response category, STAB, in patients with prostatic cancer still is not settled. Proponents for including patients who achieve STAB in the overall response rate maintain that the meager, yet statistically significant, prolongation in survival substantiates its clinical benefit.[117, 120, 133, 145-147] Opponents point out that (1) the inability to accurately document STAB, (2) the many different definitions of STAB—sometimes seeming to accommodate a longer patient survival or the whim of the investigator(s), (3) the unknown and variable patient selection factors, and (4) the absence of a clear cut "natural history" of the disease invalidate the extensive use of this category in determining the efficacy of a chemotherapeutic regimen.[118] Nevertheless, with careful interpretation of patient selection factors and the use of more rigid response criteria, an overview of the "state of the art" of chemotherapy for patients with prostatic cancer can be achieved.

Several single agents initially have been reported to show modest activity against prostatic carcinoma. Lerner and Malloy[148] noted responses in 15 of 30 patients given hydroxyurea (HU) 60 mg/kg every 3 weeks, but all patients were concurrently receiving the synthetic estrogenic compound, chlorotrianisene (Tace), or had an orchiectomy (14 cases). Although two responses persisted for more than 2 years, it is uncertain if such responses can be attributed to HU alone. The National Prostatic Cancer Project (NPCP) noted only a 15% objective response rate (CR + PR + STAB) with HU.[149]

Franks[122] evaluated melphalan (MEL) in 12 patients, and reported partial remission in 4 patients for a median duration of 43 weeks (range, 18 to 51 weeks). The Ancillary Scoring System employed in this study included changes in pain, performance status, weight, and hemoglobin and serum acid phosphatase values. No objective responses—based on measurable disease parameters—were noted.

Despite the widespread antitumor activity of doxorubicin (ADM) as a single agent in various malignant diseases, the drug has limited single-agent activity in prostatic carcinoma.[120, 126, 128, 135, 150-152] DeWys[135] summarized the course of 12 patients given 60 mg/m^2 every 3 weeks. One patient achieved a CR and 2 patients achieved a PR—defined as a 50% decrease in the size of a measurable lesion and a decrease in an abnormal serum acid phosphatase level. The median duration of response was 26 weeks. All patients had prior ablative and hormonal therapy. Eagan et al.[128] noted no partial or complete remissions in 14 adequately treated patients. The median duration of survival for patients with "stabilization or subjective improvement" was 9 months for responders versus 5 months for nonresponders. No objective response in measurable tumor masses occurred. O'Bryan et al.[152] evaluated a "high" versus "low" dose regimen of ADM. Patients (38) were stratified as good or poor risk based on performance status and extent of prior irradiation. Partial remission was reported in 14 cases in the good risk group given 60 mg/m^2 i.v. every 3 weeks, while none occurred in 5 cases in the good-risk group given 45 mg/m^2 or in 19 cases in the poor-risk category given less than 50 mg/m^2. The median duration of remission was only 3 months. Such results suggested that response to ADM was dose-dependent. A subsequent study by DeWys et al.[120] observed 9 responses (>50% tumor reduction) in 37 patients who received 60 mg/m^2 i.v. every 3 weeks. When response and its relationship to the serum acid phosphatase was examined, 5 patients demonstrated regression without change in levels and 7 had a decrease without change in tumor size. Such discordance in response evaluation has been noted in several studies, suggesting that the sole reliance for response on either variable can be misleading. At best, such patients should be separated from the overall remission rates and placed in the category, mixed response. In a recently completed trial at Memorial Sloan-Kettering Cancer Center, of ADM, 30, 45, and 60 mg/m^2 i.v. every 3 weeks, in a highly selected series of patients who had bidimensionally measurable prostatic tumor masses, regression was documented in only 2 of 46 patients.

Merrin[153, 154] utilized *cis*-platin (DDP) in a dose of 1 mg/kg every week in a 6- to 8-hour infusion. Employing response criteria similar to the NPCP, the PR + CR rate was 31% (17/54). Two responders had a decrease in ascites, 2 patients had a normalization of bone scans, and 7 patients had a decrease in lymphatic obstruction. STAB was noted in 7 (13%) additional cases. Prior chemotherapy did not appear to influence response to DDP since 9/13 (69%) responders and 22/29 (76%) nonresponders had no prior cytotoxic drugs. Similarly, 6/12 (50%) responders and 8/32 (25%) nonresponders had prior irradiation in excess of 2000 rads. In another trial by Merrin[155] utilizing a similar dosage schedule of DDP combined with diethylstilbesterol (DES), 1 mg daily, and an orchiectomy, objective response was noted in 13/32 (41%) for a median duration of 11 months (range, 6 to 28 months). Survival of those patients who progressed on therapy was not reported. Since hormonal manipulation was used simultaneously, it is unclear whether concurrent chemotherapy was of benefit. Rossof et al.[156] who used a different dose and schedule of DDP, 75 mg/m^2 every 3 weeks, noted a response rate of 21% (4/19): response criteria included simply a >50% decrease in serum acid phosphatase levels. In contrast, Yagoda and colleagues[118, 157] using a similar dosage schedule described only 3 (15%) responses in 20 adequately treated patients with bidimensionally measurable disease. STAB was observed in one additional patient. Comparison of survival in responding *versus* nonresponding groups was 11 months (range, 2- to 15-plus months) *versus* 4 months (range, 1 to 9 months). Crucial to this analysis, however, was stratification on the basis of "lead time." In comparing the responding *versus* nonresponding groups, the former had a shorter time from symptom to diagnosis (5 *versus* 12 months), a longer time from diagnosis to identification of metastatic disease (30 *versus* 1 months), and a longer interval from diagnosis to protocol (48 *versus* 26 months. Differences in remission rates between the studies of Yagoda and associates,[118, 157] and Rossof et al.,[156] and Merrin[154] may represent differences in dosage and schedules of DDP, patient selection, and response criteria. However, combining the data from all studies, 22% of 91 patients have obtained some benefit with DDP.

The most extensive single-agent trials have been carried out by the NPCP[124, 137, 158] (Table 11.5). After initial separation of patients on the basis of prior irradiation, cases were assigned to protocols involving myelosuppressive therapy with cyclophosphamide (CTX), 5-fluorouracil

(5-FU), dacarbazine (DTIC), semustine (Me-CCNU), procarbazine (MH) and HU. In the initial study (Protocol 100), CTX and 5-FU were compared to standard therapy—prednisone, estrogens, and analgesics.[124] After a therapeutic advantage was demonstrated for chemotherapy, standard therapy was discontinued. CTX proved to have greater efficacy and less toxicity than 5-FU, and became the new "standard" in future studies. The *objective regression* rates (CR + PR in the NPCP response system) for both drugs were very low: 7% (3/41) for CTX, and 12% (4/33) for 5-FU. However, utilizing a new term, *objective response* (CR + PR + STAB in the NPCP response system), 46% (19/41) of cases given CTX and 36% (12/33) given 5-FU, respectively, responded.[124] The median survival in all three arms of the study were comparable.

In Protocol 300, 165 patients were randomized to receive either CTX, DTIC or MH.[137, 161] Partial remission was noted in only 4% (2/55) of evaluable cases given DTIC. However, STAB was observed in 26% (9/35) of patients administered CTX; 26% (5/19) given MH, and 24% (13/55) given DTIC. Twenty-eight percent of cases could not tolerate the prescribed dose and schedule of MH, and were deemed inevaluable. A survival advantage for responders *versus* nonresponders was identified in all three groups: 48 *versus* 38 weeks for MH, 64 *versus* 28 weeks for DTIC, and 64 *versus* 22 weeks for CTX. No response was observed in patients who did not have a prior orchiectomy. Protocol 700 employed CTX, Me-CCNU, and oral HU.[149] Once again, the highest response rate occured in the CTX group.

Summarizing Protocols 100, 200, and 300 of the NPCP,[115, 116, 137, 161] *objective responses* (CR + PR + STAB) were noted in 35% (38/110), 29% (27/94), and 37% (18/49) of cases, respectively. When the category *objective regression* (CR + PR) was used, however, tumor regression was achieved in only 6% (7/110), 2.1% (2/94), and 6.1% (3/49) of cases, respectively.

Other single agents which have been evaluated, either by the NPCP or other investigators, include neocarsinostatin,[169] piperazinedione[123] and streptozotocin.[161] No demonstrable therapeutic benefit has been obtained with these agents used singly. Although Natale *et al.*[167] found no antitumor activity with *m*-AMSA (4'-[9-acridinylamino]-methanesulfon-*m*-anisi-dide) in patients with advanced bidimensionally measurable prostatic cancer, Drelichman *et al.*[168] described 7 of 15 patients with osseous lesions who seemed to achieve STAB. An antiviral compound, acyclovar, has recently been evaluated, and while no tumor regression was noted, a transient decrease in serum acid phosphatase levels were observed.[174]

A new development has included the formation of a class of agents which combine a hormone with a cytotoxic agent.[121, 171, 175] Theoretically, such agents might transport or preferentially localize cytotoxic agents in prostatic tumor cells. Of note, many studies have indicated that less than 1% of total radioactive-labeled androgen administered to animals localizes in the prostate, and most steroids are metabolized by other tissues.[141, 176] In fact, the number of steroid receptors on prostatic tumor cells may be few, and thus, the carrier concept may not enhance transportation of cytotoxic agents to target organs.[176] The relationship of the cellular

Table 11.5
Chemotherapy of prostatic carcinoma[a]

Drug	References	No. Cases	Number CR + PR	Number CR + PR + STAB	Comments
CTX					
No prior RX	159	15	0	0	Objectively stable or subjectively improved; 3/11 had decrease SAP; overall survival 17 wk
	160	17	0	9	Responders lived 10 mo vs. 2 mo for nonresponders; low dose CTX
	124	41	3	19	9/35 had decrease SAP; 12/39 decrease in tumor masses
	161	35	0	9	
Prior Rx	137, 161	63	1	11	Responders lived 64 vs. 22 wk for nonresponders
5-FU					
No prior Rx	147	39	7	16	
	124	33	4	12 (15%)	
	150	14	5	12	Ancillary scoring system
Prior Rx	161	20	0	6	
5-FU + CTX + MTX	146	15	1	7	Responders lived 19 mo vs. 3 mo for nonresponders
5-FU + CTX + VCR + MTX + Pred.	119	16	5 (37%)	6	Prednisone will affect subjective and evaluable response criteria
5-FU + MTX + VCR + MEL + Pred.	132, 145	84	6	33 (40%)	Responders lived 76 wk vs. 28 wk for nonresponders; Prednisone will affect subjective and evaluable criteria
ADM	135	8	1	6	
	120	12	3	6 (12%)	
	151, 152	38	5	5	
	128	14	0	3	
	150	26	6		Ancillary scoring system; responders lived 9 mo vs. 5 mo for nonresponders
ADM + CTX	5	48	2	8	Recently completed trial
	162	20	3	5	Responders lived 40 wk vs. 17 wk for nonresponders
	131	20	0		Low dose of drugs employed
ADM + CTX + BCNU	163	22	7	11	Responders lived 14 mo vs. 5 mo for nonresponders
ADM + CTX + 5-FU	164	27	7	13	Responders lived 9 mo vs. 4 mo for nonresponders
	147	8	1	7	6 STAB (2 to 6-plus mo)
ADM + CTX + MTX	136	44	12	22	No survival advantage compared to 5-FU
ADM + CTX + DDP	165	16	9	8	Responders lived 24 wk vs. 11 wk for nonresponders; patients received no prior hormonal Rx
	166	17	0	12	No prior hormones vs. chemotherapy
ADM + Mito-C + 5-FU	140	42	21	21	

Drug	Ref.	No. Patients	CR	PR	Comments
m-AMSA	167	18	0	0	Excludes two early deaths
DDP	168	10	0	7	Responders lived 11 mo vs. 4 mo for nonresponders; 3 of 4 PRs alive at 52 wk; 11 patients had prior chemotherapy
	118	25	3	4	Responders lived 90 wk vs. 21 wk for nonresponders
DTIC	156	21	4	4	Concurrently received DES and orchiectomy
	154	54	17	24	55 unpretreated; responders lived 64 wk vs. 28 wk for nonresponders
	127	35	23	29	30 patients concurrently received Tace; NPCP study now evaluating drug in a randomized trial
HU	137	64	2 (3%)	15	
	123, 148	35	16	20	
Me-CCNU	149	?	?	? (15%)	Part of randomized trial in 70-plus cases
	149	?	?	? (30%)	Part of randomized trial in 70-plus cases
MEL	122	20	4 (20%)	14	Responders lived 40 wk vs. 38 wk for nonresponders
MH					
Prior Rx	137, 161	5	0	0	Poor patient tolerance
No prior Rx	169	39	0	5	14 unpretreated
Neocarsinostatin	123	20	0	0	
Piperazinedione	161	3	0	3	
Streptozotocin	170	38	0	12	Overall survival 48 wk; heavily pretreated with irradiation
Vincristine	121	8	?	? (18%)	Randomized trial in 70-plus cases; 4/8 had decrease in tumor
Estramustine	171	44	0	8	Responders lived 10 ms vs. 5.2 mo for nonresponders
	161	72	0	7	
	130	44	10	27	Responders lived more than 30 mo vs. 10 mo for nonresponders; most responses via bone scans
Prednimustine	172	62	0	8	
	171	8	1	6	
Estramustine + prednimustine	172	54	1	7	Responders lived 60 wk vs. 30 wk for nonresponders
	171, 173	21	5	12	
Estramustine + VCR	170	?	?	27	Part of randomized trial in 70-plus cases

[a] The abbreviations used are: CR, complete remission; PR, partial remission; STAB, stabilization of disease; CTX, cyclophosphamide; SAP, serum acid phosphatase; Rx, therapy; 5-FU, 5-fluorouracil; MTX, methotrexate; VCR, vincristine; Pred, prednisone; MEL, melphalen; ADM, doxorubicin; BCNU, carmustine; DDP, diamminedichoroplatinum(II) (cis-platin); Mito-C, mitomycin-C; m-AMSA, 4'-[9-acridinylamino]-methanesulfon-m-anisidide; DES, diethylstilbesterol; DTIC, dacarbazine; HU, hydroxyurea; NPCP, National Prostatic Cancer Project; Me-CCNU, semustine; MH, procarbazine.

estrogen-binding protein receptor to estramustine phosphate (estracyst) is unclear. In the human uterus, estracyst can competively inhibit the cytoplasmic binding of [^{3}H] estradiol,[177] while in the ventral prostatic gland of the male rat, the binding protein appears to be specific for estracyst alone.[178] Although the drug circulates as an intact molecule, there is no evidence that the alkylating portion is specifically released at the estrogen-dependent site. In fact, estrogen-like side effects have been demonstrated in patients, and such effects may explain most of the biological activity of the drug.[175] Agents such as estracyst (a combination of nitrogen mustard linked to the 17-β phosphate of esterdiol *via* a carbonate linkage), estradiol mustard (*bis*-chlorethyl mustard linked to estradiol *via* an ester linkage), and prednimustine (Leo 1031) (a combination of chlorambucil and prednisolone), have been brought into clinical trials. Initial reports were encouraging, especially in hormonally pretreated patients,[121, 134] but a large randomized trial by the NPCP has found the incidence of tumor regression to be low whether such agents were used singly, in sequence, or in combination.[143, 171, 173] In fact, STAB was reported in only 10% of patients. In a recent trial with estracyst in patients with prior hormone manipulation, the overall response rate was 26% and, suprisingly, only 40% in unpretreated cases.[170] Estracyst also has been combined with Me-CCNU, and DDP + MTX with some evidence of objective remission, but with marked toxicity.[179]

The role of estracyst and prednimustine still needs to be defined. Available data indicate little clinical benefit in previously hormone-treated patients, and questions whether estracyst is superior to any other estrogenic compound in unpretreated cases. Protocol 800 of the NPCP[170] which has utilized estracyst, 600 mg/m^2 by mouth, daily, with or without vincristine, 1 mg/m^2 i.v. every 2 weeks, has found minimal efficacy. Protocols 900 and 1000, however, are utilizing estracyst in patients with stages B$_2$, C, and D (without distant metastases) in a randomized "adjuvant" trial.[180]

Various combination chemotherapy protocols also have been tried and while *objective response* has been reported in 5 to 37% of cases, in many instances, such rates simply reflect the activity of a single agent. Most protocols have used CTX or ADM combination regimens.[5, 119, 131, 136, 147, 159, 160, 162–166]

The combination, CTX + ADM, has been reported to induce a CR + PR rate in 0/20, 3/21 (14%), and 6/22 (27%) of cases.[5, 131, 162] Ihde *et al.*[131] studied 22 patients with extrapelvic adenocarcinoma of the prostate, evaluated by "direct" ((abnormalities on prostatic examination (7 cases), skeletal surveys (20 cases), computerized transaxial tomograms (3/6 cases), intravenous pyelograms with hydronephrosis (10 cases), lymphangiograms (8/19 cases), chest x-rays (3 cases), and elevated serum acid phosphatase levels (18 cases)), and "indirect" (bone scans, marrow biopsies and pain, and hemoglobin, carcinoembryonic antigen, alkaline phosphatase, and lactic dehydrogenase isoenzyme levels) parameters. However, no patient was treated solely on the basis of an abnormal bone scan. The dose of ADM was 30 mg/m^2 days 1 and 8, and of CTX, 100 mg/m^2 days 1 and 14. PR was defined as improvement in one or more direct parameters for more than 1 month without deterioration in other parameters. New radiographic osteoblastic lesions which appeared after 1 to 4 months of therapy were not considered disease progression. Partial response was noted in 7/22 (32%) patients: 1 only on the basis of a serum acid phosphatase level; 4/8 in improvement on lymphangiograms; 2/22 in digital prostatic examination measurements; and 1/11 in abnormal intravenous pyelograms cases. Overall survival was 11 months with responders living a median of 14 months (range, 7 to 30 months) *versus* 5 months (range, 2 to 15 months) for nonresponders. The mean time to PROG was 13 months for patients demonstrating a partial response, 7 months of STAB, and 3 months for PROG. A recent report by Ihde *et al.*[166] evaluated ADM and CTX in patients who had no prior hormonal or cytotoxic therapy. A response rate as high as 43% was noted. The addition of DDP in their study resulted in no partial remissions in 16 adequately treated patients, although STAB was throught to have occured in 8/16 (50%) of cases. Of 29 cases given ADM + CTX, with or without DDP, 7/29 (24%) had a PR for a median duration of 8 months (range 2 to 23), and 7/29 (24%) had STAB for a median duration of 6 months (range 5 to 16 months). Strauss *et al.*[136] described a decrease in prostatic size in 3/8 patients given ADM + CTX and methotrexate (MTX). Prior therapy was variable, and 4 patients were excluded from analysis. Another study[163] combined ADM, 30 mg/m^2 day 2, and CTX, 300 mg/m^2 day 2, and carmustine (BCNU), 100 mg/m^2, day 1. Of 27 evaluable cases, 1 obtained a CR, 6 (22%) a PR, and 2 had improvement. Median survival, however, was only 9.3 months for responders *versus* 3.9 months for nonresponders. A recent report[140] has described the efficacy of ADM, 50 mg/m^2, plus mitomycin C, 10 mg/m^2 day 1, plus 5-FU, 750 mg/m^2, days 1 and 2, every 3 to 6 weeks. Initially, 20 (62%) of 32 patients responded: 10/15 in bone lesions 1/1 in nodes, 3/5 in lung lesions, 4/6 in an obstructive uropathy, and 1/1 in malignant ascites. In an updated report (presented at the American Society of Clinical Oncologists meeting in Washington, D.C., by Logothetis *et al.*,[140] 21/42 (50%) cases responded with 11/25 (44%) in osseous and 10/17 (59%) in visceral lesions. In addition, 8/16 cases had a greater than 50% decrease in abnormally elevated serum acid phosphatase levels. Of note, there have been no trials with mitomycin C, used singly, in patients with prostatic cancer.

Various CTX-containing regimens also have been tried. Resnick *et al.*[160] employed a combination of CTX + MTX + 5-FU and noted one partial response in 15 adequately treated patients. Merrin[115] reported one complete remission of 8 months duration with CTX + 5-FU. Buell *et al.*[119] employed a 5-drug regimen with CTX + MTX + 5-FU + vincristine + prednisone, and described 6 responders in 16 patients: 4/6 with a decrease in the size of a tumor masses; and 2/10 with improvement in osseous lesions (median duration, 13 months). Overall survival was not reported. Kane *et al.*[145] described 6 "objective responses" in 25 patients given 5-FU + MTX + vincristine + MEL + prednisone. Responders lived 68 weeks *versus* 32 weeks for nonresponders. Later, Paulson *et al.*[132] reported normalization of alkaline or acid phosphatase, or weight gain of 10%—factors that correlate with increased survival—in 33/84 (39%)

patients with a survival advantage of 76 weeks *versus* 28 weeks. A subsequent study in 14 cases who had bleomycin substituted for MEL[181] described 1 response in 8 evaluable patients who had all five drugs. Of 14 patients treated, 3 patients could not receive bleomycin because of chronic obstructive pulmonary disease, and 5 patients were inevaluable because of toxicity. Lastly, Smalley *et al.*[147] noted no survival advantage or increase in the incidence of tumor regression when 5-FU was compared to CTX + ADM + 5-FU, 2/12 *versus* 2/12.

Hormonal manipulation of the hypothalamic-pituitary-testicular axis, which remains the primary therapy of prostatic carcinoma, is directed at eliminating the facilitory effect of testosterone on prostatic growth.[143] This can be accomplished by: orchiectomy; surgical or medical adrenalectomy[182, 182a]; hypophysectomy[183]; and the administration of exogenous estrogens,[184] progestins,[143] and synthetic antiandrogens such as: cyproterone acetate (Androcur)[185]; the nonsteroidal, 4'-nitro-3'-trifluoromethylisobutyranilide (flutamide)[186]; a progestational antiandrogen, megestrol acetate[187, 188]; or the antiesterogen, tamoxifen.[189, 190] At the cell membrane, testosterone is activated by 5-α-reductase to dihydrotestosterone and transported to a nuclear receptor site on chromatin. Although the exact androgen receptor has yet to be identified, prostatic tumors are composed of a mixture of cells with differential sensitivity.[142, 143, 176] Androcur is postulated to inhibit formation of the dihydrotestosterone-receptor complex thereby indirectly decreasing testicular androgen synthesis and prostatic secretory hormonal activity.[143] The therapeutic advantage of cyproterone acetate over DES is questionable, although one study does claim therapeutic benefit.[185] Flutamide, a pure antiandrogen, blocks dihydrotestosterone binding at the nuclear receptor, and has the potential advantage of less cardiovascular toxicity and feminization—a complication so frequent with DES. The drug probably possesses marginal activity in previously hormonally treated cases and is comparable to DES in unpretreated cases.[143] Tamoxifen has proven dissappointing as a therapeutic modality.[189, 190] Major ablative procedures such as hypophysectomy and adrenalectomy have been reserved for patients with severe disabling bone pain.[143, 182, 183] Subjective responses have been noted in approximately 25% (to as high as 70%), but are usually of very short duration. It is possible that the effect—decrease in pain and analgesic requirements—is mediated *via* the enkephalin system and not *via* a hormonal basis. A relationship between hormonal sensitivity and receptor content has been demonstrated for breast cancer but, as yet, is unproven for prostatic cancer, and is still under active investigation.[191]

Exogenous estrogen administration has multiple effects; not only does it decrease 5-α-reductase and DNA polymerase activity, but probably it acts centrally with the hypothalmus to inhibit leutinizing hormone releasing factor (LHRF). The resulting decrease in pituitary LH secretion would remove a potent stimulus for testosterone synthesis in the Leydig cells.[141] The results of extensive clinical trials by the Veterans Administration Cooperative Urologic Research Group[192] (VACURG) indicate that (1) there is no benefit to early therapy, and survival statistics are equivalent when therapy is delayed until symptoms appear; (2) estrogen administration in doses of greater than 1 mg daily—DES—will inhibit testosterone levels to the precastration state (rebound may occur in 40% of patients and serum testosterone levels can be brought back to castration level with 3 mg daily); (3) the role of adrenal androgen synthesis, which in normal patients contributes 10% of the serum testosterone levels, has not been defined; (4) doses in excess of 5 mg daily result in an increase in cardiovascular deaths, particularly in the 1st year, that outweigh any potential antineoplastic benefit; and (5) doses of 0.2 mg daily are marginally effective. Presently, randomized studies are evaluating the 3-mg dosage level. There is no evidence that orchiectomy is more effective than exogenous estrogen administration in inducing remission, although it may be beneficial in patients who cannot tolerate estrogens or who have problems with drug compliance. Karr et al.[193] have studied levels of testosterone-estradiol-binding globulin plus total testosterone levels in patients treated with orchiectomy plus estramustine phosphate plus DES. The latter two modalities produced elevations of testosterone-binding globulin with a resultant decrease in available testosterone when compared to an orchiectomized group. The clinical correlations of these findings are under study.

Once failure to an initial hormone manipulation has occurred, no increase in survival or significant objective tumor regression has been demonstrated with subsequent hormonal therapy.[117, 143, 184, 194] White et al.[195] observed tumor regression in only 2/25 hormone-resistant patients treated with DES diphosphate (Stilphostrol). In such cases, responses are usually subjective and very short-lived. The need for an orchiectomy to insure a subsequent response to chemotherapy still is debatable.

Only recently has there been a concerted effort to utilize cytotoxic chemotherapy in patients with advanced and early stage adenocarcinoma of the prostate.[180, 196] A large part of the credit is due the NPCP. While controversy remains concerning response criteria and efficacy of presently available single- and multidrug regimens, there is little doubt that new agents, drug combinations, and innovative techniques such as hyperthermia,[197] which may potentiate the effects of cytotoxic chemicals, will take precedence over standard—hormonal—manipulation.

BLADDER CANCER

During the past 5 years, some cytotoxic chemotherapeutic agents have shown efficacy against urothelial tract tumors (transitional cell carcinoma of the renal pelvis, ureter, urinary bladder and urethra).[198] With improved response rates in patients with advanced measurable bladder cancer, clinical trials of adjuvant chemotherapy in high risk cases also have been initiated.[199]

Major advances have included (1) the delineation of selected cases for standard phase II disease-oriented trials—bidimensionally measurable parameters which can be utilized to objectively document a clear end point of response[144, 200]; (2) the extensive use of N-[4-(5-nitro-2-furyl)-2-thiazolyl]formamide (FANFT)[201] and now the soft agar technique to define potentially useful agents and drug combinations[2, 12]; (3) the interest and initiation of randomized trials by large cooperative groups such as the National Bladder Cancer Project (NBCP), the Southwest Oncology Group (SWOG) the Eastern Cooperative Oncology Group (ECOG), the EORTC, and others, which combine a multidisciplinary team of urologists and medical oncologists; and (4) the introduction of DDP[202] which has induced clinically useful responses in patients with advanced bladder cancer, leading to a resurgent interest to define new agents and drug combinations in this tumor. Basically, chemotherapy trials have fallen into four separate areas of interest; DDP and its combination regimens, ADM and its regimens, MTX, and other single agent trials (Table 11.6).

The potential efficacy of DDP for urothelial tract tumors was noted in the FANFT model.[201] In the initial clinical study in 24 patients by Yagoda et al.,[202] objective tumor regression was observed in 33% of cases with bidimensionally measurable metastatic disease given 1.6 mg/kg or 75 mg/m² daily for 3 weeks. Although the median duration of response was only 3 months from attainment of a PR status, the majority of patients in that study refused subsequent therapy because of nausea and vomiting. However, responses were rapid, generally within 1 to 2 doses or 2 to 4 weeks, and occasionally persisted for 9-plus months. Of note, all responders were in the previously untreated group, and all progressors have received prior CTX therapy. Tannock et al.[203] also observed no responses in 10 previously treated cases, all of whom had received a CTX-containing regimen.

Table 11.6
Chemotherapy of bladder cancer[a]

	Number of Patients	CR + PR[b]		Number of Patients	CR + PR[b]
		%			
DDP	320	30	MTX	121	28
+ CTX	102	26	PALA	18	0
+ ADM	72	46	NCS	19	5
+ ADM + CTX	207	47	Mito-C	42	13
+ ADM + 5-FU	44	44	VP-16	29	0
			VLB	27	19
ADM	223	18	VM-26	108	16
+ CTX	37	18	Bleomycin	58	5
+ 5-FU	103	39	m-AMSA	19	11
+ VM-26	27	19	5-FU	(158+)[c]	(23)
+ CTX + MTX	26	38	CTX	(98+)	(31)
+ CTX + BLEO	23	35			
+ 5-FU + CTX	24	21			

[a] The abbreviations used are: CR, complete remission; PR, partial remission; DDP, diamminedichloroplatinum II (cisplatin); CTX, cyclophosphamide; ADM, doxorubicin; 5-FU, 5-fluorouracil; VM-26, 4'-dimethyl-epipodophyllotoxin 9-(4,6-O-2-thenylidene β-D-glucopyranoside); MTX, methotrexate: BLEO, bleomycin; PALA, N-(phosphonacetyl)-L-aspartate; NCS, neocarzinostatin; Mito-C, mitomycin-C; VP-16, etiopside; and VLB, vinblastine sulfate.
[b] The number of patients and % CR + PR are summation of published trials, and studies from Memorial Sloan-Kettering Cancer Center.
[c] ( ), summation of small numbers of cases from multiple trials using variable doses, schedules and response criteria.

Soloway[204] using a similar dose schedule, obtained 8 remissions (47%) in 17 adequately unpretreated patients. A recent update[205] in 27 consecutive patients with locally advanced or metastatic urothelial tract tumors showed an overall response rate of 33% with 12 (45%) patients remaining stable for an average duration of >6 months. Fourteen of 27 patients had metastatic disease while 13 had disease confined to the pelvis. The average duration of response was 8 months for patients with metastatic disease and 5.5 months for patients with locoregional tumors. Using a life table method for analysis of survival, patients who achieved PR + STAB *versus* PROG had clear-cut evidence of clinical benefit with 78 to 84% *versus* 17%, respectively, surviving 6 months. At 12 months, 57% of responders were alive *versus* 0% of nonresponders. In addition, in selected cases in which remaining disease rendered itself to surgical resection, some patients had remained in remission for more than 33 months. The longest survivor in the literature is a patient described by Higby *et al.*[44] and subsequently by Merrin[206] who presented with disseminated disease and after receiving DDP has had no evidence of tumor recurrence for 48-plus months. Merrin[206] who utilized a different schedule, 1 mg/kg every week for 6 weeks and thereafter every three weeks, has recently updated his preliminary report[154]: the overall response rate was 35% (18/51) for an average duration of 5 months.

In another study,[207] of 21 patients who received DDP, 75 mg/m^2 every 3 weeks, 3 (14%) obtained a CR and 6 (29%) a PR. CR status (inguinal nodes, pulmonary metastases and a pelvic recurrence) persisted for 13-plus to 24-plus months. One patient who presented with inguinal nodes, liver, and osseous metastases remained in CR for 26 months—13 months after the last dose of DDP. The average duration of PR status was 5.7 months. The majority of responses occurred rapidly and thus DDP was stopped usually after the third dose in the absence of a response. A definite increase in survival was noted for responders *versus* nonresponders. Other investigators who employed similar dosage schedules have reported partial remissions in 4 of 8,[208] 5 of 11,[209] and 3 of 9[156] adequately treated patients. The median survival time has been approximately 30 weeks for responders *versus* 12 for nonresponders. Oliver[210] using 50 mg/m^2 every 3 weeks noted 2 responses in 10 patients and, in a recent cooperative study from Great Britain,[211] described 8 (31%) in 26 cases.

In a prospectively randomized trial by the ECOG,[212] 98 patients received either DDP or DDP + ADM + CTX. The overall response rate for both arms was 29% (26/91) with 9 complete and 17 partial remissions persisting 26-plus weeks. Although the code has not yet been broken, the rate between the two treatments were not statistically significant: 23% (11/47) *versus* 34% (15/44). In contrast, a randomized trial of DPP *versus* DDP + CTX by the NBCP-cooperative group-A noted only a 13% response rate for DDP + CTX and 21% for DDP alone.[213] The number of remissions increased slightly (24%) when patients with bidimensionally measurable disease were evaluated separately. The NBCP results which falls outside the 95% confidence limits of DDP[198] are distinctly inferior to that which has been reported by other investigators.

Most studies with DDP have obtained remissions in 24 to 43% of cases for a median duration of 5 months.[154, 198, 205, 209, 211] Remissions occur rapidly—within 14 to 50 days—and may persist without maintenance therapy. In selected patients, long term remissions have been achieved with DDP singly and, overall, responders to DDP have lived longer than nonresponders.[198, 200, 205, 207]

Based on data in the FANFT model suggesting synergism when CTX and DDP are combined,[201] clinical trials were undertaken at Memorial Sloan-Kettering Cancer Center.[200, 214] The response rate was 43% in 35 patients (46% in unpretreated and 33% in previously treated cases): a rate which fell within the 95% confidence limits of DDP using singly.[198] In the NBCP stratified (performance status and measurable or evaluable disease) randomized study[213] which evaluated DDP *versus* DDP + CTX, 90 of 123 patients were evaluable and, thus far, no significant difference has been found between the two treatments: DDP 21% (9/43) *versus* DDP + CTX 13% (6/47). The median duration of response for DDP was greater than 14 months compared to only 4.5 months for DDP + CTX. Of interest, the combination was distinctly superior, 57% (8/14), than DDP alone 8% (1/12) for controlling the primary bladder tumor.[215] In two other studies only 2 of 10[216] and 3 of 11 patients given DDP + CTX responded (presented at poster session Abstract C-500, American Society of Clinical Oncologists, Washington, D.C., May 1, 1981 by Khandekar.[212])

ADM also has been combined with DDP.[144, 157, 198, 200, 217-220] Initially, the combination was reported to induce responses in 14 (48%) of 29 adequately treated patients.[144, 157, 200] While the rate seemed slightly higher than that which could be achieved with DDP alone, the lack of a randomized study precluded any conclusion concerning enhanced efficacy of the two-drug regimen. In a randomized study[217] in 94 patients (of whom 76 have thus far been evaluated) given either ADM alone, or ADM as 50 mg/m^2 on day 1 + DDP as 50 mg/m^2 on day 2, 8/40 (20%), *versus* 13/36 (36%) cases given single or the combination therapy, respectively, responded. Of note, 10 (45%) of 22 patients who had no prior irradiation responded, *versus* only 3 (21%) of 14 patients who did. Other studies[218, 220] noted no responses in two cases.

The combination, DDP + ADM + CTX, in a variety of dosages and schedules, also has been extensively evaluated against transitional cell carcinoma. In one study,[198, 200] 14 (48%) of 29 adequately treated patients responded to a sequential regimen of DDP, CTX, and ADM on days 1, 2, and 3, respectively. In three consecutive reports,[221-223] the three-drug combination, CISCA (utilizing CTX, 650 mg/m^2, and ADM, 50 to 60 mg/m^2 on day 1, followed by DDP, 100 mg/m^2 on day 2), induced responses in 10/12 (83%), 17/41 (41%), and 25/50 (50%) adequately treated patients. As stated previously, a recent ECOG randomized study[212] in 91 cases given DDP or the three-drug combination found no statistically significant difference between the two treatments: 23% *versus* 34%. The average duration of response, thus far, is 26 weeks. While one study[224] in 37 cases, which utilized DDP 60 mg/m^2, ADM 40 mg/m^2, and CTX 400 mg/m^2 all given as a single dose every 4 weeks, obtained CR in 11% and

PR in 67% for an average duration of 13 months, another has described only a 17% (2/12) response lasting 7 months.[225] Tumor regression also was noted in 13 (38%) of 34 cases with the same three-drug combination, except for different dosages—DDP 40 mg/m^2, ADM 50 mg/m^2, and CTX 500 mg/m^2.[226] Lastly, DDP has been combined with ADM + 5-FU in 44 patients, and the overall CR + PR rate was 44%.[227, 228]

DDP combination protocols, particularly three-drug regimens which seem to induce a higher response rate than that which can be obtained with DDP singly, show marginal statistical significance.[198]

ADM has been the most thoroughly studied drug for treatment of advanced bladder cancer.[151, 152, 198, 229, 230] Initial trials had indicated a response rate between 35 to 55%,[151, 218, 231] but subsequent studies by other investigators find objective tumor regression in only 10 to 20% of cases for a mean duration of 3 months.[152, 198, 229, 230] ADM-induced remissions seem to be dose dependent—patients receiving 60 and 75 mg/m^2 have obtained a higher remission rate than patients given doses of 30 to 45 mg/m^2,[152, 230] occur somewhat more frequently in unpretreated cases,[230] and in nonirradiated cases—4/16 versus 4/24.[217] In an overall review of the ADM literature combining all dose schedules, 39 (17.5%) of 223 patients have achieved CR + PR status.[198]

The addition of ADM to CTX[232, 233] or to 4'-dimethyl-epipodophyllo-toxin 9-(4, 6-O-2-thenylidene β-D-glucopyranoside) VM-26[234] has resulted in an 18% and 19% response rate in 39 and 27 patients, respectively. However, two studies found a higher remission rate when ADM + CTX was combined with MTX (38% in 26 cases[203]) or bleomycin (35% of 23 cases[235]). In the latter study, the median duration of survival for responders was 30 weeks (range, 19 to 75-plus weeks) versus 18 weeks, (range of 2 to 54 weeks). Although the authors concluded that their results were not superior to single-agent DDP therapy, the slightly higher response rate than that which has been obtained with ADM alone was not explained. Another combination, ADM + 5-FU, has been evaluated in four studies.[236-239] Remissions were reported in 39% of 103 adequately treated patients—a response rate distinctly higher than that which has been reported with ADM alone. However, not all patients had bidimensionally measurable disease, and two studies[147, 164] which combined both drugs with CTX described only 5 (21%) responses in 24 cases. In addition, Williams et al.,[227, 228] who combined both drugs in an identical dosage schedule with DDP, reported a response rate of 44% which was attributed mostly to the action of DDP—indicating that ADM + 5-FU did not significantly enhance the therapeutic benefit of DDP alone. At best, ADM alone must be considered to be inferior to DDP as a single agent.[198]

An old drug, MTX, has recently been re-evaluated in patients with advanced disseminated bladder cancer and found to be extremely effective.[198, 199, 240-244] Dose schedules have varied—the most frequent schedule used is 1 mg/kg i.v. every week, or 50 to 100 mg i.v. every 2 weeks, and 200 mg citrovorum factor (CF) i.m. every 2 weeks. Responses occur rapidly—generally within 2 to 4 doses—and persist for a duration similar to that of DDP. Four reports from the same institution[199, 241, 242, 244] find an overall response rate of 38% in 61 patients with higher rates when larger doses are used. In addition, Oliver, and associates[210, 211] have suggested that MTX may be more effective than DDP against loco-regional disease. Recently, MTX has also been tried after partial cystectomy (2000 mg i.v. every 3 weeks for 6 months) and 17/17 patients have survived more than 2 years.[199] A recent trial at Memorial Hospital[243] described a 27% response rate in 42 patients with bidimensionally measurable metastatic urothelial tract tumors: responses in unpretreated patients were 36% *versus* 19% in previously treated cases. Thus, MTX is an effective agent against transitional cell carcinoma of the urothelial tract with the number and duration of remissions comparable to DDP. Of importance, systemic toxicity has been minor compared to the difficulties usually encountered with DDP in this older patient population. Because of easy patient acceptance and evidence of good antitumor activity, MTX needs to be evaluated in an adjuvant or preadjuvant setting.[199, 243]

A variety of other single agents have had some clinical trials against bladder tumors.[198, 245, 246] While responses have been noted with neocarcinostatin in patients with intravesical lesions,[247, 248] only 1 of 19 patients with disseminated disease have responded.[169] The response rate in 42 cases given mitomycin-C, and in 58 cases given bleomycin, was 14% and 5%, respectively.[198, 231, 245] A recent report[249] has described a 19% response rate in 27 adequately treated patients, most of whom had extensive prior chemotherapy, given vinblastine sulfate (VLB) in doses of 0.1 to 0.15 mg/kg i.v. every week. In an additional arm of the previously reported ECOG study (see Ref. 212) only 1 of 29 (26 unpretreated) and 0/11 adequately treated cases had tumor regression with VM-26 and etiopside (VP-16), respectively. Other studies with VP-16 noted no antitumor activity 18 additional cases.[198, 250, 251] In contrast to the ECOG study, previous trials[231, 252, 253] have described antitumor activity with VM-26, particularly in patients with T_3 lesions (20% in 79 adequately treated patients).

While 5-FU has been noted to induce remission in 35% of 74-plus cases—the majority of whom received various dosages and schedules, and did not have bidimensionally measurable disease[198, 254]—and a recent trial by the Southeastern Cooperative Oncology Group described a 27% response rate,[147] Ducheck *et al.*[255] observed only 2 PRs in 30 adequately treated patients given two different dose schedules. In addition, a randomized study[256] in nonresectable bladder tumor found 5-FU no better than a placebo.

New drugs which, in limited studies, have shown minimal activity include *N*-(phosphonacetyl)-L-aspartate (PALA) and m-AMSA.[257]

The most active agents for the treatment of patients with metastatic urothelial tract tumors include DDP and MTX.[198] Marginally effective agents include ADM, VLB and, possibly, CTX and 5-FU. While there has been some suggestion that DDP-combination regimens are slightly more effective than DDP used singly, no randomized study has yet shown a statistically significant difference. Adjuvant chemotherapy trials have been instituted with DDP (NBCP), DDP + ADM + CTX, and MTX.[199] Hopefully, such studies will show some effect on overall survival and increase the tumor-free interval.

RENAL CANCER

Many single and hormonal agents, and combination drug regimens have been tried in treatment of patients with disseminated hypernephroma, yet none have been found to be predictably and consistently efficacious.[258, 259] Marginal response rates have been obtained with VLB, various progestins, and, in limited trials, almost all other drugs. Overall, remission rates remain in the 5 to 10% range (when one excludes the category, stabilization): a range which probably represents "background noise." Recent trials have included chlorozotocin, vindesine, piperazine dione, VP-16, actinomycin-D, ADM, Baker's antifol, DDP, dianhydrogalacticol, m-AMSA, PALA, lomustine, and semustine.[154, 157, 257-266] Recently, an old drug, methyl-GAG (methylglyoxal bis(guanylhydrazone) seemed promising,[267, 268] but the overall results now indicate only 8 remissions in 64 adequately treated patients.[269, 270] Another new agent, carboxyaldahyde anthracenedione (CL-216, 942), which exhibited excellent antitumor activity against human hypernephroma cells in the soft agar technique,[2, 271] was reported to have induced remission in 3 patients in early phase I-phase II studies.[271, 272] Phase II trials have been initiated to define more accurately its efficacy.

At this time, there appears to be no single-agent immunological approach, or combination regimen which is useful in controlling disseminated renal cancer and, thus, adjuvant therapies are unwarranted.

ADRENAL CANCER

Cytotoxic agents have had limited trials in patients with disseminated adrenal cortical carcinoma.[273, 274] Mitotane (o, p′-DDD), a drug which is difficult to administer in a high-dose schedule because of major, toxic, psychologic sequellae, will induce objective tumor regression in approximately a third of cases and decrease steroid synthesis in 50 to 86% of patients.[275-278] Tumor regression with mitotane also has been observed in patients whose tumors do not produce abnormally elevated steroid levels.[276, 277] Response in some patients have produced cures with unmaintained remissions persisting for more than 4 to 7 years.[279] Of importance, Wortsman and Soler[280] have described inactivation of the effect of mitotane with the concommitant administration of spirolactones. Another agent, aminoglutethimide, can be useful too in controlling biochemical abnormalities but has no direct antitumor effects.[281]

Remissions with cytotoxic chemotherapeutic agents such as 5-FU and adriamycin have been infrequent and, in the majority of reports, such agents have been combined with mitotane.[274] Thus, it is difficult to ascribe any efficacy to the cytotoxic agent. Recently,[273] some adriamycin combination regimens have induced objective tumor regression. A complete remission for 11 months duration was observed in one case given methyl-mitomycin-C,[282] and recently transient remissions (6/12) also have been noted with DDP.[154, 274, 283]

PENILE CANCER

Penile cancer is uncommon in the United States and chemotherapy trials have therefore been limited.[284] Bleomycin has been the standard drug in patients with penile cancer.[284-286] Ichikawa[286] noted excellent antitumor activity against low grade lesions (T_{1-2} and regional lesions): 39 of 59 patients had evidence of tumor regression. However, in a trial at Memorial Hospital[284] only 2 of 12 cases with disseminated disease responded.

Recently,[154, 157, 287] clinically significant responses (5 in 12 cases) have been observed with various dosages and schedules of DDP, particularly 120 mg/m² i.v. every 3 weeks. MTX also has been found to be efficacious: 4/9 patients responded to doses of 0.5 to 1.5 mg/kg i.v. every week, and 2/3 to a higher dose schedule.[157, 284, 288, 289] Both DDP and MTX induce tumor regression within 2 to 4 weeks, and responses have persisted for 3 to 11-plus months.

At this time, the first-line drugs in patients with disseminated penile cancer are MTX and DDP, and in patients with loco-regional disease, bleomycin is the drug of choice.

CONCLUSION

There has been increasing recognition of the role of chemotherapy for treatment of urological malignancies. The dramatic results in patients with testicular tumors has led to the use of cytotoxic agents as primary therapy in patients with stage III disease, and as secondary, adjuvant therapy for patients with stage IIB disease. Strides also have been made in the treatment of patients with transitional cell carcinoma and, hopefully, within the next few years an effective multidrug regimen can be developed which also could be utilized in an adjuvant fashion. While reasonably active antitumor drugs are presently available against penile tumors, only marginally effective agents, as yet, have been found for therapy of hypernephroma and adrenal cortical tumors. The role for cytotoxic, nonhormonal chemotherapy in treatment of patients with advanced prostatic adenocarcinoma remains problematical.

Acknowledgments—This paper was supported in part by the National Institutes of Health grant CA-05826, Public Health Service grant CA-09207, National Cancer Institute contract 1-CM-57043, and the Aaron Miller-Solid Tumor Service Fund.

The authors gratefully acknowledge the excellent technical, research and editorial assistance of Mrs. Isa Irvin.

REFERENCES

1. Yagoda, A. Non-hormonal cytotoxic agents in the treatment of prostatic adenocarcinoma. *Cancer 32:*1131, 1973.
2. Von Hoff, D. D., Page, C., Harris, G., Clark, G., Cowan, J., Coltman, C. A., and The South Central Texas Human Tumor Cloning Group. Prospective clinical trials of a human tumor cloning system. *Proc. Am. Assoc. Cancer Res. 22:*154, 1981.

3. Bosl, G. J., Lange, P. H., Fraley, E. E., Nochomovitz, L. E., Rosai, J., Vogelzang, N. J., Johnson, K., Crokmann, A., and Kennedy, B. J. Vinblastine, bleomycin and *cis*-diamminedichloroplatinum in the treatment of advanced testicular carcinoma. Possible importance of longer induction and shorter maintenance periods. *Am. J. Med. 68:*492, 1980.

4. Spitzer, G., Dicke, K. A., Litam, J., Verma, D. S., Zander, A., Lanzotti, V., Valdivieso, M., McCredie, K. B., and Samuels, M. L. High-dose combination chemotherapy with analogous bone marrow transplantation in adult solid tumors. *Cancer 45:*3075, 1980.

5. Izbicki, R. M., Amer, M. H., and Al-Sarraf, M. Combination of adriamycin and cyclophosphamide in the treatment of metastatic prostatic carcinoma: a phase II study. *Cancer Treat. Rept. 63:*999, 1979.

6. Reynolds, T. F., Yagoda, A., Vugrin, D., and Golbey, R. Chemotherapy of mediastinal germ-cell tumors. *Semin. Oncol. 6:*113, 1979.

7. Fox, R. M., Woods, R. L., Tattersall, M. H. N., and McGovern, V. J. Undifferentiated carcinoma in young men: The atypical teratoma syndrome. *Cancer 43:*316, 1979.

8. Greco, F. A., Fer, M. F., Richardson, R. L., Houde, K. R., Oldham, R. K., and Forbes, J. T. The unrecognized extragonadal germ-cell cancer syndrome. *Proc. Am. Assoc. Cancer Res. 21:*149, 1980.

9. Anderson, T., Waldmann, T. A., Javadpour, N., and Glatstein, E. Testicular germ-cell neoplasms: recent advances in diagnosis and therapy. *Ann. Intern. Med. 90:*373, 1979.

10. Fraley, E. E., Lange, P. H., and Kennedy, B. J. Germ-cell testicular cancer in adults. *N. Engl. J. Med. 301:*1370, and 1420, 1979.

11. Javadpour, N., and Bergman, S. Recent advances in testicular cancer. *Curr. Probl. Surg. 15:*5, 1978.

12. Natale, R. B., Yagoda, A., and Molander, D. *In vitro* and *in vivo* sensitivity of human bladder carcinoma: correlation with Phase II trials of AMSA, PALA and Methotrexate (MTX). *Proc. Am. Assoc. Cancer Res. 21:*297, 1980.

12a. Malkin, A., Malkin, D. G., Comisarow, R. H., and Sturgeon, J. F G. Lactic dehydrogenase (LDH), 2-hydroxybutyrate dehydrogenase (HBO), and 3,3′,5′-triiodothyronine (reverse T_3; rT_3) in testicular cancer. *Proc. Am. Assoc. Cancer Res. 22:*333, 1981.

13. Vaitukaitis, J. L., Braunstein, G. V., and Ross, G. T. A radioimmunoassay which specifically measures human chorionic gonadotropin in the presence of human luteinizing hormone. *Am. J. Obstet. Gynecol. 113:*751, 1972.

14. Braunstein, G. D., Vaitukaitis, J. L., Carbone, P. P., and Ross, G. I. Ectopic production of human chorionic gonadotropin by neoplasms. *Ann. Intern. Med. 78:*39, 1973.

15. Javadpour, N., McIntire, K. R., and Waldmann, T. A. Human chorionic gonadotropin (HCG) and α-fetoprotein (AFP) in sera and tumor cells of patients with testicular seminoma. A prospective study. *Cancer 42:*2768, 1978.

16. Abelev, G. T., Assecritova, I. V., Kraevsky, N. A., Perova, S. D., and Perevodchikova, N. I. Embryonal serum α-globulin in cancer patients: diagnostic value. *Int. J. Cancer 2:*551, 1967.

17. Waldmann, T. A., and McIntire, K. R. The use of radioimmunoassay for α-fetoprotein in the diagnosis of malignancy. *Cancer 34:*1510, 1974.

18. Friedman, A., Vugrin, D., and Golbey, R. B. Prognostic significance of serum tumor biomarkers (TM), α-fetoprotein (AFP), β-subunit of human chorionic gonadotropin (bHCG) and lactate dehydrogenase (LDH) in nonseminomatous germ-cell tumors (NSGCT). *Proc. Am. Assoc. Cancer Res. 21:*323, 1980.

19. Kohn, J. The value of apparent half-life assay of α-1-fetoprotein in the management of testicular teratoma In *Carcino-Embryonic Proteins*, pp. 383–386. Edited by F. G. Lehmann, Elsevier-North Holland Biomedical Press, 1979.

20. Lange, P. H. Calculations of serum marker decay in testicular tumor. *Proceedings of the American Urological Association*, p. 13, New York, May 11–15, 1979.

21. Lange, P. H., and Fraley, E. E. Serum α-fetoprotein and human chorionic gonadotropin in the treatment of patients with testicular tumors. *Urol. Clin. North Am. 4:*393, 1977.

22. Rizkallah, T., Gurpide, E., and van de Wiele, R. L. Metabolism of HCG in man. *J. Clin. Endocrinol. Metab. 29:*92, 100, 1969.

23. Perlin, E., Engeller, J. E., Edson, M., Karp, D., McIntire, K. R., and Waldman, T. A. The value of serial measurement of both human chorionic gonadotropin and α-fetoprotein for monitoring germinal cell tumors. *Cancer 37:*215, 1976.

24. Knecht, M., and Hertz, R. Relationship between plasma levels of human chorionic gonadotropin and tumor growth during chemotherapy for human choriocarcinoma maintained in the cheek pouch. *Cancer Treat. Rept. 62:*2101, 1978.

25. Vogelzang, N. J., Lange, P. H. G., Bosl, G. J., Fraley, E. E., Johnson, K., and Kennedy, B. J. Paradoxical tumor-marker elevations during induction chemotherapy for testicular tumor (TT). *Proc. Am. Assoc. Cancer Res. 21:*431, 1980.

26. Garnick, M. B. Spurious rise in human chorionic gonadotropin induced by marijuana in patients with testicular cancer. *N. Engl. J. Med. 303:*1177, 1980.

27. Bosl, G. J., Lange, P. H., Fraley, E. E., Johnson, K., and Kennedy, B. J. Multiple biologic markers in the management of testis cancer. *Proc. Am. Assoc. Cancer Res. 20:* 102, 1979.

28. Boyle, L. E., and Samuels, M. L. Serum LDH activity and the isozyme patterns in non-seminomatous germinal (NSG) testis tumors. *Proc. Am. Assoc. Cancer Res. 18:* 278, 1977.

29. Zondag, H. A., and Klein, F. Clinical applications of lactate dehydrogenase isozymes: Alterations in malignancy. *Ann. N. Y. Acad. Sci. 151:*578, 1968.

30. Wilkinson, J. H. Lactate dehydrogenase isoenzymes. In *Isoenzymes*, pp 135–203. Edited by J. H. Wilkinson. J. B. Lippincott, Philadelphia, 1970.

31. Siciliano, M. J., Bordelon-Riser, M. E., Freedman, R. S., and Kohler, P. O. A human trophoblastic isozyme (lactate dehydrogenase-Z) associated with choriocarcinoma. *Cancer Res. 40:*287, 1980.

32. Bosl, G. J., Lange, P. H., Nochomovitz, L. E., Goldman, A., Fraley, E. E., Rosai, J., Johnson, K., and Kennedy B. J. Tumor markers in advanced nonseminomatous testicular cancer. *Cancer 47:*572, 1981.

33. Scardino, P. T., Cox, H. G., Waldmann, T. A., McIntire, K. R., Mittemeyer, B., and Javadpour, N. The value of serum tumor markers in the staging and prognosis of germ-cell tumors of the testis. *J. Urol. 118:*994, 1977.

34. Talerman, A., van der Pompe, W. V., Haije, W. G., Baggerman, L., and Bockestein-Tjahjadi, H. M. Alpha-fetoprotein and carcinoembryonic antigen in germ cell neoplasms. *Br. J. Cancer 35:*288, 1977.

35. Lange, P. H., Bremner, R. E., Horne, C. H. W., Vesella, R. L., and Fraley, E. E. Is SP-1 a marker for testicular cancer? *Urology 15:*251, 1980.

36. Horne, C. H. W., and Nisbet, A. D. Pregnancy proteins: a review. *Invest. Cell Pathol. 2:*217, 1979.

37. Li, M. C., Whitmore, W. F., Golbey, R., and Grabstald, H. Effects of combined drug therapy on metastatic cancer of the testis. *JAMA 174:*1291, 1960.

38. Kennedy, B. J. Mithramycin therapy in advanced testicular neoplasms. *Cancer 26:*755, 1970.

39. Samuels, M. L., and Howe, C. D. Vinblastine in the management of testicular cancer. *Cancer 25:*1009, 1970.

40. Blom, J., and Brodovsky, H. S. Comparison of the treatment of metastatic testicular tumors with actinomycin-D or actinomycin-D, bleomycin and vincristine. *Proc. Am. Assoc. Cancer Res. 16:*247, 1975.

41. Samuels, M. L., Holoye, P. Y., and Johnson, D. E. Bleomycin combination chemotherapy in the management of testicular neoplasia. *Cancer 36:*318, 1975.

42. Samuels, M. L., Lanzotti, V. J., Holoye, P. Y., Boyle, L. E., Smith, T. L., and Johnson, D. E. Combination chemotherapy in germinal cell tumors. *Cancer Treat. Rev. 3:*185, 1976.

43. Wittes, R. E., Yagoda, A., Silvay, O., Magill, G. B., Whitmore, W. F., Krakoff, I. H., and Golbey, R. B. Chemotherapy of germ-cell tumors of the testis: induction of remission with vinblastine, actinomycin-D and bleomycin. *Cancer 37:*637, 1976.

44. Higby, D. J., Wallace, H. J., Albert, D. J., and Holland, J. F. Diamminedichloroplatinum: a Phase I study showing responses in testicular and other tumors. *Cancer 33:* 1219, 1974.

45. Bosl, G. J., Kwong, R., Lange, P., Fraley, E. E., and Kennedy, B. J. Vinblastine, intermittent bleomycin and single-dose *cis*-platinum in the management of Stage III testicular carcinoma. *Cancer Treat. Rept. 64:*331, 1980.

46. Cheng, E., Cvitkovic, E., Wittes, R. E., and Golbey, R. B. Germ cell tumors (II). VAB II in metastatic testicular cancer. *Cancer 42:*2162, 1978.

47. Einhorn, L. H., and Donohue, J. *Cis*-diamminedichloroplatinum (II) vinblastine, and bleomycin combination chemotherapy in disseminated testicular cancer. *Ann. Intern. Med. 37:*293, 1977.

48. Cvitkovic, E., Spaulding, J., Betheune, V., Martin, J., and Whitmore W. F. Improvement of *cis*-dichlorodiammineplatinum (NSC-119875): therapeutic index in an animal model. *Cancer 39:*1357, 1977.

49. Hayes, D. M., Cvitkovic, E., Golbey, R. B., Scheiner, E., Helson, L., and Krakoff, I. H. High-dose *cis*-platinum diamminedichloride: amelioration of renal toxicity of mannitol diuresis. *Cancer 39:*1372, 1977.

50. Buckner, C. D., Clift, R. A., Fefer, A., Funk, D. D., Glucksberg, P. H., Neiman P. E., Paulson, A., Storb, R., and Thomas E. D. High-dose cyclophosphamide (NSC-26271) for treatment of metastatic testicular neoplasms. *Cancer Chemother. Rept. 58:*709, 1974.

51. MacKenzie, A. R. Chemotherapy of metastatic testis cancer. *Cancer 19:*1369, 1966.

52. Cvitkovic, E., Cheng, E., Whitmore W. F., and Golbey, R. B. Germ cell tumor: chemotherapy update. *Proc. Am. Assoc. Cancer Res. 18:*324, 1977.

53. Golbey, R. B., Reynolds, T. F., and Vugrin, D. Chemotherapy of metastatic germ-cell tumors. *Semin. Oncol. 6:*82, 1979.

54. Vugrin, D., Dukeman, M., Whitmore, W. F., and Golbey, R. B. VAB-6: Progress in chemotherapy of testicular germ-cell tumors. *Proc. Am. Assoc. Cancer Res. 21:*426, 1980.

55. Vugrin, D., Herr, H., Sogani, P. C., Whitmore, W. F., and Golbey R. B. VAB-6 without maintenance: progress in chemotherapy of testicular germ-cell tumors. *Proc. Am. Assoc. Cancer Res. 22:*474, 1981.

56. Vugrin, D., Herr, H. W., Whitmore, W. F., Sogani, P. C., and Golbey, R. B. VAB-6 combination chemotherapy in disseminated cancer of the testis. *Ann. Intern. Med. 95:* 56, 1981.

57. Hong, W. K., Wittes, R. E., Hajdu, S. T., Cvitkovic, E., Whitmore, W. F., and Golbey, R. B. The evolution of mature teratoma from malignant testicular tumors. *Cancer 40:* 2987, 1977.

58. Einhorn, L. H. The role of surgery in disseminated testicular cancer. *Proc. Am. Assoc. Cancer Res. 21:*159, 1980.

59. Sogani, P. C., Vugrin, D., Whitmore, W. F., Bains, M., Herr, H., and Golbey, R. B. Experience with combination chemotherapy and surgery with management of advanced germ-cell tumors. *Proc. Am. Assoc. Cancer Res. 21:*401, 1980.

60. Lange, P. H., Hekmat, K., Bosl, G. J., Kennedy, B. J., and Fraley, E. E. Accelerated growth of testicular cancer after cytoreductive surgery. *Cancer 45:*1498, 1980.

61. Anderson, T., Javadpour, N., Schilsky, R., Barlock, A., and Young, R. C. Chemotherapy for testicular cancer: current status of the National Cancer Institute combined modality trial. *Cancer Treat. Rept. 63:*1687, 1979.

62. Einhorn, L. H. Combination chemotherapy with *cis*-dichlorodiammineplatinum (II) in disseminated testicular cancer. *Cancer Treat. Rept. 63:*1659, 1979.

63. Samson, M. K., Stephens, R. L., Rivkin, S., Opipari, M., Maloney, T., Groppe, C. W., and Fisher, R. Vinblastine, bleomycin, and *cis*-dichlorodiammineplatinum (II) in disseminated testicular cancer: preliminary report of a Southwest Oncology Group Study. *Cancer Treat. Rept. 63:*1663, 1979.

64. Einhorn, L. H. and Williams, S. D. Chemotherapy of disseminated testicular cancer. *Cancer 46:*1339, 1980.

65. Samuels, M. L., Johnson, D. E., Brown, B., Bracken, R. B., Moran M. E., and von Eschenback, A. Velban plus continuous infusion of bleomycin (VB-3) in Stage III advanced testicular cancer: results in 99 patients with a note on high-dose Velban and sequential *cis*-platinum. In *Cancer of the Genitourinary Tract*, pp. 169–172. Edited by D. E. Johnson and M. L. Samuels, Raven Press, New York, 1979.

66. Maier, J. G., Sulak, M. H., and Mittemeyer, B. T. Seminoma of the testis: an analysis of treatment success and failure. *AJR 102:*596, 1968.

67. Batata, M. A., Chu, F. C. H., Hilaris, B. S., Whitmore, W. F., Grabstald, H., and Golbey, R. B. TNM staging of testis cancer. *Int. J. Radiat. Oncol. Biol. Phys. 6:*291, 1980.

68. Yagoda, A., and Vugrin, D. Theoretical considerations in the treatment of seminoma. *Semin. Oncol. 6:*74, 1979.

69. Samuels, M. L., Logothetis, C., Trindade, A., and Johnson, D. E. Sequential weekly pulse-dose *cis*-platinum for far-advanced seminoma. *Proc. Am. Assoc. Cancer Res. 21:* 423, 1980.

70. Einhorn, L. H., and Williams, S. D. Chemotherapy of disseminated seminoma. *Cancer Clin. Trials 3:*307, 1980.

71. Bradfield, J. S., Hagen, R. O., and Ytredal, D. O. Carcinoma of the testis: an analysis of 104 patients with germinal tumors of the testis other than seminoma. *Cancer 31:*633, 1973.

72. Fraley, E. E., Kedia, K., and Markland, C. The role of radical operation in the management of nonseminomatous germinal tumors of the testicle in the adult. In *Controversies in Surgery*, pp. 479–488. Edited by R. L. Varco and J. R. Delaney. W. B. Saunders, Philadelphia, 1976.

73. Hussey, D. H., Luk, K. H., and Johnson, D. E. The role of radiation therapy in the treatment of germinal tumors of the testis other than pure seminoma. *Radiology 123:* 175, 1977.

74. Maier, J. G., Van Buskirk, K. E., Sulak, M. H., Perry, R. H., and Schamber, D. T. An evaluation of lymphadenectomy in the treatment of malignant testicular germ cell neoplasm. *J. Urol. 11:*356, 1969.

75. Maier, J. G., and Mittemeyer, B. Carcinoma of the testis. *Cancer 39:*981, 1977.

76. Nicholson, T. C., Walsh, P. C., and Rotner, M. B. Lymphadenectomy combined with preoperative and postoperative cobalt 60 teletherapy in the management of embryonal carcinoma and teratocarcinoma of the testis. *J. Urol. 112:*109, 1974.

77. Slawson, R. G. Radiation therapy for germinal tumors of the testis. *Cancer 42:*2216, 1978.

78. Staubitz, W. J., Early, K. S., Magoss, I. V., and Murphy, G. P. Surgical management of testis tumor. *J. Urol. 111:*205, 1974.

79. Tyrell, C. J., and Peckham, M. J. The response of lymph node metastases of testicular teratoma to radiation therapy. *Br. J. Urol. 48:*363, 1976.

80. van der Werf Messing, B. Radiotherapeutic treatment of testicular tumors. *Int. J. Radiat. Oncol. Biol. Phys. 1:*235, 1976.

81. Walsh, P. C., Kaufman, J. J., Coulson, W. F., and Goodwin, W. E. Retroperitoneal lymphadenectomy for testicular tumors. *JAMA 217:*309, 1971.

82. Whitmore, W. F. Germinal tumors of the testis. In *Proceedings of the Sixth National Cancer Conference*, pp 219–245. Lippincott, Philadelphia, 1970.

83. Vugrin, D., Cvitokovic, E., Whitmore, W. F., and Golbey, R. B. Prophylactic chemotherapy of testicular germ-cell carcinoma (non-seminomas) Stage II following orchiectomy and retroperitoneal dissection. *Proc. Am. Assoc. Cancer Res. 19:*352, 1978.

84. Vugrin, D., Cvitkovic, E., Whitmore, W. F., and Golbey, R. B. Adjuvant chemotherapy and resected non-seminomatous germ cell tumors of the testis: Stages I and II. *Semin. Oncol. 6:*94, 1979.

85. Vogelzang, N., and Kennedy, B. J. Personal communication.

86. Williams, S. D., Einhorn, L. H., and Donohue, J. P. High cure rate of Stage I or Stage II testicular cancer with or without adjuvant therapy. *Proc. Am. Assoc. Cancer Res. 21:* 421, 1980.

87. Jacobs, E. M., and Muggia, F. M. Testicular cancer: risk factors and role of chemotherapy. *Cancer 45:*1782, 1980.

88. Beattie, E. J. Mediastinal germ cell tumors (surgery). *Semin. Oncol. 6:*109, 1979.

89. Goldiner, P. L., and Schweizer, O. The hazards of anesthesia and surgery in bleomycin-treated patients. *Semin. Oncol. 6:*121, 1979.

90. Fossa, S. D., Klepp, O., and Aakraag, A. Testicular function after combined chemotherapy for metastatic testicular cancer. *Int. J. Androl. 3:*59, 1980.

91. Banerjee, A., and Benedict, W. F. Production of sister chromatid exchanges by various cancer chemotherapeutic agents. *Cancer Res. 39:*797, 1979.

92. Arsenau, J. C., Sponzo, R. W. Levin, D. L., Schnipper, L. E., Bonner, H, Young, R. C., Canellos, G. P., Johnson, R. E., and De Vita, V. T. Nonlymphomatous malignant tumors complicating Hodgkin's Disease; possible association with intensive therapy. *N. Engl. J. Med. 287:*1119, 1972.

93. Coleman, C. N., Williams, C. J., Flint, A., Glatstein, E. J., Rosenberg, S. A., and

Kaplan, H. S. Hematologic neoplasia in patients treated for Hodgkin's Disease. *N. Engl. J. Med. 297:*1249, 1977.

94. Reimer, K. K., Hoover, R., Fraumeni, J. F., and Young, R. C. Acute leukemia after alkylating agent therapy of ovarian cancer. *N. Engl. J. Med. 297:*177, 1977.

95. Edwards, G. S., Lane, M., and Smith, F. E. Long-term treatment with *cis*-dichloro-diammineplatinum (II)—vinblastine-bleomycin: possible association with severe coronary artery disease. *Cancer Treat. Rept. 63:*551, 1979.

96. Rothberg, H. Raynaud's phenomenon after vinblastine-bleomycin chemotherapy. *Cancer Treat. Rept. 62:*569, 1978.

97. Teutsch, C., Lipton, A., and Harvey, A. J. Raynaud's phenomenon as a side effect of chemotherapy with vinblastine and bleomycin for testicular carcinoma. *Cancer Treat Rept. 61:*925, 1977.

98. Vogelzang, N. J., Bosl, G. J., Johnson, K., and Kennedy, B. J. Raynaud's phenomenon: a common toxicity following vinblastine, bleomycin and *cis*-platin therapy of testicular cancer. *Ann. Intern. Med.* (in press).

99. Bosl, G. J., Lange, P. H., Fraley, E. E., Johnson, K, Brown, J., and Lange, P. Is maintenance therapy necessary following complete remission of Stage III testis cancer? *Proc. Am. Assoc. Cancer Res. 20:*385, 1979.

100. Neidhart, J., Memo, R., Metz, E., and Wise, H. Probable cure of advanced testicular cancers by intensive primary chemotherapy without maintenance. *Proc. Am. Assoc. Cancer Res. 20:*383, 1979.

101. Sturgeon, J. F. G., Jewett, M. A. S., Hawkins, N. Y., Alison, R. E., Comisarow, R., Grospodarowicz, M., Rider, W. D., Herman, J., Bergslagel, D. E., and Evans, W. K. Advanced non-seminomatous testicular tumors: maintenance chemotherapy is unnecessary. Poster abstract. International Symposium on Testis Cancer; Mouse Teratocarcinoma and Oncofetal Proteins. Minneapolis, Minn., June 26–28, 1980.

102. Einhorn, L. H., Williams, S., Turner, S., Troner, M., and Greco, F. A. The role of maintenance therapy of disseminated testicular cancer: A Southeastern Cancer Study Group (SECSG) protocol. *Proc. Am. Assoc. Cancer Res. 22:*463, 1981.

103. Radice, P. A., Bunn, P. A., and Ihde, D. C. Therapeutic trials with VP-16-213 and VM-26: Active agents in small cell cancer, non-Hodgkins lymphomas, and other malignancies. *Cancer Treat. Rept. 63:*1231, 1979.

104. Williams, S. D., Einhorn, L. H., Creco, A., and Donohue, J. F. VP-16-213: Salvage therapy for refractory germinal neoplasms. *Cancer 46:*2154, 1980.

105. Cavalli, F., Klept, O., Renard, J., Renard J., Hansen, H. H., and Alberto, P. A phase II study of oral VP-16-213 in patients with non-seminomatous testicular cancer. *Proc. Am. Assoc. Cancer Res. 21:*137, 1980.

106. Fitzharris, B. M., Kaye, S. B., Saverymuttu, S., Newlands, E. S., Barrett, A., Peckham, M. J., and McElwain, T. J. VP-16-213 as a single agent in advanced testicular tumors. *Eur. J. Cancer. 16:*1193, 1980.

107. Vogelzang, N. J., and Kennedy, B. J. "Salvage" chemotherapy for refractory germ-cell tumors. *Proc. Am. Assoc. Cancer Res. 22:*471, 1981.

108. Schabel, F. M., Trader, M. W., Laster, W. R., Corbett, T. H., and Griswold, D. P. *Cis*-dichlorodiammineplatinum II: Combination chemotherapy and cross-resistance studies with tumors of mice. *Cancer Treat. Rept. 63:*1459, 1979.

109. Bosl, G. J., Cirrincione, C., Geller, N., Vugrin, D., Whitmore, W. F., and Golbey, R. Complete remission (CR) in patients (pts) with metastatic nonseminomatous germ-cell tumors of the testis (NSGCTT): Multivariate analysis of prognostic variables. *Proc. Am. Assoc. Cancer Res. 22:*393, 1981.

110. Hill, J. M., Loeb, E., Pardue, A., Khan, A., King, J. J., Aleman, C., and Hill, N. O. Platinum analogues of clinical interest. *Cancer Treat. Rept. 63:*1509, 1979.

111. Carter, S. K. The clinical evaluation of analogues-III. Anthracyclenes. *Cancer Chemother. Pharmacol. 4:*5, 1980.

112. Strickland, S., and Mahdavi, V. The induction of differentiation in teratocarcinoma stem cells by retinoic acid. *Cell 15:*393, 1978.

113. Bosl, G. J., Vogelzang, N. J., Goldmann, A., and Kennedy, B. J. Delay in diagnosis of testis cancer impact on clinical stage. *Lancet* (in press).

114. Fraley, E. E. The testicular mass and approach to diagnosis and treatment. In *Advances*

in Cancer Surgery, pp. 589–596. Edited by J. S. Najarian and J. R. Delaney, eds. Symposia Specialists, Chicago, 1976.

115. Merrin, C. E. Preliminary report on combination therapy for advanced prostatic cancer. *Cancer Treat. Rept. 61:*313, 1977.

116. Schmidt, J. D. Chemotherapy of hormone-resistant stage D prostatic cancer. *J. Urol. 123:*797, 1980.

117. Torti, F. M., and Carter, S. K. The chemotherapy of prostatic adenocarcinoma. *Ann. Intern. Med. 92:*681, 1980.

118. Yagoda, A., Watson, R. C., Natale, R. B., Barzell, W. E., Sogani, P. C., Grabstald, H., and Whitmore, W. F. A critical analysis of response criteria in patients with prostatic cancer treated with *cis*-diamminedichloride platinum II. *Cancer 44:*1553, 1979.

119. Buell, G. V., Saiers, J., Saiki, J., and Bergreen, P. Chemotherapy trial with COMP-F regimen in advanced adenocarcinoma of prostate. *J. Urol. 11:*247, 1978.

120. DeWys, W. D., Bauer, M., Colsky, J., Cooper, R., Creech, R., and Carbone, P. P. Comparative trial of adriamycin and 5-fluorouracil in advanced prostatic cancer—progress report. *Cancer Treat. Rept. 61:*325, 1977.

121. Edsmyr, F., Esposti, P., Johansson, B., and Strindberg, B. Clinical experimental randomized study of 2.6-cidiphenylhexamethylcyclotetrasiloxane and estramustine-17-phosphate in the treatment of prostatic carcinoma. *J. Urol. 120:*705, 1977.

122. Franks, C. R. Melphalan in metastatic cancer of the prostate. *Cancer Treat. Rev. 6:*121, 1979.

123. Kvols, L. K., Eagan, R. T., and Myers, R. P. Evaluation of melphalan, ICRF-159 and hydroxyurea in metastatic prostate cancer: a preliminary report. *Cancer Treat. Rept. 61:*311, 1977.

124. Schmidt, J. D., Johnson, D. E., Scott, W., Gibbons, R. P., Prout, G. R., and Murphy, G. P. Chemotherapy of advanced prostatic cancer: evaluation of response criteria. *J. Urol. 7:*602, 1976.

125. Tejada, F., and Cohen, M. Initial chemotherapeutic trials in patients with inoperable or recurrent cancer of the prostate. *Cancer Chemother. Rept. 59:*243, 1975.

126. Eagan, R. T., Utz, D. C., Myers, R. P., and Furlow, W. L. Comparison of adriamycin (NSC-123127) and the combination of 5-fluorouracil (NSC-19893) and cyclophosphamide (NSC-26271) in advanced prostatic cancer: a preliminary report. *Cancer Chemother. Rept. 59:*203, 1975.

127. Merrin, C. E. and Beckly, S. Treatment of estrogen-resistant stage D carcinoma of prostate with *cis*-diamminedichloroplatinum.*J. Urol. 13:*267, 1979.

128. Eagan, R. T., Hahn, R. G., and Myers, R. P. Adriamycin (NSC-123127) *versus* 5-fluorouracil (NSC-19893) and cyclophosphamide (NSC-26271) in the treatment of metastatic prostate cancer. *Cancer Treat. Rept. 60:*115, 1976.

129. Berry, W. R., Laszlo, J., Cox, E., Walker, A., and Paulson, D. Prognostic factors in metastatic and hormonally unresponsive carcinoma in the prostate. *Cancer 44:*763, 1979.

130. Citrin, D. L., Cohen, A. I., Harberg, J., Schlise, S., Hougen, C., and Benson, R. Systemic treatment of advanced prostatic cancer: development of a new system for defining response. *J. Urol. 125:*224, 1981.

131. Ihde, D. C., Bunn, P. A., Cohen, M., Dunnick, N. R., Eddy, J., and Minna, J. D. Effective treatment of hormonally-unresponsive metastatic carcinoma of the prostate with adriamycin and cyclophosphamide. *Cancer 45:*1300, 1980.

132. Paulson, D. F., Berry, W. R., Cox, E. B., and Laszlo, J. Chemotherapy of Prostatic Cancer. In *Cancer of the Genitourinary Tract*, pp. 261–272. Edited by D. E. Johnson and M. L. Samuels. Raven Press, New York, 1979.

133. Slack, N. H., Mittelman, A., Brady, M. F., and Murphy, G. P. The importance of the stable category for chemotherapy-treated patients with advanced and relapsing prostate cancer. *Cancer 46:*2393, 1980.

134. Nilsson, T., Jonsson, G. Clinical results with estramustine phosphate (NSC-89199): a comparison of the intravenous and oral preparations. *Cancer Chemother. Rept. 59:*229, 1975.

135. DeWys, W. D. Comparison of adriamycin (NSC-123127) and 5-fluorouracil (NSC-19893) in advanced prostatic carcinoma. *Cancer Chemother. Rept. 59:*215, 1975.

136. Straus, M. J., Parmelee, J., Olsson, C., and deVere White, R. Cytoxan, adriamycin, methotrexate (CAM) therapy of Stage D prostate cancer. *Proc. Am. Assoc. Cancer Res. 19:*314, 1978.
137. Schmidt, J. D., Scott, W. W., Gibbons, R. P., Johnson, D. E., Prout, G. T., Loening, S. A., Soloway, M., Chu, T. M., Gaeta, J. F. Slack, N. H., Saroff, J., and Murphy, G. P. Comparison of procarbazine, imidazole-carboxamide and cyclophosphamide in relapsing patients with advanced carcinoma of the prostate. *J. Urol. 121:*185, 1979.
138. Pollen, J. J., Gerber, K., Ashburn, W., and Schmidt, J. D. The value of nuclear bone imaging in advanced prostatic cancer. *J. Urol. 125:*222, 1981.
139. Pollen, J. J., and Shlaer, W. J. Osteoblastic response to successful treatment of metastatic cancer of the prostate. *AJR 132:*927, 1979.
140. Logothetis, C., von Eschenback, A., Samuels, M., Haynie, T. P., and Johnson, D. E. Doxorubicin, mitomycin C, 5-fluorouracil (DMF) in the therapy of hormonal resistant adenocarcinoma of the prostate. *Proc. Am. Assoc. Cancer Res. 22:*462, 1981.
141. Coffey, D. S., and Isaacs, J. T. Control of prostatic growth. *Urol. (Suppl.) 17:*17, 1981.
142. Sandberg, A. A. Rationale and practice of testing chemotherapeutic agents for prostate cancer. *Urol. (Suppl.) 17:*34, 1981.
143. Scott, W. W., Menon, M., and Walsh, P. C. Hormonal therapy of prostatic cancer. *Cancer 45:*1929, 1980.
144. Yagoda, A. Future implications of Phase II chemotherapy trials in ninety-five patients with measurable advanced bladder cancer. *Cancer Res. 37:*2275, 1977.
145. Kane, R. D., Stocks, L. H., and Paulson, D. F. Multiple drug chemotherapy regimen for patients with hormonally-unresponsive carcinoma of the prostate: a preliminary report. *J. Urol. 117:*467, 1977.
146. Muss, H. B., Howard V., Richards II, F., White, D. R., Jackson, D. V., Cooper, M. R., Stuart, J. J., Resnick, M. I., Brodkin, R., and Spurr, C. L. Cyclophosphamide *versus* cyclophosphamide, methotrexate, and 5-fluorouracil in advanced prostatic cancer: a randomized trial. *Cancer 47:*1949, 1981.
147. Smalley, R. V., Bartolucci, A. A., Hemstreet, G., and Hester, M. A phase II evaluation of a 3-drug combination of cyclophosphamide, doxorubicin and 5-fluorouracil and of 5-fluorouracil in patients with advanced bladder carcinoma or stage D prostatic carcinoma. *J. Urol. 125:*191, 1981.
148. Lerner, H. J., and Malloy, T. R. Hydroxyurea in stage D carcinoma of the prostate. *J. Urol. 10:*35, 1977.
149. Loening, S. A., deKernion, J. B., Gibbons, R. P., Johnson, D. E., Pontes, J. E., Prout, G. R., Schmidt, J. D., Scott, W. W., Soloway, M. S., Slack, N. H., and Murphy, G. P. Comparison of cyclophosphamide, methyl CCNU, and hydroxyurea in patients with advanced and hormone resistant cancer of the prostate. *Proceedings of The American Urological Association*, p. 144, San Francisco, May 18–22, 1980.
150. DeWys, W. D., and Begg, C. B. Comparison of adriamycin (ADRIA) and 5-fluorouracil (5-FU) in advanced prostatic cancer. *Proc. Am. Assoc. Cancer Res. 19:*330, 1978.
151. O'Bryan, R. M., Luce, J. K., Talley, R. W., Gottlieb, J. A., Baker, L. H., and Bonadonna, G. Phase II evaluation of adriamycin in human neoplasia. *Cancer 32:*1, 1973.
152. O'Bryan, R. M., Baker, L. H., Gottlieb, J. E., Rivkin, S. E., Balcerzak, S. P., Grumet, G. N., Salmon, S. E., Moon, T. E., and Hoogstraten, B. Dose response evaluation of adriamycin in human neoplasia. *Cancer 39:*1940, 1977.
153. Merrin, C. E. Treatment of advanced carcinoma of the prostate (stage D) with infusion of *cis*-diamminedichloroplatinum (II NSC 119875): a pilot study. *J. Urol. 119:*522, 1978.
154. Merrin, C. E. Treatment of genitourinary tumors with *cis*-dichlorodiammineplatinum (II): experience in 250 patients. *Cancer Treat. Rept. 63:*1579, 1979.
155. Merrin, C. E. Combination orchiectomy, estrogen therapy, and *cis*-platinum for the treatment of previously untreated Stage D adenocarcinoma of the prostate. *Proc. Am. Assoc. Cancer Res. 21:*146, 1980.
156. Rossof, A. M., Talley, R. W., Stephens, R. L., Thigpen, T., Samson, M. K., Groppe, C., Eyre, H. J., and Fisher, R. Phase II evaluation of *cis*-dichlorodiammineplatinum (II) in advanced malignancies of the genitourinary and gynecologic organs: Southwest Oncology Group Study. *Cancer Treat. Rept. 63:*1557, 1979.

157. Yagoda, A. Phase II trials with *cis*-dichlorodiammineplatinum (II) in the treatment of urothelial cancer. *Cancer Treat. Rept. 63:*1565, 1979.

158. Scott, W. W., Gibbons, R. P., Johnson, D. E., Prout, G. R., Schmidt, J. D., Saroff, J., and Murphy, G. P. The continued evaluation of the effects of chemotherapy in patients with advanced carcinoma of the prostate. *J. Urol. 116:*211, 1976.

159. Chlebowski, R. T., Hestorff, R., Sardoff, L., Weiner, J., and Bateman, J. Cyclophosphamide (NSC 26271) *versus* the combination of adriamycin (NSC 123127), 5-fluorouracil (NSC 19893) and cyclophosphamide in the treatment of metastatic prostatic cancer; a randomized trial. *Cancer 42:*2546, 1978.

160. Resnick, M. I., Muss, H. B., Howard, A., Richards, F., White, O., Stuart, I. I., and Spurr, C. L. Cyclophosphamide (C) versus cyclophosphamide, methotrexate (M) and 5-fluorouracil (F) in advanced prostate cancer. *Proc. Am. Assoc. Cancer Res. 21:*135, 1980.

161. Schmidt, J. D., Scott, W. W., Gibbons, R., Johnson, D. E., Prout, G. R., Loening, S., Soloway, M., deKernion, J., Pontes, J. E., Slack, N. H., and Murphy, G. P. Chemotherapy programs of the national prostatic cancer project (NPCP). *Cancer 45:*1937, 1980.

162. Merrin, C. E., Etra, W., Wajsman, Z., Baumgartner, G., and Murphy, G. Chemotherapy of advanced carcinoma of the prostate with 5-fluorouracil, cyclophosphamide and adriamycin. *J. Urol. 116:*86, 1976.

163. Presant, C. A., Van Amburg, A., Klahr, C., and Mette, G. E. Chemotherapy of advanced prostatic cancer with adriamycin, BCNU and cyclophosphamide. *Cancer 46:* 2389, 1980.

164. Collier, D., and Soloway, M. S. Doxorubicin hydrochloride, cyclophosphamide, and 5-fluorouracil combination in advanced prostate and transitional cell carcinoma. *J. Urol. 8:*459, 1976.

165. Al-Sarraf, M. Combination of cytoxan, adriamycin and *cis*-platinum (CAP) in patients with advanced prostatic cancer. *Proc. Am. Assoc. Cancer Res. 21:*198, 1980.

166. Ihde, D. C., Bunn, P. A., Cohen, M. H., Eddy, J. L., Dunnick, N. R., Bensimon, H., Javadpour, N., and Minna, J. D. Combination chemotherapy as initial treatment for stage D_2 prostatic cancer: response rate and results of subsequent hormonal therapy. *Proc. Am. Assoc. Cancer Res. 21:*163, 1981.

167. Natale, R. B., Yagoda, A., Watson, R. C. Phase II trial of AMSA (4′[9-acridinylamino] methanesulfon-*m*-anisidide) in prostatic cancer. *Cancer Treat. Rept.* 1981 (in press).

168. Drelichman, A., Reed, M. L., and Al-Sarraf, M. Clinical trial of m-AMSA in patients with advanced prostatic carcinoma. *Proc. Am. Assoc. Cancer Res. 22:*464, 1981.

169. Natale, R. B., Yagoda, A., Watson, R. C., and Stover, D. E. Phase II trial of neocarcinostatin in patients with bladder and prostatic cancer: Toxicity of a 5-day IV bolus schedule. *Cancer 45:*2836, 1980.

170. Soloway, M. S., deKernion, J. B., Gibbons, R. P., Johnson, D. E., Loening, S., Pontes, J. E., Prout, G. R., Schmidt, J. D., Scott, W. W., Slack, N. H., and Murphy, G. P. Comparison of estracyst and vincristine alone or in combination for patients with advanced, hormone-resistant previously radiated carcinoma of the prostate. Proceedings of the American Urological Association, p. 144, San Francisco, May 18–22, 1980.

171. Mittelman, A., Catane, R., and Murphy, G. New steroidal alkylating agents in advanced stage D carcinoma of the prostate. *Cancer Treat. Rept. 61:*307, 1977.

172. Murphy, G. P., Gibbons, R. P., Johnson, D. E., Prout, G. R., Schmidt, J. D., Soloway, M. S., Loening, A., Chu, T. M., Gaeta, J. F., Saroff, J., Wajsman, Z., Slack, N., and Scott, W. W. The use of estramustine and prednimustine vs. prednimustine alone in advanced metastatic prostatic cancer patients who have received prior irradiation. *J. Urol. 121:*763, 1979.

173. Catane, R., Kaufman, J., Mittleman, A., and Murphy, G. Combined therapy of advanced prostatic carcinoma with estramustine and prednimustine. *J. Urol. 117:*332, 1977.

174. Hemstreet, G. P., III, Adolphson, C. C., Durant, J. P., and Brenckman, W. D. Phase II study of acyclovar in patients with hormonally resistant prostate cancer. (Abst. 241) Proceedings of the American Urological Association p. 144, 1980.

175. Von Hoff, D. D., Rozencweig, M., Slavik, M., and Muggia, F. Estramustine phosphate: a specific chemotherapeutic agent? *J. Urol. 117:*464, 1977.

176. deVere White, R., and Olsson, C. Androgen receptors in prostate cancer. *Urol. (Suppl.)* *17:*24, 1981.

177. Muehler, E. K., and Kohler, D. Interaction of the cytotoxic agent estramustine phosphate (Estracyst) with the estrogen receptor of the human uterus. *Gynecol. Oncol.* *8:*330, 1979.

178. Forsgren, B., Jan-Ake, G., Ake, P., and Hogberg, B. Binding characteristics of a major protein in rat ventral prostate cytosol that interacts with estramustine, a nitrogen mustard derivative of 17-β-estradiol. *Cancer Res. 39:*5155, 1979.

179. Madajewicz, S., Catane, R., Mittelman, A., Wajsman, Z., and Murphy, G. P. Chemotherapy of advanced hormonally resistant prostate cancer. *Oncology 37:*53, 1979.

180. Gibbons, R. P. Cooperative clinical trial of single and combined agent protocols: Adjuvant protocols. *Urology (Suppl.) 17:*48, 1981

181. Paulson, D. F., Walker, R. A., Berry, N. R., Cox, E. B., and Hindshow, W. Vincristine, bleomycin, methotrexate, 5-fluorouracil and prednisone in metastatic unresponsive prostatic adenocarcinoma. *J. Urol. 17:*443, 1981.

182. Sanford, E., Drago, J., Rohner, T. Jr., Santen, R., and Lipton, A. Aminoglutethimide medical adrenalectomy for advanced prostatic carcinoma. *J. Urol. 115:*170, 1975.

182a. Worgul, J. J., Santen, R. J., Samojdik, E., Lipton, A., Harvey, H., Veldhus, J. D., Drago, J. R., and Rohner, J. J. Clinical and biochemical effect of aminoglutethimide in the treatment of advanced prostatic carcinoma. *Proc. Am. Assoc. Cancer Res. 22:* 471, 1981.

183. Levin, A. B., Benson, R. C., Jr., Katz, J., and Nilsson, T. Chemical hypophysectomy for relief of bone pain in carcinoma of the prostate. *J. Urol. 119:*517, 1978.

184. Slack, N. H., Wajsman, Z., Mittelman, A., Bruno, S., and Murphy, G. P. Relationship of prior hormonal therapy to subsequent estramustine phosphate treatment in advanced prostatic cancer. *J. Urol. 14:*549, 1979.

185. Le Guillou, M., Ferriere, J. M., L'Henaff, F., and Muret, P. Action of an anti-androgen, cyproterone acetate in advanced prostatic cancer in 31 patients. *J. Urol. 86:*487, 1980.

186. Sogani, P. C., and Whitmore, W. F. Experience with flutamide in previously untreated patients with advanced prostatic cancer. *J. Urol. 122:*640, 1979.

187. Block, M., Bonomi, P., Anderson, K., Wolter, J., Showel, J., Pessis, D., and Slayton, R. Treatment of stage D prostatic carcinoma with megestrol acetate. *Proc. Am. Assoc. Cancer Res. 22:*472, 1981.

188. Geller, J., Albert, J., Yen, S. C., Geller, S., and Loza, D. Medical castration with megestrol acetate and minidose of diethylstilbesterol. *Urology* (Suppl.) *17:*27, 1981.

189. Arnold, D. J., Marquette, M., Hallbridge, E., Rosen, N., and Usher, S. Tamoxifen therapy for metastatic prostate cancer. *Proc. Am. Assoc. Cancer Res. 22:*468, 1981.

190. Glick, J. H., Wein, A., Padavic, K., Negendank, W., Harris, W., and Brodovsky, H. Tamoxifen in refractory metastatic carcinoma of the prostate. *Cancer Treat. Rept. 64:* 813, 1980.

191. Menon, M., Tananis, C., McLoughlin, M., and Walsh, P. Androgen receptors in human prostatic tissue: a review. *Cancer Treat. Rept. 61:*265, 1977.

192. Veterans Administration Cooperative Urological Research Group. Factors in the prognosis of carcinoma of the prostate: a cooperative study. *J. Urol. 100:*59, 1967.

193. Karr, J. P., Wajsman, Z., Kirdani, R. Y., Murphy, G. P., and Sandberg, A. A. Effects of diethylstilbesterol and estramustine phosphate on serum sex hormone binding globulin and testosterone levels in prostate cancer patients. *J. Urol. 124:*232, 1980.

194. Stone, A. R., Hargreave, T. B., and Chisholm, G. D. The diagnosis of oestrogen escape and the role of secondary orchiectomy in prostatic cancer. *Br. J. Urol. 52:*535, 1980.

195. White, C., Kelly, K., and Papac, R. Stilphosterol in the treatment of advanced prostate cancer. *Proc. Am. Assoc. Cancer Res. 22:*470, 1981.

196. Johnson, D. E., Scott, W. W., Gibbons, R., Prout, G. R., Schmidt, J. D., Chu, M. T., Gaeta, J., Saroff, J., and Murphy, G. P. National randomized study of chemotherapeutic agents in advanced prostatic carcinoma: A progress report. *Cancer Treat. Rept. 61:*317, 1977.

197. Mendecki, J., Friedenthal, E., Botstein, C., Paglione, R., and Sterzer, F. Microwave applications for localized hyperthermia treatment of cancer of the prostate. *Int. J. Radiot. Oncol. Biol. Phys. 6:*1583, 1980.

198. Yagoda, A. Chemotherapy of metastatic bladder cancer. *Cancer 45:*1879, 1888, 1980.

199. Hall, R. R., and Turner, A. G. Methotrexate treatment for advanced bladder cancer: a review after 6 years. *Br. J. Urol. 52:*403, 1980.

200. Yagoda, A. Phase II trials in bladder cancer at Memorial Sloan Kettering Cancer Center, 1975–1978. In *23rd Annual Conference on Cancer of the Genitourinary Tract*, pp. 107–119. Edited by D. E. Johnson and M. L. Samuels. Raven Press, New York, 1979.

201. Soloway, M. S., and Murphy, W. M. Experimental chemotherapy of bladder cancer—systemic and intravesical. *Semin. Oncol. 6:*166, 1979.

202. Yagoda, A., Watson, R. C., Gonzalez Vitale, J. C., Grabstald, H., and Whitmore, W. F. *Cis*-dichlorodiammineplatinum(II) in advanced bladder cancer. *Cancer Treat. Rept. 60:*917, 1976.

203. Tannock, I., Gospodarowicz, M., and Evans, W. K. Methotrexate, adriamycin and cyclophosphamide (MAC) chemotherapy for transitional cell carcinoma of the urinary tract. *Proc. Am. Assoc. Cancer Res. 22:*461, 1981.

204. Soloway, M. S. *Cis*-diamminedichloroplatinum(II) (DDP) in advanced bladder cancer. *J. Urol. 120:*716, 1978.

205. Soloway, M. S., Ikard, M., and Ford, K. *Cis*-diamminedichloroplatinum(II) in locally advanced and metastatic urothelial cancer. *Cancer 47:*476, 1981.

206. Merrin, C. E. Treatment of advanced bladder cancer with *cis*-diamminedichloro-platinum II (NSC 119875): A pilot study. *J. Urol. 119:*493, 1978.

207. Herr, H. W. *Cis*-diamminedichloride platinum II in the treatment of advanced bladder cancer. *J. Urol. 123:*853, 1980.

208. Peters, P. C., and O'Neill, M. R. *Cis*-diamminedichloroplatinum as a therapeutic agent in metastatic transitional cell carcinoma. *J. Urol. 123:*375, 1980.

209. Naglas, M. The chemotherapy of bladder cancer. *Zrav. Vestn. 49:*595, 1980.

210. Oliver, R. T. D. The place of chemotherapy in the treatment of patients with invasive carcinoma of the bladder. In *Bladder Tumors and Other Topics in Urological Oncology*, pp. 381–385. Edited by M. Pavone-Macaluso, P. H. Smith and F. Edsmyr. Plenum Press, New York, 1980.

211. Oliver, R. T. D., Newlands, E. S., Wiltshaw, E., and Malpas, J. S. A phase 2 study of *cis*-platinum in patients with recurrent bladder carcinoma. *Br. J. Urol.* (in press).

212. Khandekar, J. D., Elson, P. J., DeWys, W. D., and Slayton, R. E. Comparative activity and toxicity of *cis*-diamminedichloroplatinum vs. cyclophosphamide (CTX), adriamycin (ADR) and DDP (CAD) in disseminated transitional cell carcinoma of the urinary tract (DTCUT). *Proc. Am. Assoc. Cancer Res. 22:*461, 1981.

213. Einstein, A., Soloway, M., Corder, M., Bonney, W., and Coombs, J. Diamminedichlo-roplatinum (DDP) vs. DDP plus cyclophosphamide (CY) for metastatic bladder carcinoma. A national bladder cancer collaborative group-A (NBCCGA) study. *Proc. Am. Assoc. Cancer Res. 22:*461, 1981.

214. Yagoda, A., Watson, R. C., Kemeny, N., Barzell, W. E., Grabstald, H., and Whitmore, W. F. Diamminedichloride platinum II and cyclophosphamide in the treatment of advanced urothelial cancer. *Cancer 41:*2121, 1978.

215. Bonney, W., Soloway, M., Einstein, A., Corder, M., Coombs, J., and Friedel, G. Response of the primary bladder tumor to systemic cisplatinum ± cytoxan. (Abst. 585) Proceedings of the American Urological Association, p 238, Boston, May 10–14, 1981.

216. Narayana, A. S., Loening, S. A., and Culp, D. A. Chemotherapy for advanced carcinoma of the bladder. (Abst. 122) Proceedings American Urological Association, p 104, 1980.

217. Gagliano, O. R. Adriamycin vs. adriamycin plus *cis*-platinum in transitional cell bladder carcinoma. A SWOG Study. (Abst C-110) *Proc. Am. Assoc. Cancer Res. 21:* 347, 1980.

218. Middleman, F., Luce, J., and Frei, E. Clinical trials with adriamycin. *Cancer 28:*844, 1971.

219. Ostrow, S., Egorin, M. J., Hahn, D., Markus, S., LeRoy, A., Chang, P., Klein, M., Bachur, N. R., and Wiernik, P. H. *Cis*-dichlorodiammineplatinum and adriamycin therapy for advanced gynecological and genitourinary neoplasms. *Cancer 46:*1715, 1980.

220. Vogl, S., Ohnuma, R., Perloff, M., and Holland, J. F. Combination chemotherapy with

adriamycin and *cis*-diamminedichloroplatinum in patients with metastatic disease. *Cancer 38:*21, 1976.

221. Samuels, M. L., Moran, M. E., Johnson, D. E., and Bracken, R. B. CISCA combination chemotherapy for metastatic carcinoma of the bladder. In *Cancer of the Genitourinary Tract*, pp. 11–106. Edited by D. E. Johnson, and M. L. Samuels. Raven Press, New York, 1979.

222. Samuels, M. L., Logothetis, C., Trindade, A., and Johnson, D. E. Cytoxan, adriamycin, and *cis*-platinum (CISCA) in metastatic bladder cancer. *Proc. Am. Assoc. Cancer Res. 21:*137, 1980.

223. Sternberg, J. J., Bracken, R. B., Handel, P. B., and Johnson, D. E. Combination chemotherapy (Cisca) for advanced urinary tract carcinoma. A preliminary report. *JAMA 238:*2282, 1977.

224. Kedia, K. R., Gibbons, C., and Persky, L. Management of advanced bladder carcinoma. *J. Urol. 125:*655, 1981.

225. Campbell, M., Baker, L. H., Opipari, M., and Al-Sarraf, M. Phase II trial with *cis*-dichlorodiammineplatinum, adriamycin and cyclophosphamide in the treatment of urothelial transitional cell carcinoma. *Cancer Treat. Rept.* (in press).

226. Troner, M. B., and Hemstreet, G. P. (III). Cyclophosphamide, doxorubicin, and *cis*-platin (CAP) in the treatment of urothelial malignancy: A pilot study of the Southeastern Cancer Study Group. *Cancer Treat. Rept. 65:*29, 1981.

227. Williams, S. D., Rohn, R. J., Donohue, J. F., and Einhorn, L. H. Chemotherapy of bladder cancer with *cis*-diamminedichloroplatinum (DDP), adriamycin (Adr) and 5-fluorouracil. *Proc. Amer. Assoc. Cancer Res. 19:*316, 1978.

228. Williams, S. D., Einhorn, L. H., and Donohue, J. P. *Cis*-platinum combination chemotherapy of bladder cancer. *Cancer Clin. Trials 2:*355, 1979.

229. Weinstein, S. H., and Schmidt, J. D. Doxorubicin in advanced transitional cell carcinoma. *Urology 8:*336, 1976.

230. Yagoda, A., Watson, R. C., Whitmore, W. F., Grabstald, H., Middleman, M. P., and Krakoff, I. H. Adriamycin in advanced urinary tract cancer. *Cancer 39:*279, 1977.

231. Pavone-Macaluso, M., and EORTC Genitourinary Tract Cooperative Group A. Single drug chemotherapy of bladder cancer with adriamycin, VM-26, or bleomycin. A phase II multicentric cooperative study. *Eur. Urol. 2:*138, 1976.

232. Merrin, C. E., Cartagena, R., Wajsman, Z., Baumgartner, G., and Murphy, G. P. Chemotherapy of bladder carcinoma with cyclophosphamide and adriamycin. *J. Urol. 114:*884, 1975.

233. Yagoda, A., Watson, R. C., Grabstald, H., Barzell, W. E., and Whitmore, W. F. Adriamycin and cyclophosphamide in advanced bladder cancer. *Cancer Treat. Rept. 61:*97, 1977.

234. Rodriguez, L. H., Johnson, D. E., Holoye, P. Y., and Samuels, M. L. Combination VM-26 and adriamycin for metastatic transitional cell carcinoma. *Cancer Treat. Rept. 61:*87, 1977.

235. Levi, J. A., Aroney, R. S., and Dalley, D. N. Combination chemotherapy with cyclophosphamide, doxorubicin and bleomycin for metastatic transitional cell carcinoma of the urinary tract. *Cancer Treat. Rept. 64:*1011, 1980.

236. Al-Sarraf, M., Amer, M. H., and Vaitkevicius, V. K. Chemotherapy and survival in patients with urinary bladder cancer. *Proc. Am. Assoc. Cancer Res. 18:*116, 1977.

237. Cross, R. J., Glashan, R. W., Humphrey, C. S., Robinson, M. R. G., Smith, P. H., and Williams, R. E. Treatment of advanced bladder cancer with adriamycin and 5-fluorouracil. *Br. J. Urol. 48:*609, 1976.

238. EORTC: The treatment of advanced carcinoma of the bladder with a combination of adriamycin and 5-fluorouracil. *Eur. Urol. 3:*276, 1977.

239. Martinos, Samal B., and Al-Sarraf, M. Phase II study of 5-fluorouracil and adriamycin in transitional cell carcinoma of the urinary tract. *Cancer Treat. Rept. 64:*161, 1980.

240. Altman, C. C., McCague, N. J., Ripepi, A. C., and Cardozo, M. The use of methotrexate in advanced carcinoma of the bladder. *J. Urol. 108:*271, 1972.

241. Burfield, G. D. Intravenous methotrexate in the treatment of advanced bladder cancer. *Br. J. Urol. 46:*121, 1972.

242. Hall, R. R., Bloom, H. J. G., Freeman, J. E., Nawrocki, A., and Wallace, D. M. Methotrexate treatment for advanced bladder cancer. *Br. J. Urol. 46:*431, 1974.

243. Natale, R. B., Yagoda, A., Watson, R. C., Whitmore, W. F., Blumenreich, M., and Braun, D. W. Methotrexate: an active drug in bladder cancer. *Cancer 47:*1246, 1981.

244. Turner, A. G., Hendry, W. F., Williams, G. B., and Bloom, H. J. G. The treatment of advanced bladder cancer with methotrexate. *Br. J. Urol. 49:*673, 1977.

245. Early, K., Elias, E. G., Mittelman, A., Albert, D., and Murphy, G. P. Mitomycin C in the treatment of metastatic transitional cell carcinoma of urinary bladder. *Cancer 31:* 1150, 1973.

246. Fox, M. The effect of cyclophosphamide on some urinary tract tumors. *Br. J. Urol. 37:* 399, 1965.

247. Sakamoto, S., Ogata, J., Ikegami, K., and Naeda, H. Effects of systemic administration of neocarsinostatin, a new protein antibiotic on human bladder cancer. *Cancer Treat. Rept. 62:*453, 1978.

248. Sakamoto, S., Ogata, J., Ikegami, K., and Maeda, H. Chemotherapy for bladder cancer with neocarcinostatin: *Eur. J. Cancer 16:*103, 1980.

249. Blumenreich, M., Yagoda, A., Watson, R. C., and Needles, B. Phase II trial of vinblastine sulfate (VLB) in transitional cell carcinoma. Cancer (in press).

250. Falkson, G., van Dyk, J. J., van Eden, E. B. van der Merwe, A. M., van den Bergh, J. A., and Falkson, H. C. A clinical trial of the oral form of 4'-demethyl-epipodophyllo-toxin-β-ethylidene glucoside (NSC 141540). *Cancer 35:*1141, 1975.

251. Nissen, N. E., Pajak, T. F., Leone, L. A., Bloomfield, C. D., Kennedy, B. J., Ellison, R. R., Silver, R. T., Weiss, R. B., Cuttner, J., Falkson, G., Kung, F., Bergevin, P. R., and Holland, J. F. A clinical trial of VP 16-213 (NSC 14150) i.v. twice weekly in advanced neoplastic disease. *Cancer 45:*232, 1980.

252. Mechl, Z., Rovny, F., and Sopkova, B. VM-26 (4 demethyl-epipodophyllotoxin-β-d-thenylidine glucoside) in the treatment of urinary bladder tumors. *Neoplasma 24:*411, 1977.

253. Pavone-Macaluso, M., Caramia, G., Rizzo, F. P., and Messana, V. Preliminary evaluation of VM-26, a new epipodophyllotoxin derivative in the treatment of urogenital tumors. *Eur. Urol. 1:*53, 1975.

254. Glenn, J. F., Hunt, L. D., and Lathem, J. E. Chemotherapy of bladder carcinoma with 5-Fluorouracil. *Cancer Chemother. Rept. 27:*67, 1963.

255. Ducheck, M., Edsmyr, F., and Naeslund, I. 5-Fluorouracil in the treatment of recurrent cancer of the urinary bladder. In *Bladder Tumors and Other Topics in Urological Oncology*, pp. 381–385. Edited by M. Pavone-Macaluso, H. Smith, and F. Edsmyr. Plenum Press, New York, 1980.

256. Prout, G. R., Bross, I. D. J., Slack, N. H., and Ausman, R. K. Carcinoma of the bladder, 5-fluorouracil and the critical role of a placebo. *Cancer 22:*926, 1968.

257. Yagoda, A., Watson, R. C., Blumenreich, M., and Young, C. Phase II trials in urothelial tumors with AMSA and PALA. *Proc. Am. Assoc. Cancer Res. 21:*427, 1980.

258. Bodey, G. P. Current status of chemotherapy in metastatic renal cancer. In *Cancer of the Genitourinary Tract*, pp. 67–76. Edited by D. E. Johnson and M. L. Samuels. Raven Press, New York, 1979.

259. Yagoda, A., and Macchia, R. J. Antineoplastic chemotherapy of genitourinary cancer. In *Management of the Patient with Cancer*, pp. 601–632. Edited by T. F. Nealon, W. B. Saunders, Philadelphia, 1976.

260. Bukowski, R. M. N., LoBuglio, A., McCracken, J., and Pugh, R. Phase II trial of Baker's antifol in metastatic renal cell carcinoma; a Southwest Oncology Group Study. *Cancer Treat. Rept. 64:*1387, 1980.

261. Gralla, R. J., and Yagoda, A. Phase II evaluation of chlorozotocin in patients with renal cell carcinoma. *Cancer Treat. Rept. 63:*1007, 1979.

262. Hahn, R. G., Tempkin, N. R., Savlov, E. D., Perlia, C., Wampler, G. L., Horton, J., Marsch, J., and Carbone, P. P. Phase II study of vinblastine, methyl CCNU and medroxyprogesterone in advanced renal cell cancer. *Cancer Treat. Rept. 62:*1093, 1978.

263. Hahn, R. G., Bauer, M., Wolter, J., Creech, R., Bennett, J. M., and Wampler, G. L. Phase II study of single agent therapy with megesterol acetate, VP-16-213, cyclophosphamide, and dianhydrogalatitol in advanced renal cell cancer. *Cancer Treat. Rept. 63:* 513, 1979.

264. Hahn, R. G., Berg, C. B., Davis, T., and the ECOG. Phase II trial of vinblastine-

CCNU, triazinate, and actinomycin D in advanced renal cell cancer. *Cancer Treat. Rept.* (in press).

265. Schneider, R. J., Woodcock, T. M., and Yagoda, A. Phase II trial of 4′-(9-acridinylamino)methanesulfon-*m*-anisidide (AMSA) in patients with metastatic hypernephroma. *Cancer Treat. Rept. 64:*183, 1980.

266. Wong, P. P., Yagoda, A., Currie, V. E., and Young, C. W. Phase II study of desacetyl vinblastine amide sulfate (vindesine) in the therapy of advanced renal carcinoma. *Cancer Treat. Rept. 61:*1727, 1977.

267. Knight, W. A., Livingston, R. B., Fabian, C., and Costanzi, J. Phase I-II trial of methyl-GAG. *Cancer Treat. Rept. 63:*1933, 1979.

268. Todd, R. F., Garnick, M. R., Canellos, G. P., Richie, J. P., Gittes, R. F., Mayer, R. J., and Skarin, A. T. Phase I-II trial of methyl-GAG in the treatment of patients with metastatic renal adenocarcinoma. *Cancer Treat. Rept. 64:*17, 1981.

269. Callahan, S. K., and Knight, W. A. A Phase II trial of methyl glyoxal *bis*-guanylhydrazone in renal carcinoma. *Proc. Am. Assoc. Cancer Res. 22:*164, 1981.

270. Zeffren, J., Yagoda, A., Watson, R. C., Natale, R. Blumenreich, M., Chapman, R., and Howard, J. Phase II trial of methyl-glyoxal *bis*-guanylhydrazone in advanced renal cancer. *Cancer Treat. Rept. 65:*525, 1981.

271. Myers, J. W., von Hoff, D. D. Kuhn, J., Sandback, J. F., Pocelinko, R., Clark, G., Coltman, C., and Rodriguez, V. Phase I investigation of 9,10-anthracenedicarboxaldehyde *bis*-[(4,5-dihydro-1*H*-imidazol-2-yl) Hydrazone] dihydrochloride (CL 216,942) on a single intermittent schedule. *Proc. Am. Assoc. Cancer Res. 22:*174, 1981.

272. Spiegel, R. J., Blum, R., Pinto, C., Wernz, J., Levin, M., Hoffman, K., Blank, J., and Muggia, F. Phase I trial of 9,10-anthracenedicarboxaldehyde (CL 216,942). *Proc. Am. Assoc. Cancer Res. 22:*357, 1981.

273. Haq, M. M., Legha, S. S., Samaan, N. A., Bodey, G. P., and Burgess, M. A. Cytotoxic chemotherapy in adrenal corticol carcinoma. *Cancer Treat. Rept. 64:*909, 1980.

274. Zeffren, J., and Yagoda, A. Chemotherapy of adrenal cortical carcinoma. In *Chemotherapy and Urological Malignancy.* Edited by A. S. Spiers. Springer-Verlag, Berlin, 1981.

275. Hogan, T. F., Citrin, D. L., Johnson, B. M., Nakamura, S., Davis, T. E., and Bordon, C. E. O,p′-DDD (Mitotane) therapy of adrenal cortical carcinoma. *Cancer 42:*2177, 1978.

276. Hogan, T. F., Gilchrist, K. W., Westring, D. W., and Citrin, D. L. A clinical and pathological study of adrenocortical carcinoma. *Cancer 45:*2880, 1980.

277. Hutter, A. M., and Kayhoe, D. E. Adrenal cortical carcinoma—results of treatment with o,p′-DDD in 138 patients. *Am. J. Med. 41:*581, 1966.

278. Lubitz, J., Freeman, L., and Okun, R. Mitotane use in inoperable adrenal cortical carcinoma. *JAMA 223:*1109, 1973.

279. Exelby, P. R. Adrenal cortical carcinoma in a child. *Clin. Bull. 5:*26, 1975.

280. Wortsman, J., and Soler, N. G. Mitotane-spironolactone antagonism in Cushing's syndrome. *JAMA 238:*2527, 1977.

281. Schteingart, E. D., Cask, R., and Conn, J. W. Aminoglutethimide and metastatic adrenal cancer. *JAMA 198:*143, 1966.

282. Izbicki, R. M., Al-Sarraf, M., Reed, M. L., Vaughn, C. D., and Vaitkevicius, V. K. Further clinical trials with porfiromycin. *Cancer Chemother. Rept. 56:*615, 1972.

283. Tattersall, M. H., Lander, H., Bain, B., Stocks, A. E., Woods, R. L., Fox, R., Byrne, M., Trotten, J. R., and Roos, I. *Cis*-platinum treatment of metastatic adrenal carcinoma. *Med. J. Aust. 9:*419, 1980.

284. Sklaroff, R. B., and Yagoda, A. Chemotherapy of penile cancer. In *Chemotherapy and Urological Malignancy.* Edited by A. S. Spiers. Springer-Verlag, Berlin, 1981.

285. Blum, R. H., Carter, S. K., and Agre, K. A clinical review of bleomycin—a new antineoplastic agent. *Cancer 31:*903, 1973.

286. Ichikawa, T. Chemotherapy of penis cancer. In *Tumors of the Male Genital System,* pp. 140–156. Edited by E. Grundmann, and W. Vahlensieck. Springer-Verlag, Berlin, 1977.

287. Sklaroff, R. B., and Yagoda, A. *Cis*-diamminedichlorideplatinum II in the treatment of penile cancer. *Cancer 44:*1563, 1979.

288. Frei, E., Blum, R. H., Pitman, S. W., Kirkwood, J. M., Henderson, I. C., Skarin, A. T., Mayer, R. J., Bast, R. C., Garnick, M. B., Parker, L. M., and Canellos, G. P. High dose methotrexate with leucovorin rescue. *Am. J. Med. 68:*370, 1980.
289. Sklaroff, R. B., and Yagoda, A. Methotrexate in the treatment of penile carcinoma. *Cancer 45:*2214, 1980.

12

Recent and Potential Advances in Radiotherapy of Urologic Cancer

The goals of radiotherapy are to cure the patient with cancer or to palliate symptoms caused directly or indirectly by it. The overall objectives of curative radiotherapy are (1) to eradicate the cancer locally (primary site and adjacent tissues) and, when appropriate, in regional lymph nodes; and (2) to preserve the function of the tumor-bearing organs and the integrity of adjacent normal tissues. Eradication of tumor in the primary site and regional lymph nodes is necessary for effective long-term palliation even if the tumor has disseminated. As the treatment of microscopic disease by chemotherapeutic agents becomes more effective, the local eradication of many cancers by radiotherapy will assume more importance.

In the treatment of genitourinary cancers, the loss of one of the paired organs (kidney, ureter, or testicle) is still compatible with normal existence. On the other hand, loss of the bladder, prostate, urethra or penis is a significant compromise for the patient, even if cured. Several areas of radiotherapy research are investigating methods of delivering radiation or of modifying the response of tumors and normal tissues to radiation in order to achieve higher local control rates with radiation alone. These investigations may lead to effective treatment with less aggressive surgery or even by radiotherapy alone.

Although patients with disseminated disease may benefit greatly from radiotherapy for the relief of bone pain, lymphedema, urinary outlet obstruction, or spinal cord compression, this role of radiotherapy will not be addressed in this chapter.

CONSIDERATIONS IN SELECTING A TREATMENT MODALITY AND INTERPRETING DATA

In order to improve the treatment of a specific histologic type and stage of cancer with a local treatment modality such as radiotherapy, one must understand the causes of failure with present treatment techniques and the radiation time, dose, and fractionation schedules used. For most genitourinary tumors other than seminoma, one gives the maximum radiation dose compatible with an acceptable risk of injury to normal tissues. Thus, potentially curative doses of radiation usually can be delivered only to the region of the primary tumor and to regional lymph nodes. Local and regional control rates can be a direct measure of the success of these radiation therapy treatments. The frequent development of distant metastases despite local and regional control in patients treated by either surgery or radiation therapy is an indication for systemic treatment. On the other hand, if local control cannot be attained, regional failure and distant metastases are expected consequences.

In contrast to the generally slow course of prostatic carcinoma, even after the development of distant metastases, cancers of the bladder and testis generally follow a rapid course once extensive lymph node metastases have been identified. A better understanding of the natural history of these and other gentourinary cancers is evolving through more accurate diagnostic studies as well as by surgical staging. In general, the more advanced the stage and the less well differentiated the histology, the more likely the disease has disseminated and the less likely the primary tumor can be eradicated by radiotherapy because of its size. It is well recognized that local eradication of a tumor depends more upon the volume of tumor present than on the stage. The probability of killing all tumor cells decreases as the total number of tumor cells increases and the latter is proportional to the volume. Spread of tumor to regional lymph nodes has a poor prognosis independent of stage because of the increased probability of distant metastases.

A problem in comparing the results of treatment by different modalities is the frequent discrepancy between clinical staging and pathological staging. This is true for the primary tumor, for regional lymph nodes, and for distant metastases. Even with recent improvements in diagnostic imaging by computerized tomography and ultrasound, it is difficult to detect microscopic extensions of tumor into surrounding tissues or to identify micrometastases in lymph nodes. With the rapid development of tumor markers, it is reasonable to expect to have in the near future radioactively labeled tumor-associated or tumor-specific antibodies that will be useful for detecting and possibly for treating micrometastases.

As more is learned about prognostic factors related to the extent of disease (local, regional, and distant) and for the probability of achieving local or regional control, one can more wisely select appropriate diagnostic studies for staging as well as for the treatment modalities or techniques. It is in the best interest of patients to eliminate low yield diagnostic studies and to avoid treatment that would be negated by otherwise unsuspected distant metastases. For instance, the very low incidence of lymph node metastases in a favorable prognostic group of patients with prostatic carcinoma makes it difficult to justify lymphangiography, CT scanning, or lymph node dissections in this group.[1] The eventual use of tumor-associated or tumor-specific antibodies also may reduce the number of diagnostic procedures in many patients and may modify the treatment approach as well.

In the remainder of this chapter, we will discuss briefly the results and limitations of conventional radiotherapy treatment methods and will discuss in greater detail current areas of investigation that have potential applicability in the treatment of one or more cancers of the genitourinary tract by radiotherapy.

CURRENT RADIOTHERAPY TREATMENT METHODS, RESULTS, AND LIMITATIONS

Methods

Conventional radiotherapy is delivered by external beam therapy or brachytherapy. External beam therapy employs beams of photons or of electrons directed at the tumor-containing target volume from outside the body. Brachytherapy is the use of radioisotopes to treat tumors on the surface of the body, within a body cavity (intracavitary irradiation), or directly in tissues (interstitial irradiation). Among the advantages of using brachytherapy for the treatment of well-localized tumors are the ability (1) to deliver a high radiation dose to the tumor-containing volume, and (2) to minimize the radiation dose to adjacent normal structures. This is especially true for those normal structures a few centimeters from the treatment volume which would receive a high dose if the patient received external beam radiotherapy.

Most patients are treated with external beam radiotherapy, primarily with photon beams from ^{60}Co units or linear accelerators. The latter are preferred because of their higher dose rates (shorter treatment times), sharper beam collimation (better sparing of normal tissues), and greater penetrability (better dose distribution). Although electron beams can provide advantageous dose distributions for relatively superficial treatment volumes because of their discrete ranges as a function of energy, skin reactions with large treatment ports generally limit the total radiation dose that can be delivered. Thus, in the United States, only approximately 15% of patients receive electron beam therapy as part or all of their treatment. Since the total dose is generally limited by the tolerance of normal tissue, it is often essential to use multiple field treatment techniques. The number of directions from which the radiation should be delivered depends upon the energy of the photon beam and the critical normal structures adjacent to the treatment volume.

Planned combinations of surgery and external beam radiotherapy include (1) preoperative irradiation, (2) postoperative irradiation, (3) both pre- and postoperative irradiation (so-called sandwich technique), and (4) irradiation between two surgical procedures (urinary diversion-radiotherapy-cystectomy).

Role of External Beam Therapy in Treatment of Genitourinary Malignancies

The use of external beam radiotherapy for the treatment of cancers of the bladder, prostate, and testicle has been investigated extensively over the past 25 years. Its use for other genitourinary malignancies has received less emphasis either because of a low incidence of the cancer or because of the use of alternate treatment methods.

The use of external beam radiotherapy alone for the treatment of bladder cancer is limited at present to patients with unresectable tumors. In a series of 384 patients with bladder cancer treated with 7000 rad in 7 weeks to the bladder alone or in conjunction with 5000 rad to the pelvic lymph nodes, the actuarial 5-year survival rates were 35%, 22%, and 7% for stage B_2, C, and D cancers, respectively.[2]

The preferred treatment for invasive cancers of the bladder is now preoperative irradiation. Among the many regimens used are a total dose of 4000 to 4500 rad in 4 to 4½ weeks, with cystectomy 6 to 8 weeks later,[3] and a dose of 2000 rad delivered in five treatments over 5 consecutive days with surgery a few days thereafter.[4] At this time, the two regimens appear comparable with actuarial 5-year survival rates of 40 to 50%.

With regard to the treatment of prostatic carcinoma by external beam radiotherapy, Bagshaw et al.[5] reported 5- and 10-year actuarial survival rates of 70% and 42%, respectively, for 230 patients with clinical stage A and B tumors. The rates were 37% and 29%, respectively, for 200 patients with clinical stage C tumors.[5] Perez et al.[6] reported cumulative absolute 5-year survival rates of 60% for 15 patients with clinical stage B and 42% for 97 patients with clinical stage C tumors. Absolute and disease-free survival rates of 68.2% and 58.4%, respectively, were reported by Neglia et al.[7] for 154 patients with clinical stage B or C tumors.

External beam radiotherapy is still the preferred method of treatment for patients with stage I and II seminoma and may be the only treatment needed in many patients with stage III tumors. External beam radiotherapy now is seldom used in the treatment of nonseminomatous germ cell tumors of the testis because of the excellent results of treatment with surgery and chemotherapy. Prior to the demonstration of effective treatment with chemotherapy, treatment by radiotherapy alone gave 3-year recurrence-free survival rates of 86% and 82% for carefully staged clinical stage I and II patients, respectively.[8] Combining radiotherapy and surgical removal of the lymph nodes in a sandwich approach gave 97% and 81% 3-year recurrence-free survival rates for stage I and II patients, respectively.[8] It was observed that a high percentage of testicular cancer patients with lymphangiographically abnormal lymph nodes rapidly developed disseminated disease and frequently had nodal recurrences as well.[9]

The role of radiotherapy in the management of renal cell carcinoma and of ureteral carcinoma is primarily as an adjuvant to surgery in potentially curable patients. Rafla and Parikh[10] suggest that postoperative radiotherapy is of benefit to patients with renal cell carcinoma when the capular tissues are invaded. Babaian *et al.*[11] recommend postoperative radiotherapy to the ureteral bed following nephrouretectomy for infiltrative ureteral carcinoma. In both situations, the total radiation dose which can be delivered by photons is limited by the risk of injury to the small bowel as well as to the remaining contralateral kidney. If all gross tumor has been removed, a total dose of 4500 rad, which could be delivered safely, may be sufficient to eradicate residual microscopic foci of cancer.

Radiotherapy techniques used to treat carcinomas of the penis and male urethra include (1) low energy photon beams, (2) electron beams, (3) high energy photon beams, (4) radioisotope molds, (5) interstitial implants, or (6) radioactive sources in the urethral lumen. Cancers of both sites are uncommon and present a spectrum of challenges from small focal lesions to massive involvement of the organ associated with lymph node metastases. Because of the variety of presentations, treatment has to be individualized for each patient and will depend upon the specific expertise of the radiotherapist.

Role of Brachytherapy in Treatment of Genitourinary Malignancies

Treatment of the prostate gland by ^{125}I interstitial implantation has been carried out at Memorial Hospital, New York, N.Y. since 1970.[12] The implantation technique is described by Hilaris *et al.*[12] and is generally performed following a pelvic lymph node dissection. Preliminary results suggest local control in approximately 90% of tumors and actuarial 5-year survival rates of 100% in patients with small clinical stage B tumors, and approximately 65% in patients with large clinical stage B or stage C tumors.[12] The incidence of distant metastases approached 75% in 5 years in patients who had lymph node metastases as well as in patients with large clinical stage B or stage C tumors without nodal metastases. The genitourinary and gastrointestinal morbidity of implants is generally limited to the first few months after the implant and appears to be comparable to that experienced with external beam radiation therapy when the latter is given only to the prostatic region by acceptable techniques. There appears to be a lesser incidence of impotence than has been reported with external beam radiation therapy.[13]

Combined Interstitial Implantation and External Beam Radiation Therapy

Carlton *et al.*[14] have used a combination of interstitial implantation with [198]Au seeds and external beam radiation therapy for the treatment of patients with clinical stage C prostatic cancer. The implant delivered a tumor dose of 2500 to 3500 rad following a pelvic lymph node dissection. Approximately 8 to 10 days after the implant, external beam radiotherapy is used to deliver 4000 to 5000 rad to the region of the prostate gland. Of 39 patients followed 5 to 10 years since treatment, 15 (38.5%) are alive without evidence of cancer, 17 (43.6%) are alive with cancer, 6 (15.4%) are dead with cancer, and 1 is dead without tumor.[14] Mild to moderate prostatitis and cystitis were noted in 25% and 34% of patients, respectively, but was severe in only 4% and 2% of patients, respectively.[14] Impotence following treatment was noted in only 25% of patients.[14]

In summary, there are several alternatives in the treatment of the prostate gland by radiation therapy. Whereas ^{125}I or [198]Au interstitial implants treat only the gland and the immediate periprostatic region, external beam radiotherapy (alone or in conjunction with interstitial implantation) can encompass a greater volume which includes adjacent lymph nodes. The advantages and disadvantages of each of the alternatives deserve close evaluation as experience with each increases.

Brachytherapy has not been used extensively in the treatment of bladder cancer. Van der Werf-Messing[15] reported 3- and 5-year survival rates of 45% and 35%, respectively, for patients with T_3 bladder cancer treated with three external beam doses of 350 rad on 3 consecutive days followed immediately by a suprapubic radium implant. In order to treat potential pelvic lymph node metastases, Van der Werf-Messing and colleagues[16] are evaluating a treatment regimen employing the preimplant radiation course of 1050 rad, a lower dose radium implant, and then 3000 rad in 3 weeks to the true pelvis. This attempt to improve local and regional control while preserving the bladder will be followed with interest.

Brachytherapy has not been used routinely in the treatment of cancers of the kidney, ureter, or testicle. Its uses in the treatment of cancers of the penis and male urethra were commented upon earlier.

Limitations of Treatment Methods

Despite improvements in equipment, the risk of injury to normal tissues adjacent to and occasionally within the treatment volume generally limits the total external beam radiation dose that can be delivered to a tumor. Beam shaping, the use of multiple treatment fields, the use of shrinking field techniques, and the use of electrons, when possible, can decrease the risk of normal tissue injury by decreasing the volume receiving the prescribed high dose. These considerations are especially important in the treatment of tumors in the upper abdomen (kidney, ureter, and para-aortic lymph nodes) because of the relative sensitivity of the kidneys and liver (maximum safe doses of approximately 2500 and 3000 rad, respectively) and of the spinal cord and small bowel (4500 rad) compared to the dose needed to control gross tumor from any of the genitourinary tumors except seminoma. The risk of injury to the small bowel increases significantly if the radiation is preceded by a surgical procedure or by an intra-abdominal inflammatory process which produces adhesions. In such patients, aggressive radiotherapy may lead to severe late bowel injury often requiring resection and reanastomosis.[1] In the pelvis, small bowel, colon, and rectum are the dose-limiting tissues, but the risk of injury thereto during treatment for bladder and prostatic cancer can be minimized by careful planning of the radiation treatment. The bladder can tolerate substantial doses of radiation provided that part of it is spared the full radiation dose. Limitations in the use of implants include (1) risk of injury to structures (vessel, nerve, or wall of a viscus) within or adjacent to the high dose volume, which increases with the total dose and volume irradiated; and (2) the technical difficulty of implantations adjacent to physical barriers such as bone.

Limitations Due to Tumor Characteristics

One of the greatest problems in the treatment of apparently localized tumors with radiotherapy, especially with brachytherapy, is the possible spread of the tumor beyond the volume receiving the high radiation dose either to lymph nodes or other distant sites. This problem is now being addressed in part by improved tumor localization techniques and in the future may be enhanced also by the use of tumor-specific antibodies to detect lymph node and distant metastases.

Another reason for lower-than-desired tumor cure rate relates to the tumor size and inherent resistance of some tumor cells to killing by radiation. Among the reasons given for increased resistance of some tumors to radiation are (1) the presence of foci of cells with a decreased oxygen concentration, (2) differences in a capability to repair radiation-induced injury, (3) differences in sensitivity of cells as a function of their position in the cell cycle at the time of irradiation, and (4) differences in ploidy. Since oxygen-deprived cells are 2.5 to 3.0 times more resistant to radiation than are fully oxygenated cells, a substantial number of hypoxic cells would survive a single radiation dose. If this condition persisted throughout the course of radiation therapy, it would lead to a high failure rate.

The next section discusses radiation research investigations which are attempting to improve the results of treatment and their potential applicability to the treatment of genitourinary malignancies.

POTENTIAL IMPROVEMENTS IN TREATMENT OF GENITOURINARY MALIGNANCIES WITH RADIATION

The major areas of investigation in radiotherapy can be grouped as follows:

1. Improving the results of photon and/or electron (low linear energy transfer (LET)) radiotherapy.
2. Evaluating neutron and heavy charged particle (high LET) radiotherapy.
3. Evaluating the clinical significance of modifying the response of tumors and normal tissues to radiation.
4. Evaluating the clinical effectiveness of combined modality treatment.

Inherent in each of these areas of investigation are considerations pertaining to improving tumor localization and establishing the tolerance of normal tissues to new radiation treatment schedules, to new types of radiation, and to the use of radiation with radiation modifiers, chemotherapeutic agents, and surgery either alone or in various combinations. Each of these areas of investigation and its applicability to the treatment of genitourinary malignancies will be discussed in turn.

Improved Photon or Electron (Low LET) Radiotherapy

An accumulation of preclinical and clinical information suggests that the use of alternative time, dose, and fractionation schedules may be used to exploit slight differences between the responses of tumors and normal tissues to radiation. Because these differences are not great, alternative treatment schedules, like conventional fractionation, will be very dependent upon precise tumor and normal tissue delineation for achievement of good results. Successful investigations in this area would result in increased local-regional control of cancer with even less injury of normal tissues.

Several methods of delivering radiation to the primary tumor volume (or tumor bed after surgery) are being investigated. They include (1) brachytherapy alone or as part of a surgical procedure, (2) electron beam therapy, (3) radioactively labeled antitumor antibodies for the treatment of the primary tumor as well as distant metastases, and (4) dynamic treatment which incorporates simultaneous movement of the patient, the photon beam, and the beam-shaping collimators.

It is now possible to deliver high radiation doses to the bladder and prostate gland with conventional fractionation schedules. Treatment schedules utilizing multiple daily radiation fractions may reduce the risk of normal tissue injury and result in a slight improvement in local control. The potential to increase the local control of these and other genitourinary tract cancers with high-dose/fraction radiation schedules is expected to be low primarily because of normal tissue tolerance.

With regard to the use of new or improved low LET radiation delivery methods, it is apparent that interstitial irradiation is being evaluated aggressively in the treatment of prostatic cancer. It also is being investigated for the treatment of selected patients with cancer of the bladder and for the treatment of some patients with cancer of the penis and of the urethra. Implants could be used to increase the radiation dose to inoperable tumors of the kidney and ureter; however, the risk of metastatic disease may negate the potential increase in local control. Another use of implants would be for the treatment of tumor beds postoperatively.

Electron beam therapy might best be used to advantage in an intraoperative radiotherapy role, especially for resected cancers of the kidney and ureter where there is actual or presumed residual disease. Intraoperative radiotherapy has been used for inoperable bladder cancer and for prostatic cancer.[17] However, all too frequently, patients with advanced disease will fail distantly, negating most of the benefit of improved local control with such aggressive treatment.

The simultaneous movement of the patient treatment couch, the linear accelerator gantry, and the photon beam collimators during dynamic therapy is designed to optimize confinement of the high dose to a carefully contoured target volume during external beam radiotherapy. In the treatment of genitourinary neoplasms, this technique would be most useful for treating pelvic and para-aortic lymph node regions and perhaps for the postoperative treatment of renal and ureteral tumors.

There is a potentially exciting role of tumor-specific or tumor-associated antibodies for the localization of primary tumors, for the detection of lymph node and other metastases, and for the treatment of both the primary tumor and disseminated disease. Better delineation of the extent of the primary tumor and assessment of the total extent of disease will lead to better selection of treatment methods for individual patients. The use of labeled antibodies for treatment of the primary tumor either as the only treatment or as a boost to external beam treatment will depend upon the radiation dose that can be delivered by that technique. It is an opportunity that hopefully will benefit from biological and immunological advances such as the development of monoclonal antibodies.

Although the use of radioactively labeled antibodies to treat primary tumors would be helpful for all genitourinary cancers, their greatest use may be to treat distant nodal or other metastases especially in patients with cancers of the kidney, bladder, prostate, and testicle where the incidence of distant metastases is high.

Particle Beam Radiotherapy

Radiotherapy with particles such as neutrons, protons, heavy ions, and negative pi mesons may have a major impact on the care of patients with cancer by improving the local control of tumors. Therapeutic beams of neutrons, negative pi mesons, alpha particles (helium ions), and heavy ions (carbon, neon, and argon) are more densely ionizing than beams of high energy x-rays, photons, or electrons and, therefore, have a greater biological effect. Pion, helium ion, and heavy ion beams have also physical dose distribution advantages as do proton beams which do not have an increased biological advantage. Because of their finite range in tissues compared to the exponential decrease in photon or neutron dose with tissue thickness, charged particle beams have the potential of delivering an increased radiation dose to the target volume relative to the dose in adjacent normal tissues.

Local control with radiotherapy alone is poor in clinical stage B_2 and C cancers of the bladder, and for large prostatic carcinomas may be less than the generally reported 13% to 18%.[5, 6] These are sites where 6500 to 7000 rad can be delivered with relatively low morbidity using megavoltage radiotherapy equipment. It may be possible to deliver higher biologically equivalent doses with neutron beams thereby achieving higher local control rates. It should be possible to deliver higher radiation doses with charged particle beams with less morbidity. The increased biological effect of pion, helium ion, and heavy ion beams may also improve the local control rates. This potential of high LET radiotherapy beams to increase local control rates for bladder and prostatic cancer is being evaluated in clinical trials conducted under the auspices of the National Cancer Institute.

Since there is no dose distribution advantage with neutrons compared to photons, the risk of injury to sensitive normal tissues may limit the usefulness of neutron beams for the treatment of cancers of the kidney, ureter, penis, testes, and urethra. On the other hand, therapy with charged particle beams, because of their improved dose distributions, may make it possible to deliver higher and biologically more effective radiation doses to the kidney, ureter, and para-aortic, or pelvic lymph nodes. Unfortunately, patients with tumors requiring radiotherapy to the lymph nodes are highly likely to have disseminated tumor and thus even excellent local radiotherapy may be inadequate at this time. However, the ability to reduce the volume of bone marrow irradiated will be a big advantage when there is effective adjuvant chemotherapy for genitourinary tumors other than the testis.

Radiation Modifiers

Modifying the response of tumors or the surrounding normal tissues to radiation in order to change the response of one relative to the other is a way to obtain a differential response of the normal or malignant tissue. Increasing the radiation sensitivity of the tumor relative to that of the normal tissues is one approach, while decreasing the radiation sensitivity of the normal tissues relative to that of the tumor is another. There are several ways to achieve these objectives such as (1) obtaining an increased concentration of a radiosensitizer in malignant tissues compared to the adjacent radiation dose-limiting normal tissue, (2) obtaining an increased concentration of a radioprotector in the normal tissues within or surrounding the tumor than in the tumor cells proper,[18] (3) giving an agent which sensitizes hypoxic but not oxygenated cells to radiation,[19] and (4) using potential differential effects of hyperthermia on tumors and surrounding normal tissues.[20] The development of effective radiation modifiers potentially could result in a significant improvement in the treatment of genitourinary malignancies. An effective radiosensitizer might increase the local control rates for genitourinary tumors, including large testicular cancer metastases to lymph nodes and large tumors now poorly controlled with doses of 6500 to 7000 rad with no increase in morbidity.

A good radioprotector could minimize the risk of injury to the small bowel, colon, and rectum which now compromise the total radiation dose when they are in the volume irradiated. Similarly, during irradiation of cancer of the penis and urethra, morbidity associated with the skin in the groin and perineum would be reduced. Protection of the bone marrow would be important in any treatment that encompasses part or all of the pelvic bones or lumbar spine, especially if chemotherapy has a role in the treatment of the disease.

Hyperthermia is another exciting adjuvant for the treatment of genitourinary tumors, especially for bladder, prostatic, penis, and urethral tumors. Hyperthermia could improve local control rates for present radiation schedules and may even be able to improve local control rates with radiation doses less than used conventionally. Because of difficulty in avoiding irradiation of the bowel when treating cancers of the kidney or ureter with photon beams, the role of hyperthermia in the treatment of these cancers will depend upon the relative sensitivity of the bowel to the combination of heat and radiation.

Combined Modality Treatment

A major approach to improving the cure rates of patients with solid tumors involves the integration of chemotherapy and/or immunotherapy with local treatment modalities such as surgery and/or radiotherapy. The basis for this combined modality approach is the recognition that surgery and radiotherapy eradicate tumor cells only at the sites where these modalities are applied. Thus, even when the tumor is eradicated locally and regionally, patients fail because of the dissemination of disease prior to (and perhaps during) treatment of the primary tumor and regional nodes. Incorporating chemotherapy into the treatment regimen has the potential of enhancing local and regional control, and hopefully, will eradicate disseminated microscopic foci of cancer cells.

Another objective of combined modality therapy is to decrease the morbidity associated with curative treatment by any one modality alone in order to improve the quality of life. If combining a less radical surgical procedure and a modified (lower) radiation dose provide the same or better local tumor control, the treatment sequelae and functional deficiencies should be reduced.

The rationale for using combined modality therapy will depend upon (1) the relative incidence of local and distant failure of each type of tumor, (2) the morbidity associated with each treatment modality, and (3) the efficacy of each of the treatment methods. The development of each treatment strategy will require careful consideration of these factors on a site-by-site basis.

There is much interest presently in intraoperative radiotherapy wherein a single high dose of radiation is delivered during the surgical procedure. The purpose is to expose the region to be irradiated, to displace insofar as possible critical normal organs, and to deliver a high dose of radiation to the exposed tumor or preferably to the tumor bed after gross surgical resection of the tumor. By using an electron beam or low energy x-ray machine, the radiation dose to structures behind the treatment volume can be minimized. Intraoperative radiotherapy may be extremely useful in the treatment of patients who have presumed or documented incomplete resections of cancers of the kidney or ureter or of grossly enlarged lymph nodes in testicular cancer. If there is only microscopic disease, the single intraoperative radiation dose may be sufficient by itself. If there is more extensive but minimal residual tumor, a combination of intraoperative radiotherapy and external beam radiotherapy may be appropriate.

The possibility of combining intraoperative radiotherapy with one or more radiation modifiers is exciting but is dependent upon the efficacy of the modifiers. An effective radiosensitizer could greatly enhance cell killing by the single radiation dose and a hypoxic cell sensitizer would decrease the risk of failure due to hypoxic cells. A radioprotector could decrease the risk of injury to critical normal structures which cannot be removed from the treatment volume. Intraoperative hyperthermia could be used in conjunction with the single high radiation dose perhaps increasing control rates, especially for inoperable tumors, with less morbidity.

SUMMARY

Although improvements in the use of radiotherapy alone or in combination with surgery over the past decade have been gradual, preclinical and limited clinical studies during that period have generated optimism for significant advances in this decade. Brachytherapy and intraoperative radiotherapy may prove effective in the eradication of microscopic residual disease after surgical removal of tumors of the kidney, ureter, or retroperitoneal lymph nodes without great risk of injury to adjacent normal tissues.

Radiosensitizers and hyperthermia hold promise for higher rates of local and regional control of cancer of the bladder, prostate, penis, and urethra. Radioprotectors may decrease the risk of injury to normal tissues thereby allowing higher rates of local control. If significantly higher rates of local control can be achieved with radiation modifiers, one could explore the possibility of preserving organs totally or in part with limited surgical procedures.

More effective chemotherapeutic agents such as are now available for the treatment of nonseminomatous testicular cancers are needed for the adjuvant treatment of cancers of the bladder, prostate, and kidney. When this goal is realized, the benefits of potential improvements in the treatment of these malignancies with radiotherapy discussed in this chapter will be extended to thousands of persons who would otherwise succumb to their cancers because of disseminated disease at the time of initial treatment despite local control. An advantage of this improved radiotherapy also would be preservation of the unpaired organs in a large number of patients to improve their quality of life.

REFERENCES

1. Pistenma, D. A., Bagshaw, M. A., Freiha, F. S. *Extended-Field Radiation Therapy for Prostatic Adenocarcinoma: Status Report of a Limited Prospective Trial.* Proceedings of the 23rd Clinical Conference, M. D. Anderson Hospital and Tumor Institute, Houston, Tex. 1978.
2. Goffinet, D. R., Schneider, M. J., Glatstein, E. J., Ludwig, H., Ray, G. R., Dunnick, N. R., Bagshaw, M. A. Bladder cancer; results of radiation therapy in 384 patients. *Radiology 117*:149, 1975.
3. Miller, L. S. Bladder cancer: superiority of preoperative irradiation and cystectomy in clinical stages B_2 and C. *Cancer 39*:973, 1977.
4. Whitmore, W. F., Batata, M. A., Hilaris, B. S., Reddy, G. N., Unal, A., Ghoneim, M. A., Grabstald, H., Chu, F. A comparative study of two preoperative radiation regimens with cystectomy for bladder cancer. *Cancer 40*:1077, 1977.
5. Bagshaw, M. A., Ray, G. R., Pistenma, D. A. *et al.* External beam radiation therapy of primary carcinoma of the prostate. *Cancer 36*:723, 1975.
6. Perez, C. A., Bauer, W., Garza, R. *et al.* Radiation therapy in the definitive treatment of localized carcinoma of the prostate. *Cancer 40*:1425, 1977.
7. Neglia, W. J., Hussey, D. H., Johnson, D. E. Megavoltage radiation therapy for carcinoma of the prostate. *Int. J. Radiat. Oncol. Biol. Phys. 2*:873, 1977.
8. Klein, K. A., Maier, J. G. Positive nodes and treatment failures in testicular carcinomas. *Int. J. Radiat. Oncol. Biol. Phys. 2*:1229, 1977.
9. Tyrell, C. J., Peckham, M. J. The response of lymph node metastases of testicular teratoma to radiation therapy. *Br. J. Urol. 48*:363, 1976.
10. Rafla, S., Parikh, K. J. Role of adjuvant radiotherapy in management of renal cell

carcinoma. *Int. Radiat. Oncol. Biol. Phys. 6:*1418, 1980.

11. Babaian, R. J., Johnson, D. E., Chan, R. C. Combination nephroureterectomy and postoperative radiotherapy for infiltrative ureteral carcinoma. *Int. J. Radiat. Oncol. Biol. Phys. 6:*1229, 1980.

12. Hilaris, B. S., Whitmore, W. E., Batata, M. *et al.* Behavioral patterns of prostate adenocarcinoma following an ^{125}I implant and pelvic node dissection. *Int. J. Radiat. Oncol. Biol. Phys. 2:*631, 1977.

13. Fowler, J. E., Barzell, W., Hilaris, B. S. *et al.* Complications of iodine[125] implantation and pelvic lymphadenectomy in the treatment of prostatic cancer. *J. Urol. 121:*1979.

14. Carlton, C. E., Hudgins, P. T., Guerriero, W. G. *et al.* Radiotherapy in the management of stage C carcinoma of the prostate. *J. Urol. 116:*206, 1976.

15. van der Werf-Messing, B. H. P. Cancer of the urinary bladder treated by interstitial radium implant. *Int. J. Radiat. Oncol. Biol. Phys. 4:*373, 1978.

16. van der Werf-Messing, B., Star, W. M., Menon, R. S. $T_3N_xM_o$ carcinoma of the urinary bladder treated by the combination of radium implant and external irradiation: a preliminary report. *Int. J. Radiat. Oncol. Biol. Phys. 6:*1723, 1980.

17. Abe, M., Takahashi, M., Yabumoto, E., Adachi, H., Yoshii, M., Mori, K. Clinical experiences with intraoperative radiotherapy of locally advanced cancers. *Cancer 45:*40, 1980.

18. Stratford, I. J., Adams, G. E., Horsman, M. R., Kandaiya, S., Rajaratnam, S., Smith, E., Williamson, C. The interaction of misonidazole with radiation, chemotherapeutic agents, or heat: a preliminary report. *Cancer Clin. Trials 3:*231, 1980.

19. Yuhas, J. M., Spellman, J. A., Culo, F. The role of WR 2721 in radiotherapy and/or chemotherapy. *Cancer Clin. Trials 3:*211, 1980.

20. Marmor, J. B., Pounds, D., Hahn, G. M. Treatment of superficial human neoplasms by local hyperthermia induced by ultrasound. *Cancer 43:*196, 1979.

13

Immunotherapy of Genitourinary Cancer

Manipulations of the immune system of tumor-bearing hosts in attempts to restrict tumor growth can be classified into two general categories: active or passive immunotherapy. Active immunotherapy refers to those approaches in which the immunologic responses of the host are modified directly. Active immunotherapy can be further subclassified as being either specific or nonspecific.

Specific active immunotherapy denotes approaches that attempt to boost the antitumor immune response directed against a particular type of tumor. Examples of specific active immunotherapy are immunization with either tumor cells or extracts of tumor cells and procedures for releasing endogenous tumor antigens into the host's circulation such as angioinfarction or cryodestruction of tumor cells growing *in situ*.

Nonspecific active immunotherapy refers to procedures that enhance the general immune responses of the host. Examples of nonspecific active immunotherapy are the administration of bacteria or bacterial products (*e.g.* Bacillus Calmette-Guérin (BCG), *Corynebacterium parvum (C. parvum)*, *Streptomyces* (OK-432), and nonspecific immunomodulators (*e.g.* levamisole, thymosin, and interferon or interferon inducers such as poly(I: C) or pyran copolymer).

Passive immunotherapy refers to approaches in which serum, lymphoid cells or cell products thought to have antitumor activity are transferred into tumor-bearing hosts. Passive immunotherapy is usually tumor antigen specific. An example of passive immunotherapy is the transfer of immune serum or lymphocytes into tumor-bearing hosts. Passive transfer of products of immune lymphocytes such as transfer factor or immune RNA to confer tumor antigen-specific immunity on host lymphoid cells also qualifies as specific passive immunotherapy.

Clinical trials of immunotherapeutic regimens that have been shown to have some immunologic activity in animal studies or preliminary screening studies are generally carried out in three phases. Phase I trials are designed primarily to evaluate toxicity and dose-response relationships of the immunotherapeutic agent so that appropriate dose schedules can be used in phase II trials. However, phase I trials also can provide some information about the efficacy of the treatment if there is objective evidence of tumor regression.

Phase II trials are designed to document and quantitate the therapeutic value of the treatment relative to no treatment at all. Ideally, in phase II trials, patients should be prospectively and randomly assigned to control and experimental groups. When the results of such trials are tabulated, these groups should be evaluated to ensure that patients with important prognostic features of the disease are equally distributed between the control and experimental groups. For example, the distribution of histologic grades of tumors, the sites and extent of metastases, and the performance status of the patients should be comparable in control and experimental groups as should general supportive measures for the patients. Only if these stratification requirements are met can differences in survival be attributed to differences in treatments.

Phase III trials are designed to compare the relative values of different proven effective treatments or combinations of treatments.

Appropriate statistical analysis must be employed in evaluating the results of phase II and phase III trials. Moreover, in phase II trials, it is essential to recognize that the more treatments being compared, the greater the probability that the results of one treatment will differ significantly from those of another by chance alone. It is also important to realize that although careful statistical analysis can help detect and correct for some potential sources of bias, statistical analysis alone is not an adequate substitute for appropriate controls.

A number of studies of immunotherapy of urologic cancer in experimental animals and man have been published in recent years. Unfortunately, among these only a few have been designed, executed, and analyzed in a meaningful manner. In this presentation, we have attempted to review these studies in detail and integrate the conclusions that might logically be drawn from them.

PROSTATIC CARCINOMA

Animal Studies

Pollard and co-workers[1] (Table 13.1) evaluated the effects of killed C. parvum administered in doses of 1.4 mg intravenously at weekly intervals on the development of metastases from the spontaneous adenocarcinoma in Lobund-Wistar rats. C. parvum-treated animals had significantly fewer pulmonary metastases (1.3/lung) than controls (13/lung). Pollard concluded that C. parvum protects against the development of metastases in this experimental tumor model.

The only other reported animal study (to our knowledge) of immunotherapy for prostatic cancer was reported by Weissman and co-workers[2]. These studies using R3327 AT prostate cancer in F_1 hybrids of Copen-

Table 13.1
Immunotherapy of prostatic cancer, animal studies

Authors	Host	Tumor	Agent	Route	Results
Pollard et al.[1]	Lobund-Wistar rats	Spontaneous adenocarcinoma	*Corynebacterium parvum*	i.v.[a]	Fewer metastases
Weissman et al.[2]	Copenhagen rats	R3327-AT	Irradiated tumor cells	s.c.	No response
			Pyran copolymer		Fewer local recurrences after excision of small tumors

[a] The abbreviations used are: i.v., intravenous, and s.c., subcutaneous.

hagen and Fischer rats included active specific immunotherapy with irradiated tumor cells and active nonspecific immunotherapy with injections of the interferon inducer, pyran copolymer. In these studies, neither pyran copolymer (25 mg/kg) nor vaccination with 10^7-irradiated R3327 AT cells 7 days before challenge conferred protection against the outgrowth of a 1.5×10^6 subcutaneous tumor cell inoculum. Similarly, neither pyran copolymer nor irradiated cells prevented local recurrences of surgically resected large tumors (25 to 30 cc volume). However, pyran copolymer treatment 1 week before and 5 days after surgical excision of small tumors (exact size not specified) prevented tumor recurrences, while animals treated by surgical excision alone had a 40% recurrence rate. This study suggests no beneficial effects from active immunotherapy with irradiated tumor cells but a possible slight beneficial effect of pyran copolymer treatment in hosts with small tumor burdens, although it is not possible to rule out the apparent effects of pyran copolymer being alternatively due to complete excision of the tumor.

Human Studies

SPECIFIC ACTIVE IMMUNOTHERAPY

Two studies reported in the literature could be categorized as specific active immunotherapy for prostatic carcinoma[3, 4] (Table 13.2). Both deal with cryotherapy of the prostate to induce a specific immunologic response in the host. Based on previous animal studies[9] suggesting that cryodestruction of the prostate induced the production of antibodies directed against prostatic antigens. Soanes and co-workers[3] in 1970 reported on three prostatic cancer patients whose metastatic lesions regressed several months following transurethral cryotherapy of the prostate. Proofs of regression were: a lessening of cervical spine metastases on ^{85}Sr bone scan in one patient, a decrease in the size of pulmonary metastases in another

Table 13.2
Immunotherapy of prostatic cancer, human studies

Authors	Agent	Route	No. of patients	Tumor stage	No. of controls	Results
Soanes et al.[3]	Cryotherapy	t.u.r.[a]	3	D	None	3 PR
Gursel et al.[4]	Cryotherapy	t.p.	11	D	None	1 PR
Merrin et al.[5]	BCG (? type)	i.pr.	17	D	None	5 PR
Robinson et al.[6]	BCG (Galaxo)	i.pr.	6	D	None	4 PR
Robinson et al.[7]	BCG (Galaxo)	i.pr.	8	C, D	None	(See text)
Guinan et al.[8]	BCG (Tice)	i.m.	19	A, B, C, D	14	No difference in survival

[a] The abbreviations used are: t.u.r., transurethral; PR, partial regression; t.p., transperineal; i.pr., intraprostatic; and i.m., intramuscular, BCG, bacillus Calmette-Guérin.

patient, and a decrease in the size of biopsy-proven supraclavicular lymph node metastases in a third patient.

In 1972, Gursel and co-workers[4] reported on the results of transperineal cryotherapy in 11 patients who were in relapse of metastatic prostatic cancer following endocrine therapy for the disease. Ten of these patients received cryotherapy treatments three times, with 4-week intervals between treatments, and the remaining patients received two treatments. Eight of the 11 patients reported relief of pain; however, there was no correlation between pain relief and acid phosphatase activity or levels of serum proteins. One patient had evidence of regression of skeletal metastases on ^{85}Sr bone scan while 10 exhibited no change. Ten of the 11 patients died within 2 to 11 months of treatment.

Although both Soanes[3] and Gursel[4] believed that these uncontrolled trials suggested a systemic therapeutic benefit from cryosurgery, controlled clinical studies to confirm such a benefit have not been done. Moreover, other investigators[10, 11] have not found a measurable immunologic effect of cryodestruction of the prostate.

NONSPECIFIC ACTIVE IMMUNOTHERAPY

Early studies of nonspecific active immunotherapy of prostate cancer[12, 13] consist only of anecdotal case reports, and yield no generally applicable information. For example, in 1962, Johnstone[13] examined the effects of Coley's toxin on patients with various cancers. The toxin was administered intravenously each day in doses of 0.5 cc at a 1/20 dilution of the original preparation, with no more than five injections being given per week. One patient in this study had prostatic cancer with diffuse bony metastases and pain. Prior therapy included suprapubic prostatectomy. Alleviation of pain and weight gain were attributed to the 49 injections of Coley's toxin. No side effects other than severe chills and fever were described. This patient lived for 11 months after therapy was completed.

The first clinical trial of nonspecific active immunotherapy with BCG was reported by Merrin et al.[5] in 1975 in 17 patients with histologically-proven stage D carcinoma of the prostate. Patients were divided into two groups based upon their skin test reactions to purified protein derivative

(PPD) testing. Those with positive PPD skin tests, group 1, had received intraprostatic injections by one of the following two regimens: (1) 1 mg BCG/week (type and number of organisms were not specified) for 4 weeks (five patients); or (2) 1 mg BCG the 1st week, 2 mg the 2nd week, 4 mg the 3rd week, and 6 mg the 4th week (two patients). Group 2 patients—those with negative PPD skin tests—had been given 50 mg BCG orally on two occasions, with 1 week between doses; however, none of these patients converted their PPD skin tests to positive and therefore were not included in the results.

Five patients (71%) in group 1 were reported to have objective responses to BCG therapy as indicated by a 50% decrease in the size and induration of the prostate. There were no changes observed in measurable metastases except in one patient who demonstrated necrosis of a soft tissue metastasis that had been injected with BCG. Biopsies taken after BCG therapy showed necrosis of the tumor in three patients and no change in the remaining patients. No evidence of lymphocytic infiltration or granuloma formation at the injection sites was seen. The general condition of the seven patients following BCG injections was described as worse in four patients, stable in two patients, and improved in one patient. Although initial BCG injections were well tolerated, later injections produced fever in all patients. Two patients had an anaphylactoid reaction to the fourth injection, and one patient developed a rectoprostatic fistula.

As a phase I trial, this study provided only limited information. No useful dose-response data were generated, although some information on the toxicity of the dose schedules used was provided, and the authors did report measurable evidence of tumor regression of five patients.

In a similar, uncontrolled phase I trial of BCG immunotherapy, Robinson and co-workers[6,7] reported on two successive trials of prostate cancer patients treated with multiple intraprostatic injections of BCG. These investigators administered Galaxo BCG (number of organisms not stated) at weekly intervals beginning with a 1 cc dose and increasing the dose by 1 cc each successive week for a total of 6 weeks. Robinson's[6] initial clinical trial included six patients who were in relapse after endocrine therapy with 3 mg of diethylstilbestrol (DES)/day. Four (67%) of these patients were reported to have improvement in micturition and in their general medical condition, but all died within 2 months to 2 years of treatment. In Robinson's[6] first trial of patients, there was no clinical or postmortem evidence of massive tumor destruction and complications of therapy were minimal.

Robinson's second clinical trial[7] included eight similarly treated patients, six of whom had stage III (C) and two of whom had stage IV (D) disease. All had been treated previously with both transurethral resection of the prostate and bilateral orchiectomy, and six of the eight had shown positive tuberculin skin tests. In Robinson's second trial, unlike the first, complications of treatment were substantial. All eight patients developed fever, three developed gastrointestinal bleeding, and autopsy studies revealed widespread granulomas involving the prostate, lungs, liver, spleen, bone marrow, and myocardium. Accordingly, Robinson and associates recommended against administering more than three intra-prostatic BCG injections. Four of the six patients who had had positive tuberculin skin tests were reported to be alive 6 months to 1 year after therapy.

As a phase I trial, this study provides some useful information on dose-toxicity relationships, but not on dose-response relationships. In addition, measurable evidence of tumor regression was documented in some patients.

In a phase II trial of BCG immunotherapy, Guinan et al.[8] administered BCG (Tice) by a single left deltoid region intradermal vaccination of 4.2 $\times 10^7$ viable organisms/0.5 ml every 4 months. The BCG treatment group consisted of 19 patients—8 with stage A disease, 2 with stage B disease, 5 with stage C, and 4 with stage D. Of the 14 control patients who did not undergo BCG therapy, there were 7 with stage A disease, 2 with stage B, and 5 with stage D. The control and treatment groups were age matched but not randomly assigned. Criteria for the inclusion in the control group were not stated. Seven patients in each group were concurrently receiving endocrine therapy. Response to the therapy as assessed by mean survival time for the time of diagnosis of the disease was reported as 26.6 months for the BCG group as compared to 22.6 months for the untreated group. Morbidity of the BCG vaccinations was described as minimal, but specific details were not given.

As a phase II trial, this study deals with heterogeneous groups of patients in terms of extent of disease and other therapy. Although the authors stated that survival was prolonged in the BCG-treated patients, the difference between the mean survival times of 26.6 and 22.6 months was not statistically significant.

Taken together, the above described human studies (Table 10.2) on immunotherapy for prostatic carcinoma provide only limited, unconvincing evidence for a beneficial therapeutic effect from any agent or regimen reported. Toxicity of nonspecific active immunotherapy with BCG is documented in some of these studies, but little information regarding differences in strains of BCG and dose-toxicity relationships is provided.

There have been no studies (to our knowledge) of passive immunotherapy for prostatic cancer.

In summary, immunotherapy in carcinoma of the prostate has not been adequately evaluated. Although the limited information available suggests that prostate cancers may express antigens that are capable of eliciting immune responses in the host, much more work will need to be done to determine whether these immunologic response can be modified to the benefit of the host.

BLADDER CANCER

Bladder cancer is immunologically the most extensively studied urologic tumor and, in fact, adjunctive BCG therapy in patients with superficial bladder cancer is one of the most successful examples of immunotherapy reported to date in man.

Table 13.3
Immunotherapy of bladder cancer, animal studies

Authors	Host	Tumor	Agent	Route	Results
de Kernion et al.[14]	Mice	FANFT[a]	BCG (Chicago) Corynebacterium parvum	i.m. and i.p.	Prolonged survival, tumor inhibition
Lamm et al.[15]	Fischer rats	FANFT	BCG cell walls	i.v. and i.vsc.	Delayed carcinogenesis
				i.l.	Inhibition of tumor progression
			DNCB	i.v. and i.vsc.	No effect
Adolphs et al.[16]	Wistar rats	FANFT	BCG (Chicago)	Systemic	Tumor inhibition
				i.l.	No effect
Soloway[17]	Mice	FANFT	BCG (Trudeau)	i.p.	Tumor enhancement
Morales et al.[18]	Mice	FANFT	BCG (Pasteur)	i.p.	No effect
			irradiated, tumor cells	i.p.	Transplantation[b] resistance
			Tumor extract	i.p.	Transplantation[b] resistance
Lamm et al.[19]	Mice	FANFT	Levamisole	i.p.	Tumor inhibition, prolonged survival
Pimm and Baldwin[20]	Mice	T-24 cells	BCG (Galaxo)	Mixed with tumor cells	Transplanation[b] resistance
Collste[21]	Mice	FANFT	Irradiated tumor cells		Transplantation[b] resistance

[a] The abbreviations used are: FANFT, N-[4-(5-nitro-2-furyl)-2-thiazolyl]formamide, i.m., intramuscular; i.p., intraperitoneal; i.v., intravenous; i.vsc., intravesical; i.l. intralesional; BCG, Bacillus Calmette-Guérin, and, DNCB, dinitrochlorobenzene.
[b] Effectiveness reduced by BCG.

Animal Studies

NONSPECIFIC ACTIVE IMMUNOTHERAPY

Nonspecific active immunotherapy may include BCG, *C. parvum* dinitrochlorobenzene (DNCB), and levamisole.

De Kernion et al.[14] (Table 13.3) examined the effects of BCG (Chicago Research) and *C. parvum* on transplantation resistance and survival in the mouse N-[4-(5-nitro-2-furyl)-2-thiazolyl]formamide (FANFT)-induced bladder tumor MBT-2 which had been shown to be highly immunogenic. Tumors were carried by transplantation into the leg. BCG (5 × 10^5 viable units) injected intramuscularly into the groin or thigh of the same leg implanted with tumor on the day of tumor inoculation, and either weekly or biweekly thereafter, had no effect on tumor growth. Thirty days after inoculation, survival of the animals injected with BCG was significantly improved ($p < 0.05$) relative to that of controls.

De Kernion et al.[14] reported that a marked inhibition of tumor growth occurred following a single intraperitoneal injection of *C. parvum* as compared to control animals ($p < 0.05$). Weekly intraperitoneal injections of *C. parvum* in conjunction with Cytoxan inhibited tumor growth and prolonged survival more than either agent alone.

Lamm and co-workers[19] also examined the effect of immunization with BCG cell walls and with DNCB on the induction of bladder tumors in Fischer 344 rats who were fed with the carcinogen, FANFT. These investigators treated animals who had been placed on a carcinogen diet for a period of 1 month with a 150-mg injection of BCG cell walls that had been solubilized with mineral oil, saline, and Tween 80 detergent. Following the initial intravenous injection of BCG cell walls, they confirmed the fact that the animals were sensitized by testing with foot pad injections. Then 12, 14, and 16 weeks, and every 4 weeks thereafter, 0.5 ml of the BCG vaccine (15 mg/ml) along with PPD was given intravesically. Control animals not sensitized with BCG cell walls received intravesical injections of saline.

The results demonstrated a 44% tumor incidence in control animals, while the BCG animals had a tumor incidence of 14% 26 weeks into therapy. However, by 30 weeks, 83% of BCG-treated animals and 100% of controls had tumors. Finally, by 38 weeks, all animals had tumors. These results suggested immunotherapy with the BCG cell walls may have delayed the carcinogenic process, but statistical analysis was not provided.

DNCB studies of Lamm et al.[19] were performed on animals who also had been on a carcinogenic diet for 1 month. These animals were sensitized to DNCB with a 0.1 ml injection of 2% DNCB mixed with Freund's adjuvant 12, 14, 16 and 18 weeks later, and every subsequent month for the duration of the experiment. Controls received complete Freund's adjuvant mixed with ethylenol alone. The results revealed no beneficial effect of DNCB on the incidence of tumors. In fact, at 21 weeks, DNCB-treated animals actually had a higher incidence of tumors.

In further experiments by Lamm et al.,[19] animals were fed FANFT, tumors were allowed to grow, and then animals were given intralesional injections of BCG through the bladder wall. Animals that were not sensitized to BCG, and that received control emulsion injections into the lesions, had a 19% incidence of tumors that showed no further progression. Seventy percent of BCG-sensitized animals injected intralesionally with BCG had no further tumor progression; however, only 11% of animals not sensitized to BCG and injected intralesionally with BCG showed no further progression. This result suggested that intralesional injection of BCG in previously BCG-sensitized animals inhibited tumor progression.

Lamm et al.[19] also examined the fate of noninjected lesions and found that some regressed in the control group, in the BCG-sensitized group, and in the non-BCG-treated group.

Adolphs and co-workers[16] examined the effect of intralesional and systemic BCG on the induction of bladder tumors by FANFT, and also compared the effect of adding cyclophosphamide to BCG. Their immunotherapy protocol for systemic therapy involved the injection of approximately 2×10^7 BCG organisms from the Chicago Research Foundation weekly, and their protocol for the intralesional BCG administration involved injecting 2×10^7 bacilli through the intact bladder wall into the tumor nodule on one occasion. The efficacy of the treatment was evaluated by calculating the mean bladder weights of the animals in each group at the time of sacrifice.

Their results showed that systemic BCG alone was somewhat effective in that the mean bladder weight of BCG treated animals was 1.38 g while that of the control animals was 3.12 g. BCG given intralesionally did not seem to be effective, with the mean bladder weights of this group being 4.59 g. Cyclophosphamide alone was effective in reducing the mean bladder weight to 2.66 g while the combination of cyclophosphamide and systemic BCG gave the best results with the mean bladder weight being 0.935 g.

Adolphs and co-workers[16] also performed histological studies to determine the effects of BCG on the depth of tumor infiltration and found that it was unaltered by BCG therapy. Toxicity in BCG-treated animals was mainfested by weight loss and granulomas in the lungs. Although the authors concluded from this study that intralesional BCG is ineffective in treating superficial bladder cancer, there may be some question about the validity of comparing mean bladder weights of animals that have received intralesional injections to those who have not received injections.

Soloway[17] studied the effects of systemic BCG therapy either alone or in conjunction with cyclophosphamide treatment on FANFT-induced bladder cancer in C3H/HeJ mice. Mice ingested 0.1% FANFT for 11 months. Therapeutic trials begun at 5 and 7 months included (1) 10^7 BCG-viable organisms (Trudeau Mycobacterial Collection) every 2 months, and (2) cyclophosphamide 75 mg/kg plus 10^4 BCG organisms every 2 weeks. In addition, several different chemotherapeutic regimens were tested. BCG and cyclophosphamide were administered intraperitoneally. Mice receiving BCG therapy had significantly larger bladder tumors than appropriate controls. Moveover, BCG therapy did not potentiate the antitumor effects of cyclophosphamide; rather, tumor weights were lower in mice receiving cyclophosphamide alone than in mice receiving combined BCG-cyclophosphamide therapy.

Morales et al.[22] also examined the effects of BCG on induction of transplantation resistance to the FANFT-induced MBT-2 tumor. Pasteur BCG (10^7 viable organisms) were injected i.p. either alone or simultaneously with irradiated tumor cells or tumor cell extract 14 and 7 days before challenge with tumor cells. The results demonstrated no effect on the incidence of tumor takes by BCG immunization alone. BCG administered in conjunction with either irradiated tumor cells or tumor membrane extracts actually decrease their effectiveness in conferring host resistance (see below).

Lamm and co-workers[15] also examined the effects of levamisole in a dose of 2.5 mg/kg which had been found to be effective in clinical studies on the growth rate of the FANFT-induced MBT-2 tumor in C3H/He mice. In the experimental animals, one group was pretreated with levamisole (2.5 mg/kg) for 3 days a week for 2 weeks before the challenge with 5×10^3 viable tumor cells and then 3 days a week every 2 weeks for 8 weeks following challenge with the tumor. The other experimental group received levamisole 3 days a week every 2 weeks for 8 weeks beginning on the day of tumor challenge. Control animals received saline injections 3 days a week with the injections being repeated every 2 weeks for 8 weeks.

Lamm's results[15] revealed that about 50% of both the control and treatment groups ultimately developed tumors, but tumor appearance time was significantly delayed in the levamisole-treated mice by 2½ weeks. The survival was also significantly prolonged in the levamisole treated mice, but the growth rates were, statistically, significantly different only at one point in time (9 weeks). They mentioned no toxicity of this single dose of levamisole and provided no *in vitro* data that would corroborate an immunologic effect. From this experiment, they concluded that intraperitoneal levamisole in the dose schedule used had an inhibitory effect of growth of the MBT-2 tumor.

Pimm and Baldwin[20] examined the effect of injecting human bladder cancer cells of the T-24 cell line into athymic nude mice. In their experiments, animals who had BCG of the Galaxo type mixed in 0.5-mg quantities with 1×10^6 tumor cells without the BCG had no tumor takes, while animals injected with 1×10^6 tumor cells without the BCG had tumor takes in virtually all cases. They found that when BCG was injected at a site distant from the tumor there was no protection from the tumor takes. On the basis of these experiments they conclude that BCG acts locally to invoke non-T-cell mediated host immunologic responses, probably involving macrophages, to destroy the tumor cell inoculum. This result is also consistent with the hypothesis that tumor cells do not grow well in sites of delayed hypersensitivity reactions.

SPECIFIC ACTIVE IMMUNOTHERAPY

Using a tissue culture line developed from the FANFT-induced MBT-2, Morales *et al.*[22] examined the roles of immunization with viable tumor cells, irradiated tumor cells, and extracts from tumor cell membranes on conferring protection against subsequent tumor challenge in C3H/HeN mice. To demonstrate the immunogenicity of the tumor, mice were injected with 2×10^5 live tumor cells or phosphate buffered saline (PBS) in the hind leg. Thirty days later, tumors were resected by leg amputation. Thirteen days following amputation, animals were rechallenged with tumor cells. Tumor-resected mice showed significant protection (33% lower tumor incidence) as compared to controls when rechallenged with 2×10^3 MBT-2 cells; however, progressively less protection was afforded at higher tumor challenge doses (2×10^4, 2×10^5, 2×10^6). In addition, mice were immunized 14 and 7 days before challenge with 2×10^3 live MBT-2 cells with various dilutions of irradiated tumor cells or tumor cell membrane extracts. Results revealed that 10^7 irradiated tumor cells conferred complete protection while 5×10^6 irradiated cells also provided significant ($p < 0.005$) protection. Immunization with 100 μg of tumor cell membrane extract conferred complete protection to subsequent tumor challenge, while 200 μg of extract induced significant protection ($p < 0.005$). Specificity of the MBT-2 extract was shown by comparison to an extract prepared from another C3H tumor (mammary, 341 clone 101) which did not afford protection to subsequent challenge with the MBT-2 tumor.

Collste and colleagues[21] examined the effects of specific active immunotherapy with irradiated tumor cells in the MBT-2 FANFT-induced transitional cell carcinoma in C3H/HeJ mice. In their studies, animals were divided into immune animals, half of which were immunized by a single immunization with 5×10^6 irradiated tumor cells 14 days before tumor challenge, and the other half of which were immunized both 7 and 14 days before tumor challenge. Control animals received injections of suspensions of viable syngeneic benign bladder epithelial cells in the same number and at the same site. Animals were then challenged with 5×10^6 viable tumor cells and the results were evaluated in terms of percentage of tumor take. Nearly 100% of the nonimmune animals had tumor takes, 9 of 36 (25%) who had received only one immunization with irradiated tumor cells developed tumors, and only 5 of 36 (14%) that had received two immunizations had tumor takes. The authors conclude from this study that the MBT is immunogeneic and that it is capable of eliciting an immune response that can prevent the outgrowth of an isograft in syngeneic hosts.

Summary of Animal Studies on Immunotherapy of Bladder Cancer

The results of nonspecific active immunotherapy of transitional cell carcinoma in animals are conflicting. Positive results with BCG were reported in terms of increased animal survival by de Kernion et al.[14] using intramuscular Chicago BCG; delayed carcinogenesis and inhibition of tumor progression was reported by Lamm[15, 19] using intravenous and intravesical as well as intralesional BCG; reduction in tumor growth was reported by Adolphs and co-workers[16] using Chicago BCG; and elimination of human tumor outgrowth when tumor cells were transferred to nude mice was reported by Pimm and Baldwin[20] using Galaxo BCG mixed with the tumor cells. Negative results of BCG therapy were reported by Adolphs et al.[16] using Chicago BCG intralesionally, Soloway and co-workers[17] using Trudeau BCG intraperitoneally, and Morales and co-workers[18] using Pasteur BCG intraperitoneally. The reasons for these discrepancies are not entirely clear, but differences in the type, route of administration, and dose schedule of the BCG may be important factors. These studies also show that other agents, including C. parvum and levamisole may be effective in experimental bladder cancer while intravesical DNCB seems to be ineffective.

Studies of specific active immunotherapy with either live or irradiated tumor cells, or tumor membrane extracts, clearly indicate that the FANFT-induced bladder carcinoma is immunogeneic in syngeneic hosts,

Table 13.4
Immunotherapy of bladder cancer, human studies

Authors	Agent	Route	No. of patients	Tumor stage(s)	No. of controls	Results
Morales et al.,[18] and Morales[23]	BCG[a] Armand-Frappier	i.d. and i.vsc.	16	O, A	None	Fewer recurrences
Douville et al.[24]	BCG (? type)	i.d. and i. vsc.	6	O, A	None	Fewer recurrences, 4 PR
Lamm et al.[25]	BCG (Pasteur)	i.d. and i.vsc.	23	O, A	24	Fewer recurrences
Camacho et al.[26]	BCG (? type)	i.d. and i.vsc.	22	O, A	22	Fewer recurrences
Kagawa et al.[27]	OK-432	i.d. and i.vsc.	11	Not specified	None	3 PR
Purves et al.[28]	Corynebacterium parvum	i.m.	14	B, C	12	Reduced survival
Herr et al.[29]	Poly(I:C)	i.v.	20	O, A	15	No effect
Symes and Riddell[30]	Immune pig lymphocytes	Various routes	5	D	0	2 PR
Symes et al.[31]	Immune pig lymphocytes	i.a.	16	C, D	0	7 PR
Fenely et al.[32]	Immune pig lymphocytes	i.a.	25	C, D	None	14 PR
Symes et al.[33]	Immune pig lymphocytes	i.v. and i.a.	16	B, C, D	16	No difference in radiation response

[a] The abbreviations used are: BCG, bacillus Calmette-Guérin; i.d., intradermal; i. vsc., intravesical; i.m., intramuscular; i.v., intravenous, i.a., intraarterial; PR, partial response.

and that it confers significant protection on the outgrowth of tumor cell inocula.

Human Studies

NONSPECIFIC ACTIVE IMMUNOTHERAPY

Morales et al.[18] and Morales[23] (Table 13.4) examined the effects of BCG on superficial bladder cancer in 16 patients. No concurrent controls were included in this study. The patients' initial tumors were treated surgically. Each patient had a history of at least two tumor recurrences treated by endoscopic fulguration or resection. Six patients had received thio-TEPA or Epodyl therapy without benefit. BCG (120 mg) was given *via* an indwelling urethral catheter in 50-ml volume of saline and the patients were instructed to retain the suspension at least 2 hours. Simultaneous BCG (5 mg) (Armand-Frappier) intradermal injections were administered on alternate thighs. This protocol was carried out weekly for 6 consecutive weeks. Results were evaluated by cystoscopy performed 4 to 6 weeks after completion of therapy and at 3-month intervals thereafter. The 16 patients developed seven tumor recurrences during a period of 222 patient months compared with 53 recurrent tumors in 162 patient months for the same 16 patients during the 12 months preceding the initiation of the BCG therapy. The authors reported undesirable side effects as being minimal and self-limiting. Three patients developed fever, six had symptoms of lower urinary tract infection, and all showed a circumscribed but strong reaction at the BCG injection sites. This study suggested that combined intravesical and systemic BCG may be of value in reducing the recurrence rate in patients with superficial bladder cancer.

Douville et al.[24] also reported on a phase I trial of BCG immunotherapy for the treatment of recurrent superficial bladder tumors. They studied six patients who had had at least two recurrences of superficial bladder tumors within a period of 2 years. Their immunotherapy regimen included systemic immunization with BCG by abdominal scarification with 5 mg of BCG weekly for 6 weeks (the strain and number of organisms were not specified) followed by intravesical instillation of 120 mg of BCG in 50 ml of saline which was retained for 2 hours. Patients were cystoscoped 4 to 6 weeks after treatment. Four of the six patients exhibited regression of their tumors, and all four of the responders manifested evidence of systemic toxic reactions to the BCG, although they were not specific about the nature of these reactions. The two nonresponders had no toxic reactions. The authors postulated that the failure of therapy in these patients may have been due to the fact that they were anergic to BCG. The authors did not specify the long-term follow-up, but stated that their results suggested that the number of recurrences may have been less. This study, as a phase I study, reports only one dose of BCG and, as such, provides little information about dose response and dose toxicity relationships. It does, however, document tumor regression of established superficial tumors.

Lamm and associates[25] randomly assigned 47 patients with transitional cell carcinoma of the bladder to receive either standard surgical therapy or standard surgical therapy plus BCG. BCG (Pasteur strain) was given intravesically (120 mg) and intradermally (5 mg) weekly for 6 weeks. Both control and BCG therapy groups were matched by age, tumor grade, and previous number of recurrences. Their results showed that 11/24 (46%) of control patients developed tumor recurrences while only 5/23 (22%) of the patients who received BCG developed recurrences. There were 19 episodes of tumor recurrence in the control group with a total of 67 individual tumors occurring. Patients in the BCG group had 8 episodes of recurrence with a total of 17 tumors. The mean time to recurrence was reported as 12 months for control patients as compared to 19.4 months from the BCG group. Toxicity was manifested as cystitis for 1 to 3 days following BCG instillation but required no postponement of the BCG immunotherapy. This study seems to demonstrate clearly that combined intradermal and intravesical BCG reduces the recurrence rate in patients with recurrent superficial bladder cancer.

Camacho et al.[26] also examined the effects of BCG therapy in a phase II study on patients with multiple recurrent superficial bladder tumors. Fifty-one patients were randomized to receive either fulguration alone or fulguration plus BCG therapy. BCG therapy consisted of 6 weekly instillations of 120 mg BCG (type not specified) intravesically in 50 ml of saline which was retained for 2 hours. BCG was given by the percutaneous technique by the same schedule. Twenty-two patients in each group have had follow-up cystoscopies. Tumor recurrences/patient month for both BCG treatment and control groups before and after BCG therapy were evaluated. Patients who received BCG therapy showed 3.6 tumors/patient month *versus* 0.75 tumors/patient month after therapy. Control patients developed 2.97 tumors/patient month prior to the start of the study *versus* 2.37 after. Twenty-eight of the patients in this study had pretreatment positive urinary cytologies. Of these patients, $\frac{1}{12}$ (8%) of the control group developed negative cytologies compared to $\frac{8}{16}$ (50%) of the BCG treatment patients with negative cytologies. The authors reported that the intravesical BCG therapy was well tolerated with the only side effects being transient dysuria, mild hematuria, urinary frequency, chills, fever, and malaise. One patient had granulomatous prostatitis.

Kagawa and co-workers[27] studied the effects of the streptococcal preparation, OK-432, on 21 patients with bladder cancer (11 patients with grade 1 lesions, 5 patients with grade 2 lesions, and 5 patients with grade 3 lesions). No control patients were included in this study. OK-432 was administered first intravesically at a dose of 0.5 to 1.0 mg of dried preparation followed by intramuscular injection of 0.5 mg of dried preparation three times weekly. Transurethral resection or cystectomy was performed when the disease warranted such procedures. In three patients (14.3%) following partial or total cystectomy, indications of tumor regression were observed by macroscopic and histologic analysis of biopsy specimens. Lymphocyte infiltration was found in 47.6% of the specimens. Transient pyrexia was the only adverse reaction attributed to the therapy.

Purves and colleagues[28] studied the effects of adjunctive immunotherapy in patients with invasive bladder cancer using *C. parvum* as an immunologic adjuvant. In their study, 26 patients were randomly assigned to receive adjuvant immunotherapy with *C. parvum* or no adjuvant immunotherapy. Fourteen were randomized to the immunotherapy arm and 12 to the control group. The protocol for immunotherapy involved the i.m. injection of 1 mg of a suspension of *C. parvum* furnished by the Burroughs Wellcome Research Laboratories weekly for 2 years for their initial patients and for 1 year for subsequent patients. Patients also received methotrexate chemotherapy before the *C. parvum* and all were treated with 6000 to 6500 rads radiation therapy prior to cystectomy when cystectomy was required. Not all patients in the study were treated with cystectomy, but the proportion that underwent cystectomy was roughly the same in both groups with 5 to 14 *C. parvum*-treated patients and 4 of 12 controls undergoing cystectomy. Follow-up was 24 months. The results of this study revealed that *C. parvum*-treated patients had a poorer survival than controls, even when they were segregated into those who underwent cystectomy and those who did not. *In vitro* parameters of immunologic function were monitored including peripheral blood T-lymphocyte percentages, K-cell activity and mitogen responsiveness as well as monocyte and polymorphonuclear leukocyte chemotaxis. The only consistent difference between *C. parvum*-treated patients and controls was a slightly higher level of K-cell activity, but this did not correlate with prognosis. The authors concluded from this prospective, randomized study of adjuvant immunotherapy for invasive bladder cancer that *C. parvum* of the type and dose schedule used was not an effective therapeutic adjunct, at least in terms of patient survival.

In a prospective trial, Herr and associates[29] examined the efficacy of the interferon inducer, polyriboinosinic acid-polyribocytidylic acid (poly(I:C)) in patients with papillomas or superficial carcinoma of the bladder. Patients in this study were randomly assigned to treatment with poly(I:C) (20 patients) or no treatment (15 patients), and were stratified into pairs according to number of tumors (1 or 2 or more), histologic grade (benign papilloma or grade 1 or 2 superficial epidermoid carcinoma), number of previous tumors (1 or 2 or more), and recurrence rate (less than 6 months or greater than 6 months). Treatment group received 25 mg/kg of poly(I:C) intravenously every 2 weeks. The number of tumors were noted by cystoscopy every 2 to 3 months, and biopsy and fulguration was performed on existing lesions. After surgical removal of recurrent tumor at the initiation of the study, 5 of 15 (33%) of poly(I:C)-treated patients were free of tumor at 3 months compared with 0/11 (0%) of controls. However, later cystoscopic evaluation revealed that the number of patients free of tumor on poly(I:C) therapy at 6, 9, and 12 months following the start of the protocol was $\frac{1}{12}$ (8%), $\frac{2}{6}$ (33%), and $\frac{0}{4}$ (0%), while the respective controls free of tumor were $\frac{0}{10}$ (0%), $\frac{0}{3}$ (0%) and $\frac{0}{2}$ (0%). The authors concluded that there was no significant difference in the frequency or number of recurrent tumors between treated and untreated patients after 12 months of therapy. Despite these negative results, poly(I:C) induced significant interferon titers in most of the treated patients, although the interferon titers fell progressively with each successive treatment after 3 months of therapy. Poly(I:C) caused fever, headache, malaise, and two patients developed positive antinuclear antibody titers.

SPECIFIC PASSIVE IMMUNOTHERAPY

Symes and Riddell[30] examined the effects of immunized pig lymph node cells in the treatment of patients with various advanced cancers. All patients were refractory to conventional therapy. Included in this study were two patients with transitional cell carcinoma of the bladder and three with adenocarcinoma of the bladder. The treatment protocol was as follows: several pieces of tumor of about 3-ml volume were obtained, cut into multiple fragments, and implanted in the small bowel mesentery of a pig. Seven days following implantation, the hyperplastic lymph node chain was removed and the lymph nodes were minced into single suspensions. Patients were given between 10^9 and 2×10^{10} sensitized lymph node cells *via* different routes. Phenergan (25 mg) was given intramuscularly 30 minutes before pig cell infusion to minimize the risk of hypersensitivity reactions. The two patients with transitional cell carcinoma of the bladder showed tumor necrosis and obtained clinical benefit following the infusion of pig cells; however, the three patients with adenocarcinoma of the bladder showed no evidence of tumor regression as determined by clinical and pathological findings.

In 1973, Symes et al.[33] treated 16 patients with advanced carcinoma of the bladder by infusion of insensitized pig lymph node cells via the arterial blood supply of the tumor. In 14 patients, the tumor had spread beyond the bladder and surgical resection was considered inappropriate. Assessment of patient response was evaluated by (1) symptomatic changes, (2) cystoscopy and bimanual pelvic examination, (3) histology of biopsy material, and (4) periodic radiologic examination. The authors describe definite benefit from the pig cell infusion in $7/16$ (44%) patients. Two of these patients showed treatment benefit associated with radiotherapy, i.e. the tumor seemed to show unusual sensitivity to radiotherapy. Three patients (19%) had equivocal response to the pig cell treatment while in six patients (37%) there was no evidence of tumor regression.

To further examine the effects of radiotherapy in combination with sensitized pig lymph node cell infusions, Feneley et al.[32] studied 25 patients with transitional cell carcinoma (TCC) of the bladder. Twenty-three of these had advanced disease. The patients were divided into the following treatment groups: (1) group 1 received sensitized pig lymph node cells alone as described above (7 patients), (2) group 2 received pig lymph node cells on recurrence following a full conventional course of radiotherapy (7 patients), and (3) group 3 received sensitized pig lymph node cells followed at 4 to 8 weeks with an attenuated course (4000 rads) of radiotherapy (11 patients). The results showed evidence of tumor necrosis in $2/7$ (28%) patients in group 1, $3/7$ (43%) in group 2, and $9/11$ (82%) in group 3. Furthermore, five of the patients in group 3 were described as surviving greather than 1 year following infusion of the pig lymph node cells with no macroscopic evidence of tumor and no bladder symptoms.

To evaluate the possible syngergistic effect of radiotherapy and sensitized pig lymph node cell therapy, Symes et al.[31] treated 31 patients with invasive TCC of the bladder with either pig lymph node cells followed 6 weeks later with radiotherapy (5500 rads) only. Patients in the study were paired according to age, sex, clinical stage (T 3 or T 4) and histological grade. Criteria for positive response in this study included all of the following: (1) partial or complete remission of symptoms, (2) objective evidence of tumor reduction, and (3) evidence of histologic change. In group 1, $10/16$ (62%) showed evidence of remission while $9/15$ in group 2 (60%) showed evidence of remission. There was no significant difference in survival time between the two groups.

Summary of Human Studies on Immunotherapy of Bladder Cancer

The studies of Morales,[18, 23] Lamm et al.[25] and Camacho et al.[26] using BCG intravesically and intradermally in patients with superficial bladder cancer seem to demonstrate clearly that this form of immunotherapy significantly reduces the recurrence rate of superficial bladder cancer. Moreover, the uncontrolled study of Douville et al.[24] provides some evidence that intravesical BCG also causes the regression of established superficial tumor. The study of Kagawa et al.[27] indicates that streptococcal

OK-32 may also produce a similar beneficial effect although the available data are too limited to draw any definite conclusions. The studies by Purves and associates[28] using *C. parvum* in patients with more advanced bladder cancer indicates that this agent, in the dose schedule used, is not effective. Similarly, the study by Herr et al.[29] in patients with superficial bladder cancer would seem to indicate that poly(I:C) is also ineffective. The studies by Symes and associates,[30, 31, 33] and Feneley *et al.*[32] using specific passive immunotherapy with immune pig lymphocytes, are intriguing but would need to be confirmed by other investigators before this form of therapy can be recommended.

RENAL ADENOCARCINOMA

One of the first human immunotherapy trials for renal adenocarcinoma was reported by Nadler and Moore[34] (Table 13.5) who treated 118 patients with various types of tumors by subcutaneous implantation of a 1- to 2-cc piece of tumor from one patient to another and *vice versa*. In addition, 15 days following implantation of tumor, white blood cell exchanges between partners were conducted for 3 weeks. Although 23 of the patients had an objective response to this form of therapy, neither of the two patients with kidney tumors responded. Complications observed with this therapy included erythema, occasional regional lymph node hyperplasia and local infection at the implantation site.

Immunotherapy

NONSPECIFIC ACTIVE IMMUNOTHERAPY

A number of trials of nonspecific active immunotherapy for renal adenocarcinoma have been reported. In most of these trials, BCG was the agent used.

Lange[35] administered Tice strain BCG (number of organisms not specified) by the tine technique at weekly intervals to patients with stage D renal carcinoma. Immunotherapy patients were described as having metastatic lesions which were amenable to marked reduction of total excision by surgery or radiation therapy and who were immunocompetent by skin testing to recall and primary antigens. Patients were evaluated by responses in a lymphocyte-mediated microcytotoxicity assay against several human tumor cell lines. Ten patients were followed for a minimum of 15 months. Of the three patients who had a rise in cytotoxicity concurrent with BCG therapy, one patient had complete regression of disease, one had no recurrence of tumor, and the third patient showed no evidence of tumor progression. Conversely, those patients who did not have a rise in cytotoxic response concurrent with BCG therapy had continued progression of disease.

A phase I trial of BCG immunotherapy for patients with histologically proved adenocarcinoma of the kidney was initiated by Eidinger and Morales.[36] BCG (Institute Armand-Frappier, Montreal) was given in a single intradermal inoculation of 40 mg initially, and thereafter weekly

Table 13.5
Immunotherapy of renal adenocarcinoma, human studies

Authors	Agent	Route	No. of Patients	Stage(s)	No. of Controls	Results
Nadler and Moore[34]	Tumor homograft	s.c.[a]				
	Leukocyte exchange	i.v.	2	D	0	No effect
Lange[35]	BCG (Tice)	i.d.	10	C, D	0	1 CR
Eidinger and Morales[36]	BCG (Armand-Frappier)	i.d.	19	11 A, B, C, 8 D	0	3 PR, 1 CR
Morales et al.[37]	BCG (Armand-Frappier)	i.d.	20	A	16	4 PR
Laucius et al.[38]	BCG (Galaxo)	i.d.	16	D	0	1 PR
Tykka et al.[39]	Polymerized autologus and allogeneic tumor	i.d.	31	C, D	23	Prolonged survival
Bracken et al.[40]	Angioinfarction, plus Provera	i.m.	24	C, D	0	2 CR
Mohr and Whitesel[41]	Angioinfarction		1	D	0	CR
Horn and Horn[42]	Immune plasma	i.v.	1	D	0	CR
Skinner et al.[43]	Immune RNA	i.d.	12	2 C, 10 D	0	1 PR
Ramming and de Kernion[44]	Immune RNA	i.d.	29	9 C, 20 D	86 retrospective	7 PR
Richie et al.[45]	Immune RNA	In vitro incubation then i.v.	6	D	0	1 CR 2 PR
Montie et al.[46]	Transfer factor	Not specified	10	2 C, 8 D	0	NR

[a] The abbreviations used are: s.c., subcutaneous; i.v., intravenous; i.d., intradermal; i.m., intramuscular; BCG, bacillus Calmette-Guérin; PR, partial response; CR, complete response; NR, no response.

for 4 weeks, then twice monthly for 2 months followed by monthly immunizations which were administered by a multiple-puncture apparatus. Nineteen patients were included in this study, eight of whom had metastatic disease involving the lungs, and the remaining patients exhibited surgically resectable localized disease (adjunctive immunotherapy). BCG was administered to all 8 patients with metastatic disease and 5 of 11 patients with localized disease. The investigators reported no evidence of tumor recurrence in the 11 patients with localized disease at 14 months for the BCG-treated group and at 22 months for the untreated patients. These patients were not further considered in this study. Five of the eight patients with metastatic disease died with a mean survival of 8.6 months, while two patients were deteriorating at 17 and 27 months after their initial presentation with metastases. One patient was reportedly doing well 15 months following the initiation of BCG immunotherapy. The authors stated that five of the eight patients with metastases demonstrated objective evidence of improvement. This improvement was denoted by a reduction in size of pulmonary metastases in three patients, a complete disappearance of nodal metastases in one patient, and stabilization of lung metastases in one patient. Four of these favorable responses were described as transient. Side effects of the BCG immunotherapy were minor, local indolent ulceration and erythema at the injection sites, low grade fever, night sweats, and chills for 2 to 3 days.

In a subsequent phase II trial of BCG immunotherapy as an adjuvant to cytoreductive surgery in patients with stage IV renal cancer, Morales and associates[37] administered (10^7 organisms/ml) BCG administered with a multiple puncture apparatus intradermally. Immunizations were given at weekly intervals for 6 weeks, then given biweekly twice, and thereafter given monthly for an indefinite period of time. Medroxyprogesterone acetate also was given to therapy patients who showed evidence of disease progression, and radiotherapy was utilized in those patients with associated pain amenable to control by radiation. Twenty patients were included in the BCG therapy group. All had undergone nephrectomy before initiation of BCG immunotherapy. Metastatic sites were identified as soft tissue only in 14 (70%) patients, bony metastases in 3 (15%) patients, and mixed, soft and bone, metastases in 3 (15%) patients. Ages in this group ranged from 18 to 71 years with a mean of 52.6 years. Concurrent controls for this study were 16 patients with metastatic disease who received hormonal therapy (medroxyprogesterone acetate), several forms of systemic chemotherapy, and palliative radiotherapy for pain. Eleven (69%) of these patients underwent nephrectomy. Metastatic sites for the controls were found as soft tissue only 7 (44%) patients, bony metastases only in 3 (19%) and mixed in 6 (37%). The concurrent control patients ranged in age from 42 to 78 years of age with a mean of 64.8 years. Twenty historical control patients were included in this study. As with the concurrent controls, these patients had received various regimens of hormonal therapy, chemotherapy, and radiotherapy and 14 (70%) of these patients had undergone nephrectomy. Thirteen (65%) of these patients had soft tissue metastases only, four (20%) had bony metastases and three (15%) had mixed soft tissue and bony metastases. Their ages ranged from 35 to 73 years with a mean of 56.6 years. In terms of survival, the authors report a ratio of observed, to expected, deaths in the BCG immunotherapy groups of 0.60 as compared to 1.6 in the historical controls ($p < 0.01$); however, survival of the immunotherapy group was not significantly different from the concurrent controls. Median survival was 8.3 months for historical controls, 9 months for concurrent controls, and 15 months for the BCG-therapy group. Objective evidence for tumor regression was observed in six of the immunotherapy patients. The response in four of these patients was partial and temporary. The other two patients show no evidence of disease progression 3 and 5 years after histological documentation of metastases. Interestingly, one patient in each of the control groups showed objective evidence of tumor regression. The authors describe that the BCG immunizations were well tolerated with adverse side effects being only erythema at the injection site, low grade fever, malaise, and occasional nausea.

Tumor regression also had been reported by Krutchick et al.[47] and associates in the case of a 56-year-old man with advanced sarcomatoid renal adenocarcinoma following treatment with BCG and a sarcoma viral oncolysate in conjunction with several chemotherapeutic agents. Two months following nephrectomy for removal of the primary tumor the patient developed an abdominal mass considered surgically unresectable. The patient was treated by the following regimen: 1.5 mg/m^2 cyclophosphamide and 50 mg/m^2 Adriamycin intravenously on day 2; 250 mg/m^2 dacarbazine (DTIC) intravenously on days 1 through 5; Chicago BCG (6 × 10^8 organisms) administered by scarification on days 17 and 24; and a sarcoma viral oncolysate (prepared from virus-infected human sarcoma tumor cell membranes) given intradermally on days 17 and 24. This protocol was repeated every 28 days. The patient showed a reduction in the size of the tumor mass following chemoimmunotherapy. Residual tumor was resected 1 year following initiation of therapy and the patient remained in complete remission 2 years following diagnosis. No toxicity was described utilizing this form of therapy.

Laucius and associates[38] reported subjective improvement and objective tumor regression of pulmonary metastases in a 61-year-old woman with renal (clear cell) adenocarcinoma who was receiving megestrol acetate (20 mg twice daily) and 10 immunizations (4 to 9 × 10^6 organisms) of Galaxo BCG administered intradermally at monthly intervals. This patient died 10 months following the initiation of BCG therapy. In a follow-up study using BCG immunotherapy in 15 patients with surgically incurable renal adenocarcinoma, Laucius observed no objective tumor regression. Mean survival time was 10.6 months. Patients received 40 mg of megestrol acetate four times daily for 56 days. Galaxo BCG (2 to 4.5 × 10^6 organisms) was administered intradermally on days 1, 14, 28, 42, and 56. Six of the patients in this study had prior radiation, hormonal, and/or chemotherapeutic treatments. Nine patients had no prior treatment other than surgery. All patients developed injection-site abscesses and those undergoing extended therapy experienced significant flulike symptoms.

SPECIFIC ACTIVE IMMUNOTHERAPY

Tykka et al.[39] examined the effects of vaccination with polymerized autologous primary and metastatic tumor vaccine on patients with advanced renal cell carcinoma. Patients underwent nephrectomy and were randomly assigned postoperatively to immunotherapy (31 patients) or as control groups (23 patients). The mean age for the immunotherapy group of patients was 57.7 years (S.D. = 10.3); 4 of these patients had stage 3 disease, 27 patients had stage 4 disease; 6 patients had preoperative radiation, 4 underwent postoperative radiation and 5 had hormonal therapy (progesterone or testosterone). In the control group, the mean age was 55.7 years (S.D. = 11); 2 patients had stage 3 disease, 21 patients had stage 4 disease, 5 patients had preoperative radiation, 11 patients had postoperative radiation, and 17 patients had hormonal therapy. Excised autologous primary and metastatic tumor was polymerized with ethylchlorformide and was injected intradermally admixed with an individually tested adjuvant to which the patient exhibited delayed hypersensitivity (tuberculin-PPD or *Candida albicans* antigen). The first immunization was given 1 week following nephrectomy and once a month thereafter until all the immunization material was used or the patient succumbed. All patients in the treatment group received a supplement of vitamins, amino acids, and certain trace elements. The 5-year survival rate was reported as 23.6% (S.E. = 7.8) in the immunotherapy group as compared to 4.3% (S.E. = 4.3) in the controls. Life expectancy was also calculated which they reported as 31.1 months (S.E. = 2.5) for the treated patients and 15.8 months (S.E. = 1.3) for the controls. In the follow-up of at least 4 years following initiation of treatment, none of the controls were still alive; however, 7/31 (22%) of the immunotherapy patients were still alive. Two patients were free of symptoms, but had lung metastases and 5 were symptom free with no sign of carcinoma. The investigators reported no adverse side effects with their immunotherapy protocol.

Bracken and associates[40] performed percutaneous transfemoral renal artery angioinfarction on 24 patients for management of renal cell carcinoma. Gelfoam was utilized as the embolic material. In seven patients, preoperative infarction was performed and the authors described this procedure as facilitating surgery by eliminating the major blood supply to the tumor and inducing edema, which tended to make tissue planes more distinct, thereby making dissection of the tumor containing kidney easier. Of these patients, four had no evidence of metastatic disease and are disease free 5 to 12 months postinfarction. Two of the three patients with metastatic disease who were placed on medroxyprogesterone therapy following nephrectomy showed complete regression of their pulmonary metastases and are alive at 11 and 17 months. Seventeen patients with metastatic disease were treated with renal angioinfarction without nephrectomy. In this group of patients, five died within 7 months, three had progressive metastatic disease, six had not been followed sufficiently long enough for evaluation, and three have shown stabilization of their metastases 5, 8, and 10 months postinfarction. Side effects noted were pain, increased diastolic blood pressure, pyrexia, dehydration, and moderate gastrointestinal symptoms such as nausea, vomiting, and paralytic ileus. Renal failure from contrast material occurred in two patients.

Mohr and Whitesel[41] also reported regression of pulmonary metastases in one patient following preoperative angioinfarction of the primary renal cell carcinoma with subsequent nephrectomy. Embolization of the renal artery was performed using Gelfoam. The patient experienced fever, nausea, and severe flank pain following the embolization. Five days later the embolization was repeated and nephrectomy was performed on the next day. Steady regression of pulmonary metastases was reported, and the patient remained asymptomatic for 14 months until he developed a cerebral metastasis. This was subsequently removed and the patient reportedly was asymptomatic 22 months after initial therapy with the pulmonary metastases regressing to the point that no definitive disease was identifiable.

PASSIVE IMMUNOTHERAPY

Horn and Horn[42] reported on the use of plasma transfusions in the treatment of one patient with metastatic renal clear-cell carcinoma. Donor plasma was obtained from the uncle of the recipient patient who had a history of adenocarcinoma of the colon, renal clear-cell carcinoma, and transitional cell carcinoma of the bladder treated, respectively, by resection of the colon, nephrectomy, and fulguration of the bladder lesion. The plasma donor patient had shown no evidence of tumor recurrence. Plasma from two units of blood was given weekly for 3 months and thereafter every 2 weeks. Before the transfusions were begun, the patient had been treated for renal clear-cell carcinoma by nephrectomy and then developed lung metastases to the left upper lobe with regional lymph node involvement 1 year later. Lobectomy was performed with removal of some of the regional lymph nodes. The prognosis of this patient was considered poor; therefore, the plasma transfusions were initiated. Fifteen months following the induction of plasma-transfusion therapy no evidence of tumor recurrence in either the donor or recipient patient has been observed.

A phase I immunotherapy trial using xenogenic immune RNA was conducted by Skinner and associates.[43] Of the 12 patients entered into this study, 10 had advanced local or metastatic disease and 2 were described as having minimal residual disease (defined by the authors as having no detectable tumor postoperatively but having a greater than 50% probability of developing tumor recurrence within 24 months). All patients had histologically proven renal cell carcinoma and showed skin test reactivity to DNCB. Immune RNA was prepared by immunizing adult rams with 4 weekly intradermal injections of human renal cell carcinoma admixed with complete Freund's adjuvant. Six weeks following the initial immunization, spleen and mesenteric lymph nodes were excised and RNA was extracted from this lymphoid tissue. Patients received 1 to 12 mg/week of immune RNA injected intradermally in multiple sites in the axilla or groin. When possible, patients received RNA from rams which had been immunized with their own tumor, otherwise, RNA prepared from allogeneic tumor of the same histologic type was used. In this phase I trial, it was shown that patients treated up to 16 months with xenogeneic immune RNA showed no evidence of local or systemic toxicity. One patient on immune RNA immunotherapy was described as showing regression of a mediastinal mass from 8.6 to 7.4 cm 18 months following the diagnosis of metastatic disease. Three patients demonstrated stability of their metastatic disease and remain asymptomatic for up to 16 months. Three patients revealed no evidence of tumor recurrence following nephrectomy and two patients revealed no evidence of tumor recurrence following removal of a metastatic lesion. Three patients had been treated for less than 2 months and their response was indeterminate.

Ramming and de Kernion[44] also investigated the effects of xenogeneic immune RNA in the treatment of advanced renal cell carcinoma. Some of these may have been previously reported by Skinner. Immune RNA was prepared by injecting a sheep intradermally with human renal cell carcinoma admixed with Freund's complete adjuvant weekly for 4 weeks, removing the spleen and lymph nodes from the sheep 10 days following the last injection, and extracting the RNA by the hot phenol technique.

Patients received RNA in doses ranging from 2 to 40 mg/week injected in multiple wheels of 0.1 ml about the lymph node bearing regions of the groin or axilla. Twenty patients with advanced renal cell carcinoma and nine patients who were surgically free of gross disease received immune RNA therapy. Eighty-six retrospective patients with metastatic renal cell carcinoma were used as controls. None of the 9 patients surgically free of gross disease developed recurrence 10 to 34 months following initiation of therapy. Although none of the 20 patients with advanced disease showed objective responses, as measured by a 50% reduction in tumor volume, 7 patients showed a partial response with measurable regressions of less than 50% volume. Significantly prolonged survival time in immunotherapy patients with metastatic disease compared with historical controls was seen only in patients with metastases confined to the lungs. No significant prolongation of survival time was apparent in immunotherapy patients with metastases to organ sites outside the lungs. Mild adverse side effects reported with the therapy were transient malaise and anorexia, low-grade fever, and erythema at the injection sites. No allergic or anaphylactic reactions were observed.

A phase I study on the effects of xenogeneic immune RNA in patients with stage IV renal cell carcinoma also was conducted by Richie and associates.[45] Immune RNA was prepared by immunizing Hartley guinea pigs in the footpads with fresh tumor cells admixed with complete Freund's adjuvant. Two weeks following immunization, spleen and lymph nodes were removed and the RNA was extracted from the pooled lymphoid tissues by the hot phenol technique. Two to three weeks following nephrectomy, patients underwent leukopheresis in which approximately 10^{10} mononuclear cells were obtained. These mononuclear cells were incubated 1 hour with immune RNA (prepared from the patient's own tumor) at a concentration of 750 to 1000 mg/5 $\times$ 10^7 cells. The mononuclear cells were collected and reinfused on the same day. There were 5 treatments administered every other day. Of the six patients who received immune RNA therapy, one showed complete remission of pulmonary metastases following therapy, and two patients had a partial response to the therapy by showing a greater that 50% decrease in tumor metastases for 8 to 10 months. Two patients were described as having transient stabilization in the growth of their pulmonary metastases following therapy. Five of the six were dead from cancer within 18 months. No toxicity with immune RNA therapy was reported.

The use of transfer factor in patients with disseminated renal cell carcinoma was examined by Montie and associates.[46] Transfer factor was obtained from donors who, on the basis of microcytotoxicity assays, showed greater than 50% cell inhibition of renal cell carcinoma lines. Transfer factor was prepared by the method of Lawrence.[48] Each dose of transfer factor (equivalent to the amount obtained from 10^9 leukocytes) was administered weekly for 12 weeks and biweekly thereafter until progressive disease was documented. Ten patients were treated with transfer factor—eight patients with metastatic disease previously treated by nephrectomy, and two patients described as without clinically evident metastases but at a high risk for recurrent disease. None of the eight patients with metastatic disease showed objective evidence of tumor remissions. The authors reported stabilization of metastases at 1, 3, and 6 months in three patients and stable metastases for 4 and 5 months in two patients before rapid progression of the disease. The two patients free of metastases remained free of disease for 4 and 5 months. Problems with the use of transfer factor include donor selection and dosage. No adverse local or systemic side effects were noted except for a strong inflammatory reaction in sites of a large amount of tumor.

Summary of Immunotherapy for Renal Adenocarcinoma

We are aware of no reported animal studies on the immunotherapy of renal adenocarcinoma. The early human studies[34] using sensitization with tumor allografts and leukocyte exchange transfusions are too limited to permit any definite conclusions to be drawn, although the results in other tumors have been disappointing. Nonspecific active immunotherapy with BCG also has not produced dramatic results. Objective evidence of tumor regression has been documented in less than 20% of patients treated and complete remissions have been rare.[35–37, 47] Active specific immunotherapy with polymerized autologous and allogeneic tumor cells as reported by Tykka and associates[39] may have prolonged the survival of the treated patients, but these results need to be confirmed by other investigators. Active specific immunotherapy using angioinfarction[41] with or without Provera recently has received considerable clinical attention, but the available studies are not controlled and final evaluation of this form of treatment must await further experience. Plasma transfusion therapy[42] has not been extensively evaluated in patients with renal cell carcinoma; however, this form of therapy has been evaluated in other tumors and has yielded disappointing results. Passive specific immunotherapy using immune RNA either injected directly as described by Skinner and co-workers[43] and by Ramming and de Kernion[44] had yielded some reported responses; however, animal studies have suggested that immune RNA injected without ribonuclease inhibitors would be rapidly degraded by endogenous ribonucleases, and it is difficult to imagine how a therapeutic benefit could result in the clinical setting. Immune RNA therapy in which lymphocytes are incubated in immune RNA and then reinfused into the patient as described by Richie et al.[45] warrants further consideration; however, it is important to note that five of six of Richie's patients were dead within 18 months.

Passive specific immunotherapy with transfer factor as described by Montie and co-workers[46] has yielded disappointing results.

CONCLUSION

Immunotherapy for genitourinary malignancies has not been adequately evaluated in terms of well conceived, well executed phase I, II, and III trials. Except for active nonspecific immunotherapy with intra-dermal and intravesical BCG for superficial bladder cancer, immuno-therapy for genitourinary malignancies, like immunotherapy for most other tumors, has not provided encouraging results. Further work on the development and regulation of the underlying immune responses will need to be done before significant advances in immunotherapy can be anticipated.

There is a need for properly controlled clinical trials of immunotherapy for patients with genitourinary cancer, if for no other reason than to identify those treatments that are ineffective so that their use can be discontinued and resources diverted to other therapeutic avenues that ultimately may prove successful.

REFERENCES

1. Pollard, M., Chang, C. F., and Burleson, G. R. Investigations on prostate adenocarci-nomas in rats. *Cancer Treat. Rept. 61:*153, 1977.
2. Weissman, R. M., Coffey, D. S., and Scott, W. W. Cell kinetic studies of prostatic cancer: adjuvant therapy in animal models. *Oncology 34:*133, 1977.
3. Soanes, W. A., Ablin, R. J., and Gonder, M. J. Remission of metastatic lesions following cryosurgery in prostate cancer. *J. Urol. 104:*154, 1970.
4. Gursel, E. O., Roberts, M., and Veenema, R. J. Regression of prostatic cancer following sequential cryotherapy in the prostate. *J. Urol. 108:*928, 1972.
5. Merrin, C., Han, T., Klein, E., Wajsman, Z., Murphy, G. P. Immunotherapy of prostatic carcinoma with bacillus Calmette-Guérin. *Cancer Treat. Rep. 59:*157, 1975.
6. Robinson, M. R. G., Rigby, C. C., Pugh, R. C. B., Dumonde, D. C. Prostate carcinoma: intratumor BCG immunotherapy. *Natl. Cancer Inst. Monogr. 49:*35, 1976.
7. Robinson, M. R. G., Rigby, C. C., Pugh, R. C. B., and Dumonde, D. C. Adjuvant immunotherapy with BCG in carcinoma of the prostate. *Br. J. Urol. 49:*221, 1977.
8. Guinan, P. D., John, T., Sahadevan, V., Crispen, R., Nagale, V., McKiel, C., and Ablin, R. J. Prostate carcinoma: immunostaging and adjuvant immunotherapy with BCG. *Natl. Cancer Inst. Monogr. 49:*355, 1978.
9. Yantorno, C., Soanes, W. A., Gonder, M. J., and Shulman, S. Studies in cryo-immu-nology. I. The production of antibodies to urogenital tissue in consequence of freezing treatment *Immunology 12:*395, 1967.
10. Flocks, R. H., Nelson, C. M. K., and Boatman, D. L. Perineal cryosurgery for prostate carcinoma. *J. Urol. 108:*933, 1972.
11. Schmidt, J. D. Cryosurgical prostatectomy. *Cancer 32:*1141, 1973.
12. Villasor, R. P. The clinical use of BCG vaccine in stimulating host resistance to cancer. *J. Philippine Med. Assoc. 41:*619, 1965.
13. Johnstone, B. J. Clinical effects of Coley's toxin: a controlled study. *Cancer Treat. Rep. 21:*19, 1962.
14. de Kernion, J. B., Ramming, K. P., and Fraser, K. A bladder tumor model response to immunotherapy. *Natl. Cancer Inst. Monog. 49:*333, 1978.
15. Lamm, D. L., Yee, G. N., Reichert, D. F., and Radwin, H. M. Levamisole immuno-therapy of experimental transitional cell carcinoma. *Invest. Urol. 16:*286, 1979.
16. Adolphs, H. D., Thiele, J., and Kiel, H. Effect of intralesional and systemic BCG-application or a combined cyclophosphamide/BCG treatment on experimental bladder cancer. *Urol. Res. 7:*71, 1979.
17. Soloway, M. S. Effectiveness of long-term chemotherapy and/or BCG on murine bladder cancer. *Natl. Cancer Inst. Monogr. 49:*327, 1978.
18. Morales, A., Eidinger, D., and Bruce, A. W. Intracavitary Bacillus Calmette-Guerin in the treatment of superficial bladder tumors. *J. Urol. 116:*180, 1976.
19. Lamm, D. L., Harris, S. C., Gittes, R. F. Bacillus Calmette-Guerin and dinitrochloro-benzene immunotherapy of chemically induced bladder tumors. *Invest. Urol. 14:*369, 1977.

20. Pimm, M. V., and Baldwin, R. W. BCG treatment of human tumor xenografts in athymic nude mice. *Br. J. Cancer. 38:*699, 1978.
21. Collste, L. G., Kostyrka-Claps, M. L., Darzynkiewicz, Z., Devonec, M., Traganos, F., Whitmore, W. F., and Melamed, M. R. Lymph node reactivity to experimental bladder tumor in preimmunized animals as measured by two-parameter flow cytometry. *Invest. Urol. 17:*191, 1979.
22. Morales, A., Djeu, J., and Herberman, R. B. Immunization by irradiated whole cells or cell extracts against an experimental bladder tumor. *Invest. Urol. 17:*310, 1980.
23. Morales, A. Adjuvant immunotherapy in superficial bladder cancer. *Natl. Cancer. Inst. Monogr. 49:*315, 1978.
24. Douville, Y., Pelouze, G., Roy, R., Charrois, R., Kibrite, A., Martin M., Dionne, L., Coulonval, L., and Robinson, J. Recurrent bladder papillomata treated with Bacillus Calmette-Guerin: a preliminary report (phase I trial). *Cancer Treat. Rept. 62:*551, 1978.
25. Lamm, D. L., Thor, D. E., Harris, S. C., Stogdill, V. D., and Radwin, H. W. Intravesical and percutaneous BCG immunotherapy of recurrent superficial bladder cancer. In *Immunotherapy of Cancer: Present Status of Trials in Man* (Abstract) National Cancer Institute. Bethesda, Md. April 28–30, 1980.
26. Camacho, F., Pinsky, C., Kerr, D., Whitmore, W., and Oettgen, H. Treatment of superficial bladder cancer with intravesical BCG. In *Immunotherapy of Cancer: Present Status of Trials in Man.* (Abstract) National Cancer Institute. Bethesda, Md. April 28–30, 1980.
27. Kagawa, S., Ogura, K., Kurokawa, K., and Uyama, K. Immunological evaluation of a streptococcal preparation (OK-432) in treatment of bladder carcinoma. *J. Urol. 122:*467, 1979.
28. Purves, E. C., Snell, M., Cope, W. A., Addison, J. E., Copland, R. F. P., and Berenbaum, M. C. Subcutaneous *Corynebacterium parvum* in bladder cancer. *Br. J. Urol. 51:*278, 1979.
29. Herr, H. W., Kemery, N., Yagoda, A., and Whitmore, W. F. Poly(I:C) immunotherapy in patients with papillomas or superficial carcinomas of the bladder. *Natl. Cancer Inst. Monogr. 49:*325, 1978.
30. Symes, M. O., and Riddell, A. G. The use of immunized pig lymph node cells in the treatment of patients with advanced malignant disease. *Br. J. Surg. 60:*176, 1973.
31. Symes, M. O., Eckert, H., Feneley, R. C. L., Lai, T., Mitchell, J. P., Roberts, J. B. M., and Tribe, C. R. Adoptive immunotherapy and radiotherapy in the treatment of urinary bladder cancer. *Br. J. Urol. 50:*328, 1978.
32. Feneley, R. C. L., Eckert, H., Riddell, A. G., Symes, M. O., and Tribe, C. R. The treatment of advanced bladder cancer with sensitized pig lymphocytes. *Br. J. Surg. 61:*825, 1974.
33. Symes, M. O., Riddell, A. G., Feneley, R. C. L., and Tribe, C. R. The treatment of advanced bladder cancer with sensitized pig lymphocytes. *Br. J. Cancer 28*, (Suppl. I):276, 1973.
34. Nadler, S. H., and Moore, G. E. Immunotherapy of malignant disease. *Arch. Surg. 99:*376, 1969.
35. Lange, P. H. Lymphocyte-mediated cytotoxicity in patients with renal and transitional cell carcinoma receiving BCG. *Natl. Cancer. Inst. Monogr. 49:*343, 1978.
36. Eidinger, D., and Morales, A. BCG immunotherapy of metastatic adenocarcinoma of the kidney. *Natl. Cancer. Inst. Monogr. 49:*339, 1978.
37. Morales, A., Wilson, J. L., Pater, J. L., and Loeb, M. Cytoreductive surgery and systemic BCG therapy in metastatic renal cancer. *J. Urol.* (Submitted for publication).
38. Laucius, J. F., Patel, Y. A., Lusch, C. J., Koons, L. S., Bellet, R. E., and Mastrangelo, M. J. A phase II evaluation of Bacillus Calmette-Guerin plus Megestrol Acetate in patients with metastatic renal adenocarcinoma. *Med. Pediatr. Oncol. 3:*237, 1977.
39. Tykka, H., Oravisto, K. J., Lehtonen, T., Sarna, S., and Tallberg, T. Active specific immunotherapy of advanced renal cell carcinoma. *Eur. Urol. 4:*250, 1978.
40. Bracken, R. B., Johnson, D. E., Goldstein, H. M., Wallace, S., and Ayala, A. G. Percutaneous transfemoral renal artery occlusion in patients with renal carcinoma. *Urology 6:*6, 1975.
41. Mohr, S. J., and Whitesel, J. A. Spontaneous regression of renal cell carcinoma

metastases after preoperative embolization of primary tumor and subsequent nephrectomy. *Urology 14:*5, 1979.

42. Horn, L., and Horn, H. L. An immunological approach to the therapy of cancer? *Lancet 2:*466, 1971.
43. Skinner, D. G., de Kernion, J. B., Brower, P. A., Ramming, K. P., and Pilch, Y. H. Advanced renal cell carcinoma: treatment with xenogeneic immune ribonucleic acid and appropriate surgical resection. *J. Urol. 115:*246, 1976.
44. Ramming, K. P., and de Kernion, J. B. Immune RNA therapy for renal cell carcinoma: survival and immunologic monitoring. *Ann. Surg. 186:*459, 1977.
45. Richie, J. P., Wang, B. S., Steele, G. D., Wilson, R. E., Mannick, J. A. *In vivo* and *in vitro* effects of xenogeneic immune RNA in patients with advanced renal cell carcinoma: a phase I study. *J. Urol.* (Submitted for publication)
46. Montie, J. E., Bukowski, R. M., Doedhar, S. D., Hewlett, J. S., Stewart, B. H., and Straffon, R. A. Immunotherapy of disseminated renal cell carcinoma with transfer factor. *J. Urol. 117:*553, 1977.
47. Krutchik, A. N., Sullivan, C., Sinkovics, J. G., and Ayala, A. Chemoimmunotherapy of sarcomatoid renal cell carcinoma. *Med. Pediatr. Oncol. 5:*9, 1978.
48. Lawrence, H. S. Transfer factor. *Adv. Immunol. 11:*195, 1969.

14

Parenteral Nutrition in Cancer Patients

Nutritional support of the cancer patient has been proven to be a safe and efficacious treatment modality in rehabilitating the malnourished cancer patient and reducing the complications of oncologic therapy. The importance of adequate nutrition was demonstrated by Warren[1] in 1932 in an autopsy series of 500 cancer patients. Among the causes of death, cachexia was found to be the most frequent contributing factor in the patient's demise.

Although nutritional deficiencies in cancer patients had been recognized, their nutritional requirements had been neglected until the recent advances in parenteral and enteral nutrition. An awareness of catheter infections and the complications of glucose, amino acid, lipid, and mineral metabolism is imperative for the proper implementation of nutritional therapy. In addition to this, nutrition in malignant disease is more than the use of tubes, ostomies, and nutritional solutions. Clinical nutrition must bring the advances in immunology and biochemistry to the bedside management of the cancer patient. An understanding of the implications of nutritional alterations on host metabolism and immunocompetence is essential for improving patient care and for potentiating tumor response to the therapeutic regimen.

GLUCOSE DEPRIVATION

Starvation in man initiates a number of physiological mechanisms by which energy stores are mobilized to satisfy caloric demands.[2] In a normal 70-kg man, the potential reserves consists of hepatic and muscle glycogen (900 calories), total body protein (24,000 calories), and total body fat (141,000 calories). Because a fasting individual consumes approximately 1500 to 1800 calories under basal conditions, glycogen stores are insignificant in satisfying caloric requirements. Triglycerides and protein, therefore, become the principal potential energy sources. The primary function of fat is to serve as an energy reserve; on the other hand, there are no protein reserves as such, for all body protein exists for a functional or structural purpose.

Starvation results in the conversion of certain amino acids to glucose by the liver *via* its gluconeogenic pathways. This endogenously synthesized glucose is utilized primarily by the central nervous system. Leukocytes, erythrocytes, bone marrow, peripheral nerve, and possibly skeletal muscle also metabolize glucose but do so *via* the anaerobic glycolytic pathway producing pyruvate and lactate as end products. These products of anaerobic glycolysis can be converted back to glucose *via* the Cori cycle in the liver. Man depends upon lipid as the primary fuel with only 13% of the caloric requirements being met by the metabolism of tissue protein for gluconeogenesis.

The cancer patient receiving oncologic therapy deviates somewhat from the protein-sparing pattern described above. Operative procedures, septic episodes secondary to chemotherapeutic myelosuppression, enteritis secondary to radiation therapy, or chemotherapy may result in excessive protein losses sequestered in the abdomen, or from their gastrointestinal tract, and in accelerated protein catabolism. The caloric expenditure of patients following an operative procedure or sepsis may be as high as 3000 to 5000/day. Infusion of 2 to 3 l of 5% dextrose/day provides 400 to 600 calories, an amount which is inadequate to meet the caloric needs of these patients. However, through the use of intravenous hyperalimentation (IVH) with 20 to 25% dextrose/l (800 to 1000 calories) sufficient glucose can be supplied with the administration of 3 l/day.

GLUCOSE METABOLISM

With large amounts of hypertonic glucose being infused to fulfill the caloric needs of an individual, the rate of infusion must be regulated carefully. Infusion rates of 20% dextrose at 200 ml/hour in normal adults are usually well tolerated without significant urinary losses.[3] The average 70-kg adult can utilize glucose at an infusion rate of 0.5 gm/kg/hour with a corresponding blood sugar of about 120 mg/ml, which is far below the usual renal glucose threshold of 160 to 180 mg/ml. However, in any given patient, glucose tolerance is somewhat unpredictable with the initiation of hypertonic glucose infusions or with increases in the infusion rate. Careful and compulsive monitoring of blood glucose levels and urine sugar is essential.

The insulin response to prolonged hyperalimentation should be understood in order to avoid complications. Sanderson and Deitel[4] demonstrated that with a constant glucose infusion rate of 500 mg/minute in normal subjects, there was an immediate rise in blood glucose levels with a concomitant increase in serum insulin levels. When glucose was administered over a week at a steady rate of 500 mg/minute and then was suddenly stopped, there was an immediate fall in blood sugar from 100 to 60 mg/ml, with a subsequent rise to a steady state level of 80 mg/ml.

Sudden cessation of glucose infusion, though not recommended, did not produce symptomatic hypoglycemia. A 5% glucose infusion for a few hours after cessation of hyperalimentation should protect against rebound hyperglycemia.

It should be emphasized that the above study was done in normal subjects under rigidly controlled conditions. Sudden cessation of hyper-alimentation can result in rebound hypoglycemia secondary to high en-dogenous insulin levels. This is apt to occur particularly in infants or in malnourished patients, as both of these groups characteristically have decreased glycogen stores. Rebound hypoglycemia can result in convul-sions, coma, and permanent neurological sequelae. Hypertonic glucose infusion should not be interrupted completely for infusions of other fluids or replaced by a nonglucose containing fluid during an operation. Com-plications of hypoglycemia can be avoided by decreasing the infusion rate over a 24-hour period and infusing isotonic glucose for several hours following cessation of the hyperalimentation solution.

A serious complication of hypertonic glucose infusion is hyperosmolar, nonketotic hyperglycemic coma. The basic pathophysiology is hyperos-molarity secondary to hyperglycemia with a resultant osmotic diuresis, dehydration, and subsequent coma. This complication may arise from an excessive rate of glucose infusion, glucose intolerance secondary to sepsis, and latent or frank diabetes mellitus. In order to minimize the risk of developing the hyperosmolar state, the initial administration of hyperali-mentation solution must proceed at a slow constant rate not exceeding 1000 ml/day. If this proceeds satisfactorily without the appearance of sugar in the urine, the infusion rate can be increased gradually. Wide fluctuations in glucose infusion rates can best be prevented by the use of a mechanical infusion pump. Septic patients should always be carefully monitored with daily blood sugar levels in order to document and treat, at an early stage, the hyperglycemic syndrome.

AMINO ACID METABOLISM

Although hypertonic glucose can be administered to provide calories, positive nitrogen balance cannot be achieved unless a minimum daily requirement of the essential amino acids is given along with a calorie source. In the past, 5% protein hydrolysates of either fibrin or casein were commonly used for hyperalimentation regimens. These preparations con-tained significant quantities of free ammonia, titratable acid up to 30 mEq/l to restore the solutions to neutral pH and large quantities of oligopeptides which were poorly utilized and excreted in the urine.[5] Because of these disadvantages, hydrolysate solutions are infrequently used today.

Crystalline amino acid solutions are currently the most commonly used nitrogen source in parenteral fluids. These solutions are biologically more efficient because all of the nitrogen is in the form of amino acids. The ammonia levels are much lower at 55 to 65 mg/ml and have a titratable acidity which is considerably less than that of the protein hydrolysate solutions. The complications of amino acid infusion can include metabolic acidosis and hyperammonemia particularly in neonates and in patients with hepatic disorders.

The branch chain amino acids, leucine, isoleucine and valine, may play an important role in the future development of improved amino acid solutions. These particular amino acids can inhibit protein catabolism in muscle tissue and thereby reduce urinary nitrogen losses. This would be important in the malnourished patient with compromised liver function. Freund, et al.[6, 7] have shown that the infusion of branch chain amino acids has a major role in improving nitrogen balance.

LIPID METABOLISM

The metabolism of fat furnishes nine calories/g and meets 20 to 50% of the daily caloric requirement in normal adults. This nutrient is potentially of great importance in satisfying the nutritional requirements of malnourished patients. Fat must be in the form of an emulsion when administered intravenously. Intra-Lipid-Vitrum (Paines and Byrne) and Liposyne (Abbott) are two fat preparations that are currently available.

Many reports have shown that fat emulsions infused intravenously are metabolized and utilized biologically. Coran[8] has popularized the combined infusion of a fat emulsion with 5% amino acid-10% glucose solution through peripheral venous cannula. The peripheral catheter site is maintained with an aseptic technique to reduce the incidence of thrombophlebitis. Adequate nutritional support can be achieved with the combined use of fat emulsion, dextrose, and amino acid combinations. However, many cancer patients who are referred for oncologic therapy are already malnourished because of their disease or previous therapy. Rapid nutritional replenishment is necessary before appropriate chemotherapy, radiotherapy, or operative treatment can be undertaken. Under these circumstances, nutritional repletion is most rapidly achieved when hypertonic glucose-amino acid solutions are infused through a central venous catheter.

Although the use of intravenous fat as a caloric source is expensive, these emulsions provide a source of essential fatty acid (EFA). EFA deficiency can occur during prolonged hyperalimentation with hypertonic glucose and amino acids. Clinical signs and symptoms of EFA deficiency include a dry scaly dermatitis, impaired wound healing, and thrombocytopenia. A soybean or safflower emulsion is high in the essential fatty acid, linoleic acid, and can readily correct these clinical abnormalities. Investigations in adults have shown that the biochemical abnormalities of essential fatty acid deficiencies in patients receiving fat-free parenteral nutrition can be readily reversed with the infusion of a 10% fat emulsion twice a week.[9, 10]

ELECTROLYTE METABOLISM

Potassium, phosphorous, calcium, and magnesium deficits often coexist during periods of extreme metabolism. The reason for this increased need during early anabolism in the cachetic patient is unclear; however, these ions have a much higher concentration within the intracellular compartment than in the extracellular compartment. When infusion of hypertonic glucose and amino acids restores tissue synthesis to normal, these ions play an important role in the expansion of the intracellular compartment.

Severe hypophosphatemia during hyperalimentation can result in neurological dysfunctions. The complications of paraesthesias, weakness, lethargy, dysarthia, seizures, and abnormal respiratory patterns can be averted by the addition of 10 to 15 mEq of phosphate to each liter of hyperalimentation solution. Calcium gluconate (4.5 mEq/l) also should be added along with the phosphate supplementation in order to avoid hypocalcemia.

Hypomagnesemia is seen occasionally in both the chronically malnourished and hyperalimented patients. This deficiency is characterized by neuromuscular irritability, disorientation, tremor, and seizures. This electrolyte deficiency can be avoided by the routine addition of 10 to 20 mEq of magnesium/day to their parenteral solution.

TRACE METALS

Trace metals, such as copper and zinc, are administered as part of the hyperalimentation solution. The significance of trace metal metabolism during total parenteral nutrition has been established in adult and pediatric studies. Over a 6-week period, serum zinc and copper levels were noted to decline below the normal range of these trace-metal concentrations. However, the clinical manifestations of these deficiencies were not apparent. The development of clinical zinc deficiency is probably dependent upon the length of total parenteral nutrition and the amino acid solution used in that regimen. In both adults and infants, there is an entity known as acrodermatitis enteropathic, characterized by intractable diarrhea and by vesicular dermatitis around the mouth, anus, and extremities. These manifestations of zinc deficiency have been correlated with extremely low serum zinc levels and were readily corrected by zinc supplementation.[11] The addition of zinc sulfate 5 mg/day has been found to maintain or correct zinc deficiencies.

Clinical manifestations of copper deficiency include neutropenia and an apparent iron deficiency anemia. The role of copper in the metabolism of iron has been well established in both animals and man. The observation of copper deficiencies have been noted in cases of prolonged total parenteral nutrition (approximately 6 months). Copper deficiencies can be corrected by the addition of 1 mg of cupric sulfate to the daily hyperalimentation regimen.

METHODS OF NUTRITIONAL MANAGEMENT

Enteral Nutritional Management

Nutritional supplementation *via* the functional gastrointestinal tract always should be pursued in the cancer patient undergoing oncologic therapy.[12] Preventive nutritional maintenance often has been ignored in the past and some oncologists have allowed their patients to become progressively malnourished during and after therapy. Liquid diets are commercially available and the patients should be instructed as to the availability, cost and palatability of these diets.

In patients with head and neck malignancies, nasogastric feeding tubes have played an important role in nutritional maintenance of otherwise healthy patients who were receiving radiation therapy for malignancies of the head and neck, or in the postoperative management of these patients until normal swallowing function returned. These tubes were placed in the distal esophagus in order to prevent the complications of reflux around the tube. Many head and neck cancer surgeons have found this technique useful for many years.

Soft pliable, small diameter, nasogastric feeding tubes are now available and can be manipulated easily into the proximal duodenum. These feeding tubes have been found an efficient means for supplying either an elemental diet or standard liquid diets. Placement of these tubes in the proximal duodenum reduces the incidence of aspiration and the small diameter of the tube can prevent the complications of esophageal gastric reflux. Complications of enteral feeding include hyperglycemia, diarrhea, and electrolyte abnormalities. Tube feedings should be monitored with daily urine sugars in order to establish tolerance. If diarrhea develops, the infusion rate may be reduced or the carbohydrate or fat content of the formula may be lowered.

Gastrostomy tubes and jejunostomy feeding tubes require a moderate operative procedure and can be accomplished with safety in well nourished individuals. Severely malnourished individuals are often borderline operative candidates and these operative procedures should not be pursued in such patients. These simple procedures can result in complications such as: (1) wound dehiscence, (2) separation of the intestine from the abdominal wall, and (3) bleeding abnormalities.[13]

All enteral feedings are dependent upon an intact gastrointestinal tract. The luxury of a functional intestine is often not available in malnourished cancer patients with metastatic disease. Furthermore, nutritional replenishment *via* the gastrointestinal tract is often slow compared with the use of total parenteral nutrition.

Parenteral Nutritional Management

Hyperalimentation solutions utilizing 20 to 25% dextrose as a calorie source always must be administered through a central venous catheter. Cannulation of the superior vena cava is essential for infusing these hypertonic solutions in order to avoid thrombophlebitis.

The method of subclavian vein catheterization and care was established by Dudrick and co-workers in 1969.[14] The patient is positioned in a supine Trendelenburg position with a rolled sheet between the scapulae. The skin is carefully shaved in the infraclavicular region. An inorganic solvent (acetone or ether) is used to defat the skin followed by a generous application of an iodine-based antiseptic solution. All instruments used in the insertion of the catheter have been heat sterilized prior to insertion. In order to assure maximum patient comfort and cooperation, the skin and periosteum of both the clavicle and first rib should be anesthetized thoroughly with 1% lidocaine. A large bore needle attached to a 3-ml syringe is introduced near the point where the first rib passes beneath the clavicle just lateral to the midclavicular line. This needle is aimed toward the sternal notch and advanced beneath the clavicle. This advancement is kept parallel to the floor and is crucial for preventing the complication of pneumothorax and subclavian artery puncture. Gentle continuous suction is applied to the syringe while the needle is advanced. After the subclavian vein has been entered and free backflow of blood established, the syringe and needle are rotated so that the bevel is facing down towards the patient's feet. A hemostat is used to stabilize and fix the needle while the syringe is removed and an 18-gauge catheter is threaded into the vein. During the moment of catheter insertion, the patient is instructed to avoid inspiration and the open needle hub is occluded by the thumb so as to minimize the risk of air embolism. Once the catheter has been inserted, the needle catheter is pulled back as a unit until the needle has been withdrawn completely. The catheter and needle guard are secured to the skin with a heavy black suture. The intravenous tubing is attached securely to the catheter and the bottle should be lowered to assure once again prompt venous return through the catheter. Betadine ointment is placed around the catheter introduction site which is then covered with a sterile gauze. The sterile gauze is then secured in an occlusive manner to the anterior chest wall. A chest x-ray is taken promptly to document the proper catheter position and to assure the absence of a pneumothorax or hydrothorax before the hyperalimentation solution is started.

A carefully trained team of intravenous therapy nurses is responsible for administration of the hyperalimentation solutions. These nurses also maintain the catheter site by changing the catheter dressings and cleansing the catheter site on a regular basis (Monday, Wednesday, and Friday). Stopcocks are never inserted into the hyperalimentation line. Should supplemental solutions be required, the Y tubing method for administering additional infusions through the catheter is used. An infusion pump is incorporated into the tubing in order to maintain a constant rate even with changes in the patient's position during ambulation.

The patient is initially started on 1 l of a standard hyperalimentation solution to be infused over a 24-hour period (Table 14.1). The urine is checked for glucose every 6 hours and, if there is no glycosuria, the infusion rate can be increased at a rate of 1 additional liter/day until the desired level is reached. Temperatures are taken every 4 hours. Liver function tests, electrolytes, urea nitrogen, calcium, and phosphorus are determined on Monday, Wednesday, and Friday. Complete blood count, protime, partial thromboplastin time, and magnesium are determined on Monday.

Folic acid, 10 mg, and Vitamin K, 10 mg, are given intramuscularly every Monday. Vitamin B_{12}, 1 mg, is given every 3 weeks intramuscularly.

Table 14.1
Intravenous hyperalimentation solution

500 ml	D50W	250 g glucose
500 ml	8.5% Amino acid solution	42.5 g protein
	Sodium (chloride, acetate)	20–40 mEq
	Potassium (chloride, acetate)	20–40 mEq
	Phosphate (potassium, sodium)	10–20 mEq
	Ca gluconate	4.5 mEq
	$MgSO_4$	10–15 mEq
	MVI	5 ml
	$CuSO_4$	2 mg
	$ZnSO_4$	5 mg
	Albumin (as needed)	
	Regular insulin (as needed)	

CATHETER COMPLICATIONS

The complications of central venous catheters are related to cannulation and potential infectious contamination of the catheter. Pneumothorax and arterial puncture are the most common complications of this procedure. These complications can be avoided if the needle is inserted just below the clavicle and the direction of the insertion is parallel to the floor. Subclavian venous catheterization can be carried out safely as long as (1) there is strict adherence to the method described, (2) a chest x-ray is taken promptly following attempted insertion, and (3) there is supervision when performed by those who have done few catheterizations.[15]

Sepsis is one of the most serious complications of IVH. Constant attention should be made in maintaining the sterility of the catheter and infusion apparatus. The blood sugar should be maintained below 200 mg/ml because blood sugars above this level can be associated with granulocytic dysfunction. The sudden appearance of fever (38°C or greater) during total parenteral nutrition should be viewed as an urgent problem. Common sense should dictate the course of management. A thorough expeditious fever work-up should be performed in a search for the infectious focus. Blood cultures are essential in the work-up and cultures can be obtained through the catheter. The catheter can be maintained until the blood culture reports become available as long as the patient does not become hypotensive.

In a series of 406 cancer patients receiving oncologic therapy, Copeland and co-workers[16] found that the incidence of catheter related sepsis during hyperalimentation was 2.3%. These patients were treated by catheter removal and antibiotics when necessary. In many of these instances of catheter sepsis, removal of the catheter resulted in defervescence. Experience has shown that, if the catheter must be removed, 24 to 48 hours following a normal temperature should elapse before a new central line is inserted. This is to allow the bacteremia to clear and thus minimize the risk of the hematogenous seeding of a new line. The efficacy of strict maintenance of sterility of the catheter and intravenous tubing has been recognized by other investigators.[17]

IMMUNOCOMPETENCE AND NUTRITION

Both clinical and experimental investigations have established a relationship between dietary intake and immune responses. Most of the clinical work has come from areas of the world where malnutrition is particularly endemic in the pediatric population. A nutritional survey of hospitalized patients in a general city hospital pointed out the prevalence and often neglected problems of malnutrition in this country. Recently, attention has been focused on the effects of nutritional support of cancer patients on host immunocompetence.

Neutrophil function is important for maintaining a first line defense against bacterial infections. The adverse effects of malnutrition on neutrophil function in man have recently been reviewed by Chandra.[18] Neutrophil function against bacteria is a complex process consisting of complement, opsonins, neutrophil ingestion of bacteria, and bactericidal activity following the phagocytosis of bacteria. In general, opsonin function and the ability of polymorphonuclear leukocytes to ingest bacteria have been reported to be intact in malnourished children. However, a consistent finding of impaired neutrophil function was the killing of bacteria following phagocytosis. Intracellular killing of organisms was readily restored by nutritional repletion. Data from controlled animal experiments support the observation that malnutrition has an adverse effect on neutrophil function.[19, 20]

The effects of nutritional changes on lymphocyte function have been studied extensively. Lymphocytes are divided into two major groups, based upon their immune function. Bone marrow derived (B) lymphocytes are involved with antibody production while thymus derived (T) lymphocytes are responsible for cell mediated immune reactions and have the capability to regulate antibody production. Certain antigens (T-dependent) require cooperation between B and T lymphocytes for maximal antibody production while T-independent antigens can stimulate antibody synthesis without the presence of T lymphocytes. *In vitro* assays have been developed to study the function of these two lymphocyte populations and have been applied in investigations of nutrition and immunocompetence.

Clinical studies of malnourished children have demonstrated that the capability of B lymphocytes to differentiate into plasma cells appeared to be relatively intact. In children with reduced dietary intake, serum levels of immunoglobulins were noted to be increased[21] when specific immunoglobulin levels were studied, and only secretory IgA concentrations in nasopharyngeal secretions, tears, and saliva were found to be low.[22]

Animal studies have confirmed the clinical observations that B-lymphocyte antibody production is minimally affected by dietary intake. An important variable when evaluating the effect of protein depletion on antibody production is the type of the antigenic stimulus. Certain antigens can elicit antibody production only in presence of T lymphocytes. Experimental conditions have shown that antibody production to T-independent antigens such as *Brucella abortus* are resistant to dietary protein restriction. T-dependent antigens, such as tetanus toxoid and sheep red blood cells, require cooperation between B and T lymphocytes for maximal antibody production and protein depletion results in lower antibody-producing cells and serum antibody titers to this group of antigens.[19, 23] These results suggest that, depending upon the antigenic stimulus, defects in antibody production are a result of T-lymphocyte dysfunction.

Impairment of T-lymphocyte function with protein depletion also has been shown in animal studies using delayed hypersensitivity responses as a measure of cell-mediated immunity. Daly *et al.*[24, 25] reported that protein depletion of rats with and without transplanted tumors resulted in suppression of tuberculin skin test responses. This impairment of skin test reactivity was shown to be corrected by nutritional repletion. Other investigators have demonstrated that protein depletion of guinea pigs and mice resulted in a similar depression of delayed hypersensitivity responses.[26, 27]

However, other investigators using various assays of T-lymphocyte function have demonstrated that protein depletion could enhance T-lymphocyte responsiveness. Cooper *et al.*[19] used graft *versus* host (GVH) reactivity, skin allograft rejection, viral resistance, and phytohemagglutinin (PHA) lymphocyte blastogenic assays to assess T-cell immunity in protein-depleted mice. Their observations showed that protein malnutrition enhanced T-lymphocyte responsiveness. Bell and Hazell[28] reported similar findings of increased GVH reactivity with protein depletion. Ota *et al.*[29] utilizing the *in vitro* PHA lymphocyte blastogenic assay found enhanced responses under their tissue culture conditions.

Floyd *et al.*[30] noted that previous experimental studies[19, 29] of *in vitro* PHA lymphocyte blastogenesis involved heterologous serum sources such as human serum in mice and rat lymphocyte cultures. By using autologous serum in the PHA assay, they showed that the serum in the tissue culture media played an important role in determining the results of a nutritional study involving T-lymphocyte function. PHA blastogenesis of lymphocytes from rats fed a protein-free diet for 4 weeks cultured with autologous serum showed a significant reduction compared with PHA blastogenesis of lymphocytes from rats maintained on a 25% protein diet incubated with autologous serum. Cross serum experiments showed that PHA blastogenesis of protein free diet lymphocytes in serum obtained from well nourished rats could be restored to normal during the first 4 weeks of dietary manipulation. These results emphasized that PHA lymphocyte blastogenesis required autologous serum to correctly assess T-lymphocyte responses.

Results from various animal studies showed that malnutrition had an adverse effect on T-cell immunity. Antibody production to T-dependent antigens, delayed hypersensitivity responses and PHA lymphocyte blastogenesis were suppressed by protein malnutrition. These reports were in agreement with observations in man that malnutrition impaired T-cell immunity. Investigators using microbial antigen skin testing methods reported that malnutrition in man suppressed delayed hypersensitivity responses.[21, 31] The investigation of PHA blastogenesis of peripheral blood lymphocytes demonstrated that inadequate nutrition in children and adults reduced T-lymphocyte immunocompetence.[21, 32, 33] Quantitation of the T-lymphocyte population in peripheral blood using sheep red blood cell rosette methods showed a reduction in T-lymphocytes in malnourished pediatric patients.[34] Further studies of these lymphocytes by Chandra[32] showed that the null cell population was increased in malnourished children.

Although impairment of T-lymphocyte function in malnourished individuals has been documented, the effects of malnutrition on immunocompetence in cancer patients are more difficult to understand. Various forms of oncologic therapy are known to suppress immune function, especially cell mediated immunity.[35] Chemotherapy, operative procedures, and radiotherapy have the potential to limit host nutritional intake and can adversely affect T-lymphocyte function.

In an attempt to define the contribution of malnutrition to the suppression of immunocompetence associated with oncologic therapy, Daly et al.[36] studied 160 patients who were tested with a battery of five recall skin test antigens at 7- to 10-day intervals throughout antineoplastic therapy and nutritional support with intravenous hyperalimentation. Skin tests were read 48 hours after intradermal injection and any reaction to any of the five antigens consisting of 10×10 mm of induration was considered a positive result. Anergic skin testing, 10×10 mm of induration existed in one or more antigen sites or there was a 100% increase in the diameter of induration when compared with the pre-IVH skin test results. Of the 45 patients in the chemotherapy group who were intially skin test negative, 25 patients were converted to skin test positive in an average period of 19.2 days of IVH. Of the 20 patients in the radiation therapy group, 11 failed either to convert skin test reactions from negative to positive or to maintain positive skin test reactions during radiotherapy. These patients usually were receiving radiation therapy to T-lymphocyte bearing areas such as the thymus or larger areas of the bone marrow which may explain these observations. Although positive skin test reactivity was often difficult to achieve in this group, there were no complications secondary to radiotherapy and nutritional rehabilitation was considered adequate.

In the 49 surgical patients, the incidence of postoperative complications in patients whose skin test reaction remained negative throughout IVH, or were converted to negative despite IVH, was 69%. The incidence of postoperative complications in patients who maintained positive skin test reactivity or converted to skin test positive preoperatively was 25%. Meakins et al.[37] have reported similar results in evaluation of immunocompetence and nutritional status of patients undergoing operative therapy for various stages of colorectal cancer. Patients who manifested skin test anergy had significantly greater weight loss and a significantly higher incidence of postoperative complications compared with the skin test-positive patients. These results were consistent with experimental animal studies correlating nutritional deficiencies with skin test anergy.[24–27]

There are many attractive features of skin testing with microbial antigens in the preoperative evaluation of surgical patients. Expensive laboratory facilities were not required to perform these studies. In addition, nursing personnel were trained to apply and read the skin test battery. The microbial antigens used in the preoperative assessment of surgical patients are commercially available. Meaningful clinical information, practical solutions to correct nutritional deficits, and simplicity of immune assessment in identifying patients at risk for postoperative complications are important features of skin testing that make it an important bedside tool.

The evaluation of immunocompetence in 160 patients undergoing oncologic therapy by Daly *et al.*[36] determined the effect of IVH on cell mediated immunity in the cancer patient. The conclusions reached in this study were: (1) immune depression attributed to chemotherapy may be secondary to malnutrition; (2) skin test reactivity, in general, was depressed during radiation therapy to the mediastinum and pelvis even though nutrition was estimated to be adequate; and (3) surgical patients with negative skin test reactivity had prolonged postoperative recovery periods compared with patients who were skin test positive. Intravenous hyperalimentation was responsible for nutritional repletion in these patients and probably was responsible for or, at the very least, was associated with return of skin test reactivity in the majority of the anergic patients. This study indicated that a portion of the immunodepression associated with oncologic therapy was secondary to malnutrition and not necessarily a result of a suppressor effect on the immune system by oncologic therapy or by circulating substance liberated by the neoplasm.

METABOLISM IN CANCER PATIENT

Patients with malignant diseases are at a distinct disadvantage in their attempt to maintain their nutritional intake. A growing neoplasm extracts nutrients from the host and this can contribute to host malnutrition. Gastrointestinal involvement with a primary or metastatic neoplasm can limit sufficient caloric intake, placing the host at a disadvantage with respect to maintenance of homeostasis while, at the same time, offering the tumor the opportunity to extract substrates for growth. The subsequent treatment modality of neoplasms involves either operation, chemotherapy or radiation therapy, all of which have the potential to limit host caloric intake.

Patients harboring a growing neoplasm have unique problems in evaluating energy requirements. The utilization of energy substrates by the neoplasm has been hypothesized to result in extreme weight loss. Anerobic glycolysis might play a significant role in energy production in tumors, and studies in cancer patients have demonstrated increased lactate production.[38-40] Lactic acid occupies a fundamental position in gluconeogenesis. Neoplastic tissues convert glucose to lactic acid which then has to be reconverted to glucose in the liver. The metabolic pathway by which glucose is metabolized to lactic acid, and through the process of gluconeogenesis in the liver is recycled to glucose, is known as the Cori cycle. Holroyde *et al.*[38] have shown that the Cori cycle activity was significantly increased in malnourished patients with metastatic colon cancer compared with normal individuals. Based upon stoichiometric analysis of ATP production and consumption, this increase in the Cori cycle activity in cancer patients represented an inefficient utilization of energy substrates. The utilization of one glucose molecule to lactic acid *via* the glycolytic pathway in tumor tissues resulted in two ATP molecules for tumor utilization. The conversion of lactic acid *via* gluconeogenesis to glucose required 6 molecules of ATP. The net result of this cycling of glucose to lactic acid, back to glucose, was a loss of 8 ATP molecules from normal host tissues for each molecule of glucose metabolized by the tumor. This inefficient utilization of energy substrates is thought to place a higher energy drain on the host tissues, resulting in cachexia.

Nutritional support of the cancer patient initially raised concerns over hosts in tumor competition for nutrient substrates and for accelerated tumor growth during nutritional repletion. However, clinical observations in adult and pediatric cancer patients indicated that tumor growth was not enhanced by nutritional repletion.[13, 41] Animal studies have shown that protein calorie malnutrition inhibited tumor development and retarded tumor growth.[42, 43] Other investigators have reported that nutritional therapy in tumor-bearing malnourished rats might stimulate tumor growth.[44] Thus, in the laboratory animals, nutritional therapy may increase tumor growth to the detriment of the host.

Biochemical studies in animal tumor models have suggested that tumor biosynthetic function are unaffected by host dietary intake. In terms of total RNA and protein content, experimental hepatomas appeared to be insensitive to dietary intake while the host liver manifested fluctuations in RNA and protein levels depending on the protein level in the diet.[45, 46] These results suggested that nutritional repletion was advantageous to the host by restoring depleted cellular RNA and protein while not altering tumor levels of these components.

Nutritional changes in macromolecular synthesis in host and tumor tissues during changes in dietary intake have been studied using tracer labeling methods. Stein *et al.*[47] reported that tumor protein synthesis rates during a depleting regimen of low glucose infusion were significantly depressed compared with a standard IVH regimen. However, these investigators have published contradictory data concerning protein synthesis rates during low glucose infusion.[48] Experiments that attempt to define macromolecular synthesis in host and tumor tissues *via* tracer techniques often have produced data that are difficult to analyze because of the uncontrolled variables of tracer labeling under different nutritional conditions. Tracer studies of protein, RNA and DNA *in vivo* are dependent upon (1) pool size of the substrate, (2) tissue uptake of the substrate, (3) blood flow through the tissues, (4) distribution of the substrate within the host, and (5) alterations of the tracer substrate through various metabolic pathways.[49] Because these five indices vary with changes in host nutritional intake, data derived from tracer studies for determining the rates of tissue macromolecular synthesis in protein-depleted or starved animals cannot accurately be compared with data from a well nourished group.

Future investigations into the effects of nutritional therapy on host and tumor macromolecular synthesis in experimental models will require methods to monitor synthesis rates that are not subject to the problems encountered in interpreting data from tracer substrate labeling experiments.

CLINICAL APPLICATION OF NUTRITIONAL THERAPY IN CANCER PATIENT

Studies done at the M. D. Anderson Hospital using adjunctive nutritional support of malnourished patients undergoing oncologic therapy have demonstrated both the effectiveness and safety of total parenteral nutrition. By adhering to the proper aseptic techniques of management of the venous catheter and the IVH delivery system as described by Dudrick and co-workers,[14] septic complications from indwelling catheters in the superior vena cava in patients with depressed leucocyte counts secondary to chemotherapy or radiotherapy can be reduced to an acceptably low rate. Cachectic cancer patients who would otherwise not be considered candidates for oncologic therapy because of the complications that might result from the combination of malnutrition and the use of antineoplastic therapy have been successfully managed with intravenous nutrition and subsequently became eligible for oncologic treatment.

The nutritional complications of chemotherapy are reviewed by Ohnuma and Holland[50]; the alimentary tract is particularly vulnerable to the chemotherapeutic agents. Nausea and vomiting are commonly seen with the various alkylating agents, antimetabolites, antibiotic agents such as bleomycin and the heavy metal drugs such as cis-diaminedichloroplatinum. Stomatitis in the form of ulceration, glossitis, and pharyngitis is a manifestation of the toxic side effects of chemotherapy on the rapidly dividing epithelial surface. Patients complain of sore throat and discomfort when attempting to chew and swallow solid food. Adynamic ileus is a feature of vincristine toxicity while 5-fluorouracil and other drugs may produce diarrhea. The result of these complications is a loss of appetite and reduced oral intake of essential food stuffs; inability to consume 1500 calories/day eventually leads to malnutrition.

Most patients receiving chemotherapy can be successfully managed without adjunctive nutritional support. Nausea, vomiting and gastrointestinal complications are usually self-limiting and nutritional recovery can be achieved before the next cycle is given. This, almost always, assumes that the patient has not experienced any recent weight loss. However, patients who are candidates for chemotherapy but manifest greater than 10% body weight loss can be safely rehabilitated in order to complete a planned course of chemotherapy. In a series of retrospective and prospective studies, malnourished patients were nutritionally repleted while undergoing intensive chemotherapy and immunotherapy.[51, 52] Some of these patients had recorded weight losses of up to 20%. Proceeding with intensive chemotherapy under these situations, these physicians realized that without parenteral nutritional support their patients would not have been able to correct their own nutritional deficits.

Following nutritional repletion, these same investigators made the observation that the tumor-response rates to chemotherapy appeared to be enhanced by nutritional repletion. Studies currently sponsored by the Diet, Nutrition, and Cancer Program of the National Cancer Institute are investigating whether patients receiving IVH have higher rates of response and survival while undergoing their treatment regimen, and these studies are nearing completion. The preliminary data indicate that there may be little significant difference in survival between responding patients who received IVH and responding patients who did not. In many of these studies, patients with only marginal degrees of malnutrition have been entered into the randomization process. From both the ethical and moral standpoint, most investigators may be hesitant to deny patients suffering from malnutrition access to nutritional therapy in order to obtain randomized data. The conclusions and lessons obtained in earlier studies by Copeland and Dudrick[13] remain relevant today. IVH should be used in cancer patients as a means of nutritional rehabilitation when such a goal is desirable to optimize response to chemotherapeutic agents and to minimize their side effects.

The judicious use of parenteral nutrition in surgical practice has been well established in those situations where the gatrointestinal tract was not available for restoring nutritional deficiencies. Impairment of wound healing and immunosuppression can result in major complications following operative procedures. Copeland et al.[53] reported that malnourished cancer patients with surgically resectable lesions had higher rates of postoperative complications and mortality, attributable to an individual's inability to heal the wound and resist infections secondary to deficiencies in nutrient substrates. The use of skin testing with common microbial antigens has now been incorporated into the overall nutritional preoperative assessment of surgical candidates. These studies of skin test immunocompetence have identified anergic patients as being at risk for a higher incidence of postoperative complications. Improvement of immunocompetence with intravenous nutritional therapy, both preoperatively and postoperatively, was associated with fewer complications and a shorter hospitalization time.

Experience with intravenous nutrition in urologic cancer patients has been limited to patients with invasive bladder cancer. In a retrospective review of low concentration dextrose-amino acid infusion *versus* dextrose-saline solutions in postoperative cystectomy patients, Foster et al.[54] reported that there was no difference in mortality or hospitalization time between the two parenteral treatment regimens. Hensle,[55] however, found that preoperative assessment of patients undergoing cystectomy for bladder malignancy suggested the need for nutritional support based upon delayed hypersensitivity reactions, serum albumin levels, and recent history of weight loss. Using these criteria, he reported that almost 40% of the patient population were malnourished prior to operation. Although the incidence of nutritional depletion may seem high, 70% of these patients had received preoperative radiotherapy (4500 R). In a prospective, randomized trial of peripheral amino acid infusion *versus* dextrose-saline infusion, Hensle[55] suggested that his form of adjunctive nutritional therapy could maintain immunocompetence and reduce the postoperative complications. Severe, nutritional depletion and life-threatening complications prompted the early use of IVH in this study.

Radiotherapy, especially to the abdomen and pelvis, can interrupt normal gastrointestinal function. Goffinet et al.[56] reported a series of patients undergoing radiotherapy for carcinoma of the bladder and noted an 8% incidence of severe small bowel complications. Although Donaldson[57] suggested many alternatives for maintaining the nutritional intake of patients receiving radiotherapy, complications such as fistulae, chronic enteritis, and intestinal obstruction require total parenteral nutrition, especially with a recent weight loss history. Malnourished patients have a narrower range for tolerating complications compared with a relatively healthy individual and judicious use of IVH is important when complications related to oncologic therapy impairs the intestinal absorption of nutrient substrates.

FUTURE CONSIDERATIONS

The application of IVH to the clinical setting was initially dictated by the obvious deteriorating clinical course or by the natural history of major gastrointestinal complications. Parenteral nutrition also has been used as a preventive measure when nutritional assessment indicates the potential benefits of this therapy. A number of markers of malnutrition such as serum albumin levels, serum transferrin levels, anthropometric measurements, and skin testing with microbial antigens have been used to identify patients who are likely to benefit from aggressive nutritional support. Better, but practical, analytical methods to determine a patient's ability to synthesize cellular macromolecules such as proteins, RNA and DNA and thus, predict more accurately the need for nutritional therapy, are needed.

In the field of chemotherapy and nutrition, there is little information available concerning drug metabolism and its effect on host toxicity and tumor response. A better understanding of chemotherapy drug activation and the nutritional status of the host may potentially enhance tumor responses and reduce the side effects on the host.

REFERENCES

1. Warren, S. The immediate causes of death in cancer. *Am. J. Med. Sci. 184:*610, 1932.
2. Cahill, G. F., Jr. Starvation in man. *N. Engl. J. Med. 282:*668, 1970.
3. Geyer, R. P. Parenteral nutrition. *Physiol. Rev. 40:*150, 1960.
4. Sanderson, I., and Deitel, M. Insulin response in patients receiving concentrated infusions of glucose and casein hydrolysate for complete parenteral nutrition. *Ann. Surg. 179:*387, 1974.
5. Chan, J. C., Asch, M. J., Lin, S., and Hays, D. M. Hyperalimentation with amino acids and casein hydrolysate solutions and mechanism of acidosis. *JAMA 220:*1700, 1972.
6. Freund, H., Yoshimura, N., Lunetta, L., and Fischer, J. E. The role of branched-chain amino acids in decreasing muscle catabolism *in vivo. Surgery 83:*611, 1978.
7. Freund, H., Ryan, J., and Fischer, J. Amino acid derangements in patients with sepsis: treatment with branched amino acid rich infusions. *Ann. Surg. 188:*423, 1978.
8. Coran, A. Total intravenous feeding of infants and children without the use of a central venous catheter. *Ann. Surg. 179:*445, 1974.

9. Goodgame, J. T., Lowry, S. F., and Brennan, M. F. Essential fatty acid deficiency in total parenteral nutrition: time course of development and suggestions for therapy *Surgery 84:*271, 1978.

10. O'Neil, J. A., Caldwell, M., and Meng, H. C. Essential fatty acid deficiency in surgical patients. *Ann. Surg. 185:*535, 1977.

11. Kay, R. G., Tasman-Jones, C., Pybus, J., Whiting, R., and Black, H. A syndrome of acute zinc deficiency during total parenteral alimentation in man. *Ann. Surg. 183:*331, 1976.

12. Shils, M. E. Enteral nutrition by tube. *Cancer Res. 37:*2432, 1977.

13. Copeland, E. M., and Dudrick, S. J. Nutritional aspects of cancer. In *Current Problems in Cancer*, Vol. 1, No. 3. Editor R. C. Hickey. Year Book Medical Publishers, Chicago, 1976.

14. Dudrick, S. J., Wilmore, D. W., Vars, H. M., and Rhoads, J. E. Can intravenous feeding as the sole means of nutrition support growth in the child and restore weight loss in the adult? An affirmative answer. *Ann. Surg. 169:*974, 1969.

15. Bernard, R. W., and Stahl, W. M. Subclavian vein catheterizations: a prospective study. I. Non-infectious complications. *Ann. Surg. 173:*184, 1971.

16. Copeland, E. M., MacFadyen, B. V., McGowan, C., and Dudrick, S. J. The use of hyperalimentation in patients with potential sepsis. *Surg. Gynecol. Obstet. 138:*377, 1974.

17. Ryan, J. A., Abel, R. M., and Abbott, W. M., *et al.* Catheter complications of total parenteral nutrition. *N. Engl. J. Med. 290:*757, 1974.

18. Chandra, R. K. Interactions of nutrition, infection and immune response. *Acta Paediatr. Scand. 68:*137, 1979.

19. Cooper, W. C., Good, R. A., and Mariani, T. Effects of protein insufficiency on immune responsiveness. *Am. J. Clin. Nutr. 27:*647, 1974.

20. Wunder, J. A., Stinnett, J. D., and Alexander, J. W. The effects of malnutrition on variables of host defense in the guinea pig. *Surgery 84:*542, 1978.

21. Neumann, C. G., Lawlor, G. J., Jr., Stiehm, E. R., Swendseid, M. E., Newton, C., Herbert, J., Ammann, A. J., and Jacob, M. Immunologic responses in malnourished children. *Am. J. Clin. Nutr. 28:*89 1975.

22. McMurray, D. N., Rey, H., Casazza, L. J., and Watson, R. R. Effect of moderate malnutrition on concentrations of immunoglobulins and enzymes in tears and saliva of young Colombian children. *Am. J. Clin. Nutr. 30:*1944, 1977.

23. Law, D. K., Dudrick, S. J., and Abdou, N. Effect of dietary protein depletion on immunocompetence. *Ann. Surg. 179:*168, 1974.

24. Daly, J. M., Copeland, E. M., and Dudrick, S. J. Effects of intravenous nutrition on tumor growth and host immunocompetence in malnourished animals. *Surgery 84:*655, 1978.

25. Daly, J. M., Dudrick, S. J., and Copeland, E. M. Effects of protein depletion and repletion on cell-mediated immunity in experimental animals. *Ann. Surg.188:*791, 1978.

26. Good, R. S., Fernandez, G., Yunis, E. J., Cooper, W. C., Jose, D. C., Kramer, T. R., and Hansen, M. A. Nutritional deficiency, immunologic function, and disease. *Am. J. Path. 84:*599 1976.

27. Narayanan, R. B., Nath, I., Bhuyan, U. N., and Talwar, G. D. Depression of T-cell function and normality of B-cell response in protein calorie malnutrition. *Immunology 32:*345, 1977.

28. Bell, R. G., and Hazell, L. A. Influence of dietary protein restriction on immune competence. I. Effect on the capacity of cells from various lymphoid organs to induce graft-vs-host reactions. *J. Exp. Med. 141:*127, 1975.

29. Ota, D. M., Copeland, E. M., Corriere, J. N., Jr., Jacobson, K. A., and Dudrick, S. J. Effects of protein nutrition on lymphocyte transformation. *Surg. Forum 28:*65, 1977.

30. Floyd, C., Ota, D., Corriere, J. N., Jr., Dudrick, S. J., and Copeland, E. M. Effect of protein depletion on serum factors for lymphocyte transformation. *Surg. Forum 30:*57, 1979.

31. Edelman, R., Suskind, R., Olson, R. E., and Sirisinha, S. Mechanisms of defective delayed cutaneous hypersensitivity in children with protein-calorie malnutrition. *Lancet 1:*506, 1973.

PARENTERAL NUTRITION IN CANCER PATIENTS   313

32. Chandra, R. K. Lymphocyte subpopulations in human malnutrition: cytotoxic and suppressor cells. *Pediatrics 59:*423, 1977.
33. Reddy, V., Jagadeesan, V., Ragharamulu, C., Bhaskaram, C., and Srikantia, S. G. Functional significance of growth retardation in malnutrition. *Am. J. Clin. Nutr. 29:*3, 1976.
34. Ferguson, A. S., Lawlor, G. J., Jr., Neumann, C. G., Oh, W., and Steihm, E. R. Decreased rosette-forming lymphocytes in malnutrition and intrauterine growth retardation. *J. Pediatr. 85:*717, 1974.
35. Ota, D. M., Copeland, E. M., Corriere, J. N., Jr., and Dudrick, S. J. The effects of nutrition and treatment of cancer on host immunocompetence. *Surg. Gynecol. Obstet. 148:*104, 1979.
36. Daly, J. M., Dudrick, S. J., and Copeland, E. M. Intravenous hyperalimentation: effect on delayed cutaneous hypersensitivity in cancer patients. *Ann. Surg.* (in press).
37. Meakins, J. L., Cristou, N., Halle, C.C., and MacLean, L. D. Influence of cancer on host defense and susceptibility to infection. *Surg. Forum 30:*115, 1979.
38. Holroyde, C. P., Axelrod, R. S., Skutches, C. L., Haff, A. C., Paul, P., and Reichard, G. A. Lactate metabolism in patients with metastatic colorectal cancer. *Cancer Res. 39:* 4900, 1979.
39. Shapot, V. S. Some biochemical aspects of the relationship between the tumor and the host. *Adv. Cancer Res. 15:*253, 1972.
40. Waterhouse, C. Lactate metabolism in patients with cancer. *Cancer 33:*66, 1974.
41. Filler, R. M., Jaffee, N., Cassady, J. R., Traggis, D. G., and Das, J. B. Parenteral nutritional support in children with cancer. *Cancer 39:*2665, 1977.
42. Saxton, J. A., Jr., Boon, M. C., and Furth, J. Observations on the inhibition of development of spontaneous leukemia in mice by underfeeding. *Cancer Res. 4:*401, 1944.
43. Wiernik, P. H. Effect of starvation of intact and adrenalectomized mice bearing lymphosarcoma P1798 on tumor regression and ribonuclease activity. *Cancer Res. 30:* 280, 1970.
44. Cameron, I. L., and Pavlat, W. A. Stimulation of growth of a transplantable hepatoma in rats by parenteral nutrition. *J. Natl. Cancer Inst. 59:*597, 1976.
45. Munro, H. N., and Clark, C. M. The influence of dietary protein on the metabolism of ribonucleic acid in rat hepatoma. *Br. J. Cancer 13:*324, 1959.
46. Ota, D. M., Copeland, E. M., Strobel, H. W., Daly, J. M., Gum, E. T., Guinn, E., and Dudrick, S. J. The effect of protein nutrition on host and tumor metabolism. *J. Surg. Res. 22:*181, 1977.
47. Stein, T. P., Hargrove, W. C., III, Miller, E. E., Wallace, H. W., Buzby, G. P., and Mullen, J. L. Effect of nutritional status and 5-fluorouracil on protein synthesis in parenterally alimented LEW/Mai rats. *J. Natl. Cancer Inst. 63:*379, 1979.
48. Stein, T. P., Oram-Smith, J. C., Leskiu, M. J., Wallace, H. W., and Miller, E. E. Tumor-caused changes in host protein synthesis under different dietary situations. *Cancer Res. 36:*3936, 1976.
49. Lea, M. A. Regulation of macromolecular synthesis in Morris hepatomas. In *Advances in Experimental Biology and Medicine, Morris Hepatomas: Mechanisms of Regulation,* Vol. 92. P. 289. Edited by H. P. Morris and W. E. Criss. Plenum Press, New York, 1977.
50. Ohnuma, T., and Holland, J. F. Nutritional consequences of cancer chemotherapy and immunotherapy. *Cancer Res. 37:*2329, 1977.
51. Issell, B. F., Valdivieso, M., Zaren, H. A., Dudrick, S. J., Freireich, E. J., Copeland, E. M., and Bodey, G. P. Protection against chemotherapy toxicity by IV hyperalimentation. *Cancer Treat. Rept. 62:*1139, 1978.
52. Lanzotti, V. C., Copeland, E. M., George, S. L., Dudrick, S. J., and Samuels, M. L. Cancer chemo- therapeutic response and intravenous hyperalimentation. *Cancer Chemother. Rept. 59:*437, 1975.
53. Copeland, E. M., MacFadyen, B. V., and Dudrick, S. J. Effect of intravenous hyperalimentation on established delayed hypersensitivity in the cancer patient. *Ann. Surg. 184:* 60, 1976.
54. Foster, K. J., Alberti, K., Allen, N., Jenkins, J., MacIver, A., Smart, C. J., and Karran,

S. J. The influence of early postoperative intravenous nutrition upon recovery after total cystectomy. *Br. J. Urol. 50:*319, 1978.

55. Hensle, T. W. Protein-sparing in cystectomy patients. *JPEN 2:*519, 1978.
56. Goffinet, D. R., Schneider, M. J., Glatstein, E. J., Ludwig, H., Ray, G. R., Dunnick, N. R., and Bagshaw, M. A. Bladder cancer: results of radiation therapy in 384 patients. *Radiology 117:*149, 1975.
57. Donaldson, S. S. Nutritional consequences of radiotherapy. *Cancer Res. 37:*2407, 1977.
58. Cameron, I. L., and Rogers, W. Total intravenous hyperalimentation and hydroxyurea chemotherapy in hepatoma-bearing rats. J. Surg. Res. 23:279, 1977.
59. Copeland, E. M., Daly, J. M., and Dudrick, S. J. Nutrition as an adjunct to cancer treatment in the adult. *Cancer Res.* 37:2451, 1977.
60. Geefhuysen, J., Rosen, E. U., Katz, J., and Metz, J. Impaired cellular immunity in kwashiorkor with improvement after therapy. *Br. Med. J. 4:*527, 1971.
61. Goodgame, J. T., Lowry, S. F., Reilly, J. J., Jones, D. C., and Brennan, M. F. Nutritional manipulations and tumor growth. I. The effects of starvation. *Am. J. Clin. Nutr. 32:* 2277, 1979.
62. Law, D. K., Dudrick, S. J., and Abdou, N. I. Immunocompetence of patients with protein-calorie malnutrition. *Ann. Intern. Med. 79:*545, 1973.
63. Rose, W. C., Wixom, R. L., Lockhart, M. D., and Lambert, F. The amino acid requirements of man. XV. Valine requirements: summary and final observations. *J. Biol. Chem. 217:*987, 1955.

Index

v